Regional Intestinal Drug Absorption: Biopharmaceutics and Drug Formulation

Regional Intestinal Drug Absorption: Biopharmaceutics and Drug Formulation

Editors

Arik Dahan
Maria Isabel Gonzalez-Alvarez

MDPI • Basel • Beijing • Wuhan • Barcelona • Belgrade • Manchester • Tokyo • Cluj • Tianjin

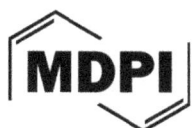

Editors
Arik Dahan
Department of Clinical Pharmacology
Ben-Gurion University of the Negev
Beer-Sheva
Israel

Maria Isabel Gonzalez-Alvarez
Dpto Ingenieria: Area de Farmacia y Tecnología Farmacéutica
Universidad Miguel Hernandez
San Juan de Alicante
Spain

Editorial Office
MDPI
St. Alban-Anlage 66
4052 Basel, Switzerland

This is a reprint of articles from the Special Issue published online in the open access journal *Pharmaceutics* (ISSN 1999-4923) (available at: www.mdpi.com/journal/pharmaceutics/special_issues/intestinal_biopharm_formul).

For citation purposes, cite each article independently as indicated on the article page online and as indicated below:

LastName, A.A.; LastName, B.B.; LastName, C.C. Article Title. *Journal Name* **Year**, *Volume Number*, Page Range.

ISBN 978-3-0365-3658-3 (Hbk)
ISBN 978-3-0365-3657-6 (PDF)

© 2022 by the authors. Articles in this book are Open Access and distributed under the Creative Commons Attribution (CC BY) license, which allows users to download, copy and build upon published articles, as long as the author and publisher are properly credited, which ensures maximum dissemination and a wider impact of our publications.

The book as a whole is distributed by MDPI under the terms and conditions of the Creative Commons license CC BY-NC-ND.

Contents

About the Editors vii

Preface to "Regional Intestinal Drug Absorption: Biopharmaceutics and Drug Formulation" . ix

Arik Dahan and Isabel González-Álvarez
Regional Intestinal Drug Absorption: Biopharmaceutics and Drug Formulation
Reprinted from: *Pharmaceutics* **2021**, *13*, 272, doi:10.3390/pharmaceutics13020272 1

Leonardo de Souza Teixeira, Tatiana Vila Chagas, Antonio Alonso, Isabel Gonzalez-Alvarez, Marival Bermejo and James Polli et al.
Biomimetic Artificial Membrane Permeability Assay over Franz Cell Apparatus Using BCS Model Drugs
Reprinted from: *Pharmaceutics* **2020**, *12*, 988, doi:10.3390/pharmaceutics12100988 7

Giang Huong Ta, Cin-Syong Jhang, Ching-Feng Weng and Max K. Leong
Development of a Hierarchical Support Vector Regression-Based In Silico Model for Caco-2 Permeability
Reprinted from: *Pharmaceutics* **2021**, *13*, 174, doi:10.3390/pharmaceutics13020174 21

Alejandro Ruiz-Picazo, Sarin Colón-Useche, Blanca Perez-Amorós, Marta González-Álvarez, Irene Molina-Martínez and Isabel González-Álvarez et al.
Investigation to Explain Bioequivalence Failure in Pravastatin Immediate-Release Products
Reprinted from: *Pharmaceutics* **2019**, *11*, 663, doi:10.3390/pharmaceutics11120663 47

Marival Bermejo, Bart Hens, Joseph Dickens, Deanna Mudie, Paulo Paixão and Yasuhiro Tsume et al.
A Mechanistic Physiologically-Based Biopharmaceutics Modeling (PBBM) Approach to Assess the In Vivo Performance of an Orally Administered Drug Product: From IVIVC to IVIVP
Reprinted from: *Pharmaceutics* **2020**, *12*, 74, doi:10.3390/pharmaceutics12010074 57

Milica Markovic, Moran Zur, Inna Ragatsky, Sandra Cvijić and Arik Dahan
BCS Class IV Oral Drugs and Absorption Windows: Regional-Dependent Intestinal Permeability of Furosemide
Reprinted from: *Pharmaceutics* **2020**, *12*, 1175, doi:10.3390/pharmaceutics12121175 85

Ana Ruiz-Garcia, Weiwei Tan, Jerry Li, May Haughey, Joanna Masters and Jennifer Hibma et al.
Pharmacokinetic Models to Characterize the Absorption Phase and the Influence of a Proton Pump Inhibitor on the Overall Exposure of Dacomitinib
Reprinted from: *Pharmaceutics* **2020**, *12*, 330, doi:10.3390/pharmaceutics12040330 101

David Dahlgren, Maria-Jose Cano-Cebrián, Tobias Olander, Mikael Hedeland, Markus Sjöblom and Hans Lennernäs
Regional Intestinal Drug Permeability and Effects of Permeation Enhancers in Rat
Reprinted from: *Pharmaceutics* **2020**, *12*, 242, doi:10.3390/pharmaceutics12030242 119

Maoqi Fu, Jozef Al-Gousous, Johannes Andreas Blechar and Peter Langguth
Enteric Hard Capsules for Targeting the Small Intestine: Positive Correlation between In Vitro Disintegration and Dissolution Times
Reprinted from: *Pharmaceutics* **2020**, *12*, 123, doi:10.3390/pharmaceutics12020123 133

Milica Markovic, Moran Zur, Noa Fine-Shamir, Ester Haimov, Isabel González-Álvarez and Arik Dahan
Segmental-Dependent Solubility and Permeability as Key Factors Guiding Controlled Release Drug Product Development
Reprinted from: *Pharmaceutics* **2020**, *12*, 295, doi:10.3390/pharmaceutics12030295 . . . . **147**

Juliane Fjelrad Christfort, Antonio José Guillot, Ana Melero, Lasse Højlund Eklund Thamdrup, Teresa M. Garrigues and Anja Boisen et al.
Cubic Microcontainers Improve In Situ Colonic Mucoadhesion and Absorption of Amoxicillin in Rats
Reprinted from: *Pharmaceutics* **2020**, *12*, 355, doi:10.3390/pharmaceutics12040355 . . . . **163**

K. Sandy Pang, H. Benson Peng and Keumhan Noh
The Segregated Intestinal Flow Model (SFM) for Drug Absorption and Drug Metabolism: Implications on Intestinal and Liver Metabolism and Drug–Drug Interactions
Reprinted from: *Pharmaceutics* **2020**, *12*, 312, doi:10.3390/pharmaceutics12040312 . . . . **179**

Cong Xie, Karen L. Jones, Christopher K. Rayner and Tongzhi Wu
Enteroendocrine Hormone Secretion and Metabolic Control: Importance of the Region of the Gut Stimulation
Reprinted from: *Pharmaceutics* **2020**, *12*, 790, doi:10.3390/pharmaceutics12090790 . . . . **203**

About the Editors

Arik Dahan

Arik Dahan is a Professor of Pharmaceutics and Biopharmaceutics at the Department of Clinical Pharmacology and the School of Pharmacy, Ben-Gurion University of the Negev, Beer-Sheva, Israel. He is also an Adjunct Professor of Pharmaceutical Sciences at the College of Pharmacy, University of Michigan. Dr. Dahan received his Ph.D. (2007) from the Hebrew University of Jerusalem. He was a Post-Doctoral Research Fellow at the University of Michigan (2007–2010) with Professor Gordon Amidon. Dr. Dahan's research interest is the integration of up-to-date molecular/cellular mechanistic investigations of drug disposition in the context of the human body. In implementing this molecular biopharmaceutical approach to ADME research, Dr. Dahan is seeking to enable mechanistic-based successful solutions to drug delivery/therapy, in challenging scenarios, e.g., low-solubility, low-permeability, extensive metabolism, poor site targeting, and various pathophysiological conditions. He has published over 115 top-notch journal papers, and contributed chapters to 10 books.

Maria Isabel Gonzalez-Alvarez

Isabel Gonzalez-Alvarez is an Assoc. Professor at the University Miguel Hernández of Elche-Alicante, Spain. She earned her B.Pharm. and Ph.D. degrees at the University of Valencia under the supervision of Prof. Bermejo. After serving as Clinical Trials Responsible Pharmacist (2002), and a Senior Researcher at University of Valencia (2005), she was appointed Academic Staff Member at University Miguel Hernández, Area of Pharmacy and Pharmaceutical Technology, in the Department of Engineering (2008). Dr. Gonzalez-Alvarez research is focused on intestinal drug absorption, including in-situ and in-vitro models for oral permeability predictions and their application in drug development, biopredictive dissolution of formulations, and the use of modeling and simulations as important tools in modern drug development; her many research projects (>20) are funded by the European Commission, or Government of Spain. Dr. Gonzalez-Alvarez performed two post-doctoral research fellowships at the University of Michigan, working with Prof. Gordon Amidon. She has authored a hundred scientific papers and 10 book chapters, and advised 9 Ph.D. students and more than 20 Master degree students.

Preface to "Regional Intestinal Drug Absorption: Biopharmaceutics and Drug Formulation"

The gastrointestinal tract (GIT) can be broadly divided into several regions: the stomach, the small intestine (which is subdivided to duodenum, jejunum, and ileum), and the colon. The conditions and environment in each of these segments, and even within the segment, are dependent on many factors, e.g., the surrounding pH, fluid composition, transporters expression, metabolic enzymes activity, tight junction resistance, different morphology along the GIT, variable intestinal mucosal cell differentiation, changes in drug concentration (in cases of carrier-mediated transport), thickness and types of mucus, and resident microflora. Each of these variables, alone or in combination with others, can fundamentally alter the solubility/dissolution, the intestinal permeability, and the overall absorption of various drugs. This is the underlying mechanistic basis of regional-dependent intestinal drug absorption, which has led to many attempts to deliver drugs to specific regions throughout the GIT, aiming to optimize drug absorption, bioavailability, pharmacokinetics, and/or pharmacodynamics. In the book "Regional Intestinal Drug Absorption: Biopharmaceutics and Drug Formulation" we aim to highlight the current progress and to provide an overview of the latest developments in the field of regional-dependent intestinal drug absorption and delivery, as well as pointing out the unmet needs of the field.

Arik Dahan and Maria Isabel Gonzalez-Alvarez
Editors

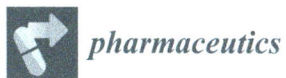

Editorial

Regional Intestinal Drug Absorption: Biopharmaceutics and Drug Formulation

Arik Dahan [1,*] and Isabel González-Álvarez [2,*]

[1] Department of Clinical Pharmacology, School of Pharmacy, Faculty of Health Sciences, Ben-Gurion University of the Negev, Beer-Sheva 8410501, Israel
[2] Engineering, Pharmacokinetics and Pharmaceutical Technology Area, Miguel Hernandez University, 03550 Juan de Alicante, Spain
* Correspondence: arikd@bgu.ac.il (A.D.); isabel.gonzalez@umh.es (I.G.-A.)

Abstract: The gastrointestinal tract (GIT) can be broadly divided into several regions: the stomach, the small intestine (which is subdivided to duodenum, jejunum, and ileum), and the colon. The conditions and environment in each of these segments, and even within the segment, are dependent on many factors, e.g., the surrounding pH, fluid composition, transporters expression, metabolic enzymes activity, tight junction resistance, different morphology along the GIT, variable intestinal mucosal cell differentiation, changes in drug concentration (in cases of carrier-mediated transport), thickness and types of mucus, and resident microflora. Each of these variables, alone or in combination with others, can fundamentally alter the solubility/dissolution, the intestinal permeability, and the overall absorption of various drugs. This is the underlying mechanistic basis of regional-dependent intestinal drug absorption, which has led to many attempts to deliver drugs to specific regions throughout the GIT, aiming to optimize drug absorption, bioavailability, pharmacokinetics, and/or pharmacodynamics. In this Editorial we provide an overview of the Special Issue "Regional Intestinal Drug Absorption: Biopharmaceutics and Drug Formulation". The objective of this Special Issue is to highlight the current progress and to provide an overview of the latest developments in the field of regional-dependent intestinal drug absorption and delivery, as well as pointing out the unmet needs of the field.

Keywords: biopharmaceutics; drug absorption; drug solubility/dissolution; intestinal permeability; oral drug delivery; regional/segmental-dependent permeability and absorption

---

Oral administration is without a doubt the most preferred and convenient way of drug delivery. Oral drug products are easy to use and usually do not require hospitalization or the assistance of medical staff. Oral intake of drugs may also prevent both the local side effects and the risk of systemic infections associated with injections. However, orally taken drugs must enter the enterocytes and cross through the gastrointestinal tract (GIT) membrane in order to reach the systemic circulation and exert their pharmacological effect. The GIT membrane acts as a barrier against the absorption of xenobiotics, and while some drugs easily overcome this barrier, many other drugs fail to penetrate through this membrane and have to be administered parenterally. These drugs include antibodies, protein/peptides, hormones, and even small molecules. Orally swallowed drugs are very much influenced by the physiological/biochemical conditions throughout the GIT, which may dictate their absorption potential, resulting in significant diversions from the predicted/desired pharmacokinetics and pharmacodynamics.

The GIT can be broadly divided to several regions: the stomach, the small intestine (which is subdivided into the duodenum, jejunum, and ileum), and the colon. The conditions and environment in each of these segments, and even within the segment, are dependent on many factors, e.g., the surrounding pH [1–6], fluid composition [7–9],

Citation: Dahan, A.; González-Álvarez, I. Regional Intestinal Drug Absorption: Biopharmaceutics and Drug Formulation. *Pharmaceutics* **2021**, *13*, 272. https://doi.org/10.3390/pharmaceutics13020272

Received: 21 December 2020
Accepted: 15 February 2021
Published: 17 February 2021

Publisher's Note: MDPI stays neutral with regard to jurisdictional claims in published maps and institutional affiliations.

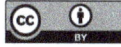

Copyright: © 2021 by the authors. Licensee MDPI, Basel, Switzerland. This article is an open access article distributed under the terms and conditions of the Creative Commons Attribution (CC BY) license (https://creativecommons.org/licenses/by/4.0/).

transporters expression [10–12], metabolic enzymes activity [13,14], tight junction resistance [15,16], different morphology along the GIT [17,18], variable intestinal mucosal cell differentiation [19,20], changes in drug concentration (in cases of carrier-mediated transport), thickness and types of mucus [21], and resident microflora [22–24]. Each of these variables, alone or in combination with others, can fundamentally alter the solubility/dissolution, the intestinal permeability, and the overall absorption of various drugs [25–28]. This is the underlying mechanistic basis of regional-dependent intestinal drug absorption, which has led to many attempts to deliver drugs to specific regions throughout the GIT, aiming to optimize drug absorption, bioavailability, pharmacokinetics and/or pharmacodynamics.

The objective of this Special Issue is to highlight the current progress and to provide an overview of the latest developments in the field of regional-dependent intestinal drug absorption and delivery, as well as pointing out the unmet needs of the field.

Nowadays, the "3R's Principle", that is, replacement, reduction, and refinement, has greatly influenced scientific research in oral drug development, and several preclinical models have been developed to predict intestinal absorption process, aiming to reduce or even replace human/animal experiments. These methods are thoroughly evaluated in this Special Issue. The differences in anatomical and physiological features along the GIT complicate absorption predictions. Rezende's group demonstrated that the BAMPA (biomimetic artificial membrane permeability assay) over Franz cell apparatus showed acceptable log-linear correlation (R^2 = 0.664) with fraction of dose absorbed in humans (F_a%), as seen for P_{app} in Caco-2 cells (R^2 = 0.805), and, thus, both methods are acceptable for BCS classification [29]. Caco-2 cell predictability has been widely studied, and several authors demonstrated the correlation between Caco-2 cells and structure–activity of the drug [30–32]. In this issue, Huong Ta et al. developed a QSAR model (quantitative structure–activity relationship) using a machine learning-based hierarchical support vector regression (HSVR) scheme [33]. This tool allowed for the development of a model to predict Papp in Caco-2 cells permeability for drugs that are transported across the intestinal membrane not only in passive diffusion but also in transporter-mediated active transport. The group of Bermejo and González-Álvarez demonstrated that in vitro permeability studies in Caco-2 can be used to compare formulation performance and even to explain bioequivalence failures associated with excipient effect on the intestinal membrane [34]. In this study, Ruiz-Picazo et al. showed that permeability differences in rat vs. Caco-2 cells of pravastatin formulations (a BCS class III compound) can explain the bioequivalence failure and the higher C_{max} due to excipient effects on the intestinal membrane in the nonequivalent formulation. In the same article, the authors demonstrated non-similar dissolution profiles with USP apparatus and the relevance of using 500 mL instead of 900 mL [34]. A great research effort is focused on the development of new dissolution systems, mono- and multi-compartmental dynamics models. The adequate in vitro model should be chosen depending on the BCS classification of the studied drug and its physicochemical properties. These in vitro systems combine dissolution and absorption processes and simulate pH or peristaltic changes in luminal conditions; therefore, a mechanistic, physiologically based biopharmaceutics modeling (PBBM) approach to assess the in vivo performance of orally administered drug products (IVIVC) should be used to model the obtained data. These models are more complicated and require adequate software but generate better correlations between in vitro and in vivo values, as demonstrated by Bermejo at al. in their study of different ibuprofen formulations [35]. Several absorption models can be tested with different software, such as Phoenix WinNonlin® [35] or the GastroPlus™ simulator, as was demonstrated by Dahan's group [36], studying the rather complicated intestinal permeability of the BCS class IV drug furosemide that shows high dependency on many biochemical/physiological variables. Another common piece of software in the population pharmacokinetic area is NONMEM, which can be used in modelling absorption due to the flexibility of using custom-made empirical, semi-mechanistic, or physiological-based absorption approaches. Transit compartment models, absorption with and without lag time, or passive/active absorption kinetics models can be applied. In this context, Ruiz-Garcia et al. modeled dacomitinib absorption differences in the presence/absence of a proton pump inhibitor by comparing several physiologically based absorption models [37].

The behavior of controlled release formulations and the difficulties in predicting the human situation are studied in this Special Issue. Lennernäs et al. thoroughly discuss the predictive ability of rat colon studies in relation to human data and conclude that improved predictability is needed for controlled release formulations, and the use of permeation enhancers to increase colonic permeability could have higher risks than potential rewards [38]. Langguth's group studied the relevance of dissolution and disintegration of controlled release (CR) dosage forms, obtaining good correlations between the two processes [39]. This work may have significant regulatory impact, as it opens the way to extend the dissolution-based waiver concept beyond immediate-release dosage forms. However, the authors conclude that the extrapolation of these results to the in vivo situation should be done with caution due to additional factors that should be considered, e.g., transporter saturation effects, interplay with food and gastric emptying effects, and different hydrodynamics or mechanical stresses; these factors may complicate the correlation between disintegration and bioavailability [39]. Dahan's group investigated the role of segmental-dependent intestinal absorption in controlled release (CR) drug product development. The studied drug was carvedilol due to its zwitterionic nature; thus, this compound changes solubility in different conditions throughout the GIT [40]. The solubility, permeability, and dissolution of the drug were investigated in silico, in vitro, and in vivo, focusing on location-dependent effects. The authors demonstrated that a CR product could modify the drug solubility behavior from class II to I; these results are highly relevant in the decision-making process regarding the development of new CR drug products. The increased interest in drug delivery to the last segments of the GIT has led to new insights in the design of colonic delivery devices; Christfort et al. studied cylindrical, triangular, and cubic microcontainers with amoxicillin and showed that shape and surface texture of microcontainers influence the ex vivo mucoadhesion (cubic microcontainers are more adhered to intestinal mucus than cylindrical microcontainers), and the absorption of amoxicillin was higher from cubic microcontainers than from cylindrical or triangular microcontainers [41].

This Special Issue also includes two highly relevant review articles: the group of K. Sandy Pang focus on intestinal and liver metabolism and drug–drug interactions [42], and Tongzhi et al. focus on regional gut stimulation, concluding that the region of the gut exposed to intraluminal stimuli is of major relevance to the secretion profile of gastrointestinal hormones and associated metabolic responses [43].

Conflicts of Interest: The authors declare no conflict of interest.

References

1. Dahan, A.; Miller, J.M.; Hilfinger, J.M.; Yamashita, S.; Yu, L.X.; Lennernäs, H.; Amidon, G.L. High-Permeability Criterion for BCS Classification: Segmental/pH Dependent Permeability Considerations. *Mol. Pharm.* **2010**, *7*, 1827–1834. [CrossRef]
2. Fairstein, M.; Swissa, R.; Dahan, A. Regional-Dependent Intestinal Permeability and BCS Classification: Elucidation of pH-Related Complexity in Rats Using Pseudoephedrine. *AAPS J.* **2013**, *15*, 589–597. [CrossRef]
3. Kataoka, M.; Fukahori, M.; Ikemura, A.; Kubota, A.; Higashino, H.; Sakuma, S.; Yamashita, S. Effects of gastric pH on oral drug absorption: In vitro assessment using a dissolution/permeation system reflecting the gastric dissolution process. *Eur. J. Pharm. Biopharm.* **2016**, *101*, 103–111. [CrossRef]
4. Zur, M.; Cohen, N.; Agbaria, R.; Dahan, A. The biopharmaceutics of successful controlled release drug product: Segmental-dependent permeability of glipizide vs. metoprolol throughout the intestinal tract. *Int. J. Pharm.* **2015**, *489*, 304–310. [CrossRef] [PubMed]
5. Zur, M.; Gasparini, M.; Wolk, O.; Amidon, G.L.; Dahan, A. The Low/High BCS Permeability Class Boundary: Physicochemical Comparison of Metoprolol and Labetalol. *Mol. Pharm.* **2014**, *11*, 1707–1714. [CrossRef]
6. Zur, M.; Hanson, A.S.; Dahan, A. The complexity of intestinal permeability: Assigning the correct BCS classification through careful data interpretation. *Eur. J. Pharm. Sci.* **2014**, *61*, 11–17. [CrossRef] [PubMed]
7. Figueroa-Campos, A.; Sánchez-Dengra, B.; Merino, V.; Dahan, A.; González-Álvarez, I.; García-Arieta, A.; González-Álvarez, M.; Bermejo, M. Candesartan Cilexetil In Vitro–In Vivo Correlation: Predictive Dissolution as a Development Tool. *Pharmaceutics* **2020**, *12*, 633. [CrossRef]

8. Kostewicz, E.S.; Aarons, L.; Bergstrand, M.; Bolger, M.B.; Galetin, A.; Hatley, O.; Jamei, M.; Lloyd, R.; Pepin, X.; Rostami-Hodjegan, A.; et al. PBPK models for the prediction of in vivo performance of oral dosage forms. *Eur. J. Pharm. Sci.* **2014**, *57*, 300–321. [CrossRef] [PubMed]
9. Mudie, D.M.; Amidon, G.L.; Amidon, G.E. Physiological Parameters for Oral Delivery and in Vitro Testing. *Mol. Pharm.* **2010**, *7*, 1388–1405. [CrossRef] [PubMed]
10. Dahan, A.; Amidon, G.L. Segmental Dependent Transport of Low Permeability Compounds along the Small Intestine Due to P-Glycoprotein: The Role of Efflux Transport in the Oral Absorption of BCS Class III Drugs. *Mol. Pharm.* **2009**, *6*, 19–28. [CrossRef]
11. Dahan, A.; Sabit, H.; Amidon, G.L. Multiple Efflux Pumps Are Involved in the Transepithelial Transport of Colchicine: Combined Effect of P-Glycoprotein and Multidrug Resistance-Associated Protein 2 Leads to Decreased Intestinal Absorption Throughout the Entire Small Intestine. *Drug Metab. Dispos.* **2009**, *37*, 2028–2036. [CrossRef]
12. Jappar, D.; Wu, S.-P.; Hu, Y.; Smith, D.E. Significance and Regional Dependency of Peptide Transporter (PEPT) 1 in the Intestinal Permeability of Glycylsarcosine: In Situ Single-Pass Perfusion Studies in Wild-Type and Pept1 Knockout Mice. *Drug Metab. Dispos.* **2010**, *38*, 1740–1746. [CrossRef] [PubMed]
13. Tubic-Grozdanis, M.; Hilfinger, J.M.; Amidon, G.L.; Kim, J.S.; Kijek, P.; Staubach, P.; Langguth, P. Pharmacokinetics of the CYP 3A Substrate Simvastatin following Administration of Delayed Versus Immediate Release Oral Dosage Forms. *Pharm. Res.* **2008**, *25*, 1591–1600. [CrossRef]
14. Vaessen, S.F.C.; Van Lipzig, M.M.H.; Pieters, R.H.H.; Krul, C.A.M.; Wortelboer, H.M.; Van De Steeg, E. Regional Expression Levels of Drug Transporters and Metabolizing Enzymes along the Pig and Human Intestinal Tract and Comparison with Caco-2 Cells. *Drug Metab. Dispos.* **2017**, *45*, 353–360. [CrossRef] [PubMed]
15. Jung, K.; Eyerly, B.; Annamalai, T.; Lu, Z.; Saif, L.J. Structural alteration of tight and adherens junctions in villous and crypt epithelium of the small and large intestine of conventional nursing piglets infected with porcine epidemic diarrhea virus. *Vet. Microbiol.* **2015**, *177*, 373–378. [CrossRef] [PubMed]
16. Ozawa, M.; Tsume, Y.; Zur, M.; Dahan, A.; Amidon, G.L. Intestinal Permeability Study of Minoxidil: Assessment of Minoxidil as a High Permeability Reference Drug for Biopharmaceutics Classification. *Mol. Pharm.* **2015**, *12*, 204–211. [CrossRef]
17. Dahan, A.; Lennernäs, H.; Amidon, G.L. The Fraction Dose Absorbed, in Humans, and High Jejunal Human Permeability Relationship. *Mol. Pharm.* **2012**, *9*, 1847–1851. [CrossRef] [PubMed]
18. Lennernäs, H. Regional intestinal drug permeation: Biopharmaceutics and drug development. *Eur. J. Pharm. Sci.* **2014**, *57*, 333–341. [CrossRef] [PubMed]
19. Lennernäs, H. Human in Vivo Regional Intestinal Permeability: Importance for Pharmaceutical Drug Development. *Mol. Pharm.* **2014**, *11*, 12–23. [CrossRef]
20. Olivares-Morales, A.; Lennernäs, H.; Aarons, L.; Rostami-Hodjegan, A. Translating Human Effective Jejunal Intestinal Permeability to Surface-Dependent Intrinsic Permeability: A Pragmatic Method for a More Mechanistic Prediction of Regional Oral Drug Absorption. *AAPS J.* **2015**, *17*, 1177–1192. [CrossRef]
21. Markovic, M.; Zur, M.; Dahan, A.; Cvijić, S. Biopharmaceutical characterization of rebamipide: The role of mucus binding in regional-dependent intestinal permeability. *Eur. J. Pharm. Sci.* **2020**, *152*, 105440. [CrossRef]
22. Bisanz, J.E.; Spanogiannopoulos, P.; Pieper, L.M.; Bustion, A.E.; Turnbaugh, P.J. How to Determine the Role of the Microbiome in Drug Disposition. *Drug Metab. Dispos.* **2018**, *46*, 1588–1595. [CrossRef]
23. Clarke, G.; Sandhu, K.V.; Griffin, B.T.; Dinan, T.G.; Cryan, J.F.; Hyland, N.P. Gut Reactions: Breaking Down Xenobiotic–Microbiome Interactions. *Pharmacol. Rev.* **2019**, *71*, 198–224. [CrossRef]
24. Spanogiannopoulos, P.; Bess, E.N.; Carmody, R.N.; Turnbaugh, P.J. The microbial pharmacists within us: A metagenomic view of xenobiotic metabolism. *Nat. Rev. Microbiol.* **2016**, *14*, 273–287. [CrossRef] [PubMed]
25. Dahan, A.; Beig, A.; Lindley, D.; Miller, J.M. The solubility–permeability interplay and oral drug formulation design: Two heads are better than one. *Adv. Drug Deliv. Rev.* **2016**, *101*, 99–107. [CrossRef] [PubMed]
26. Fine-Shamir, N.; Beig, A.; Dahan, A. Adequate Formulation Approach for Oral Chemotherapy: Etoposide Solubility, Permeability, and Overall Bioavailability from Cosolvent- vs. Vitamin E TPGS-Based Delivery Systems. *Int. J. Pharm.* **2021**. [CrossRef]
27. Lozoya-Agullo, I.; Zur, M.; Beig, A.; Fine, N.; Cohen, Y.; González-Álvarez, M.; Merino-Sanjuán, M.; González-Álvarez, I.; Bermejo, M.; Dahan, A. Segmental-dependent permeability throughout the small intestine following oral drug administration: Single-pass vs. Doluisio approach to in-situ rat perfusion. *Int. J. Pharm.* **2016**, 201–208. [CrossRef]
28. Wolk, O.; Markovic, M.; Porat, D.; Fine-Shamir, N.; Zur, M.; Beig, A.; Dahan, A. Segmental-Dependent Intestinal Drug Permeability: Development and Model Validation of In Silico Predictions Guided by In Vivo Permeability Values. *J. Pharm. Sci.* **2019**, *108*, 316–325. [CrossRef] [PubMed]
29. Teixeira, L.d.; Chagas, T.V.; Alonso, A.; Gonzalez-Alvarez, I.; Bermejo, M.; Polli, J.; Rezende, K.R. Biomimetic Artificial Membrane Permeability Assay over Franz Cell Apparatus Using BCS Model Drugs. *Pharmaceutics* **2020**, *12*, 988. [CrossRef]
30. Lozoya-Agullo, I.; Gonzalez-Alvarez, I.; Zur, M.; Fine-Shamir, N.; Cohen, Y.; Markovic, M.; Garrigues, T.M.; Dahan, A.; Gonzalez-Alvarez, M.; Merino-Sanjuán, M.; et al. Closed-Loop Doluisio (Colon, Small Intestine) and Single-Pass Intestinal Perfusion (Colon, Jejunum) in Rat—Biophysical Model and Predictions Based on Caco-2. *Pharm. Res.* **2017**, *35*, 2. [CrossRef] [PubMed]
31. Pham-The, H.; Cabrera-Pérez, M.Á.; Nam, N.-H.; Castillo-Garit, J.A.; Rasulev, B.; Le-Thi-Thu, H.; Casañola-Martin, G.M. In Silico Assessment of ADME Properties: Advances in Caco-2 Cell Monolayer Permeability Modeling. *Curr. Top. Med. Chem.* **2018**, *18*, 2209–2229. [CrossRef]

32. Pham-The, H.; Garrigues, T.; Bermejo, M.; González-Álvarez, I.; Monteagudo, M.C.; Cabrera-Pérez, M.Á. Provisional Classification and in Silico Study of Biopharmaceutical System Based on Caco-2 Cell Permeability and Dose Number. *Mol. Pharm.* **2013**, *10*, 2445–2461. [CrossRef] [PubMed]
33. Ta, G.H.; Jhang, C.-S.; Weng, C.-F.; Leong, M.K. Development of a Hierarchical Support Vector Regression-Based In Silico Model for Caco-2 Permeability. *Pharmaceutics* **2021**, *13*, 174. [CrossRef]
34. Ruiz-Picazo, A.; Colón-Useche, S.; Perez-Amorós, B.; González-Álvarez, M.; Molina-Martínez, I.; González-Álvarez, I.; García-Arieta, A.; Bermejo, M. Investigation to Explain Bioequivalence Failure in Pravastatin Immediate-Release Products. *Pharmaceutics* **2019**, *11*, 663. [CrossRef]
35. Bermejo, M.; Hens, B.; Dickens, J.; Mudie, D.; Paixão, P.; Tsume, Y.; Shedden, K.; Amidon, G.L. A Mechanistic Physiologically-Based Biopharmaceutics Modeling (PBBM) Approach to Assess the In Vivo Performance of an Orally Administered Drug Product: From IVIVC to IVIVP. *Pharmaceutics* **2020**, *12*, 74. [CrossRef]
36. Markovic, M.; Zur, M.; Ragatsky, I.; Cvijić, S.; Dahan, A. BCS Class IV Oral Drugs and Absorption Windows: Regional-Dependent Intestinal Permeability of Furosemide. *Pharmaceutics* **2020**, *12*, 1175. [CrossRef] [PubMed]
37. Ruiz-Garcia, A.; Tan, W.; Li, J.; Haughey, M.; Masters, J.; Hibma, J.; Lin, S. Pharmacokinetic Models to Characterize the Absorption Phase and the Influence of a Proton Pump Inhibitor on the Overall Exposure of Dacomitinib. *Pharmaceutics* **2020**, *12*, 330. [CrossRef]
38. Dahlgren, D.; Cano-Cebrián, M.-J.; Olander, T.; Hedeland, M.; Sjöblom, M.; Lennernäs, H. Regional Intestinal Drug Permeability and Effects of Permeation Enhancers in Rat. *Pharmaceutics* **2020**, *12*, 242. [CrossRef]
39. Fu, M.; Al-Gousous, J.; Blechar, J.A.; Langguth, P. Enteric Hard Capsules for Targeting the Small Intestine: Positive Correlation between In Vitro Disintegration and Dissolution Times. *Pharmaceutics* **2020**, *12*, 123. [CrossRef] [PubMed]
40. Markovic, M.; Zur, M.; Fine-Shamir, N.; Haimov, E.; González-Álvarez, I.; Dahan, A. Segmental-Dependent Solubility and Permeability as Key Factors Guiding Controlled Release Drug Product Development. *Pharmaceutics* **2020**, *12*, 295. [CrossRef]
41. Christfort, J.F.; Guillot, A.J.; Melero, A.; Thamdrup, L.H.E.; Garrigues, T.M.; Boisen, A.; Zór, K.; Nielsen, L.H. Cubic Microcontainers Improve In Situ Colonic Mucoadhesion and Absorption of Amoxicillin in Rats. *Pharmaceutics* **2020**, *12*, 355. [CrossRef] [PubMed]
42. Pang, K.S.; Peng, H.B.; Noh, K. The Segregated Intestinal Flow Model (SFM) for Drug Absorption and Drug Metabolism: Implications on Intestinal and Liver Metabolism and Drug–Drug Interactions. *Pharmaceutics* **2020**, *12*, 312. [CrossRef] [PubMed]
43. Xie, C.; Jones, K.L.; Rayner, C.K.; Wu, T. Enteroendocrine Hormone Secretion and Metabolic Control: Importance of the Region of the Gut Stimulation. *Pharmaceutics* **2020**, *12*, 790. [CrossRef] [PubMed]

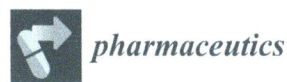

Article

Biomimetic Artificial Membrane Permeability Assay over Franz Cell Apparatus Using BCS Model Drugs

Leonardo de Souza Teixeira [1,†], Tatiana Vila Chagas [2,†], Antonio Alonso [3], Isabel Gonzalez-Alvarez [4], Marival Bermejo [4], James Polli [5] and Kênnia Rocha Rezende [2,*]

1. Institute of Pharmaceutical Sciences, Goiânia, Goiás 74175-100, Brazil; leonardo.teixeira@icf.com.br
2. Laboratory of Biopharmacy and Pharmacokinetics (BioPK), Faculty of Pharmacy, Federal University of Goiás, Goiânia, Goiás 74175-100, Brazil; tatianavchagas@gmail.com
3. Institute of Physics, Federal University of Goiás, Goiânia, Goiás 74175-100, Brazil; alonso2233@gmail.com
4. Department of Engineering, Pharmacy Section, Miguel Hernandez University, 03550 Alicante, Spain; isabel.gonzalez@goumh.umh.es (I.G.-A.); mbermejo@umh.es (M.B.)
5. Faculty of Pharmacy, University of Maryland, Baltimore, MD 21021, USA; jpolli@rx.umaryland.edu
* Correspondence: kennia@ufg.br; Tel.: +55-(62)-98117-9445
† These authors contribute equally to this paper.

Received: 8 September 2020; Accepted: 10 October 2020; Published: 19 October 2020

Abstract: A major parameter controlling the extent and rate of oral drug absorption is permeability through the lipid bilayer of intestinal epithelial cells. Here, a biomimetic artificial membrane permeability assay (Franz–PAMPA Pampa) was validated using a Franz cells apparatus. Both high and low permeability drugs (metoprolol and mannitol, respectively) were used as external standards. Biomimetic properties of Franz–PAMPA were also characterized by electron paramagnetic resonance spectroscopy (EPR). Moreover, the permeation profile for eight Biopharmaceutic Classification System (BCS) model drugs cited in the FDA guidance and another six drugs (acyclovir, cimetidine, diclofenac, ibuprofen, piroxicam, and trimethoprim) were measured across Franz–PAMPA. Apparent permeability (Papp) Franz–PAMPA values were correlated with fraction of dose absorbed in humans (Fa%) from the literature. Papp in Caco-2 cells and Corti artificial membrane were likewise compared to Fa% to assess Franz–PAMPA performance. Mannitol and metoprolol Papp values across Franz–PAMPA were lower (3.20×10^{-7} and 1.61×10^{-5} cm/s, respectively) than those obtained across non-impregnated membrane (2.27×10^{-5} and 2.55×10^{-5} cm/s, respectively), confirming lipidic barrier resistivity. Performance of the Franz cell permeation apparatus using an artificial membrane showed acceptable log-linear correlation ($R^2 = 0.664$) with Fa%, as seen for Papp in Caco-2 cells ($R^2 = 0.805$). Data support the validation of the Franz–PAMPA method for use during the drug discovery process.

Keywords: Franz–PAMPA; BCS drugs; biomimetic membrane; Franz cell; passive drug transport

1. Introduction

Favorable absorption, distribution, metabolism, and excretion (ADME) of orally administered drugs are essential for therapeutic activity in vivo. Poor oral bioavailability contributes to a very high failure rate during pre-clinical drug development [1,2]. In this regard, the Biopharmaceutic Classification System (BCS) proposed by Amidon and co-workers [3] have been widely used as an important tool to support early drug development [4–6]. For orally administered drugs, gastrointestinal physiology is a key factor impacting on the rate and extent of drug absorption [7]. Transcellular passive diffusion across membranes is the major route and is governed by several molecular properties such as partition and distribution coefficient, as well as molecular weight [8,9].

Currently, important tools based on physicochemical properties and in vitro assays are used to predict in vivo gastrointestinal absorption [10]. In vitro methodologies include animal [11,12] or human tissues [13], cultured cells [14,15] and artificial membranes [16–18]. The Caco-2 cell monolayers in vitro model is thoroughly studied and generally mimics major transport pathways in the gastrointestinal tract [19]. However, this method is limited by long cell growth and differentiation cycles, risks of microbial contamination, and high implementation costs [19–21].

Cell-free permeation systems using artificial membranes are gaining progressively more interest as an alternative model to cell-based systems that can be simpler, less time consuming, and cost-effective [22,23]. Depending on the composition of the barrier, it can be classified as biomimetic barrier which is constructed from (phospho)lipids or, alternatively, from non-biomimetic barrier containing dialysis membrane [24].

Particularly, there is a growing interest in PAMPA studies with direct comparisons to Caco-2 cells using a consistent number of drugs displaying equally well prediction of in vivo data between them [25]. In this regard, major differences of key components amid cell-free membranes currently used in permeability systems was highlighted by Berben et al. (2018) [23].

Here, a previously validated biomimetic artificial permeability membrane comprising of a microfilter impregnated by a phospholipid solution [5] was mounted on horizontal Franz-cells diffusion chambers (Microette™, Hanson Research) [20]. This new setup approach, herein called Franz–PAMPA (Figure 1), was challenged to assess permeability of BCS model drugs simulating gastrointestinal permeation. Therefore, the aim of this study was to validate this Franz–PAMPA system by evaluating the correlation power between apparent permeability (Papp) for BCS model drugs to their fraction of drug absorbed (Fa%) in humans for rapid and reliable information about passively transported drugs [25,26].

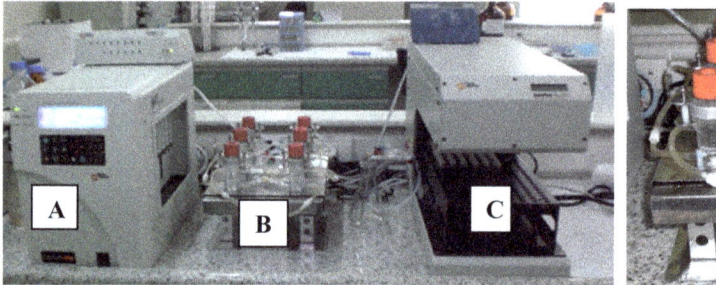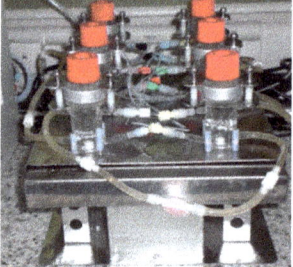

Figure 1. Franz cells apparatus (Microette™, Hanson Research) mounted with a previously validated PAMPA membrane from Corti et al. [5,16] for simulating gastrointestinal permeation. (**A**) System control for injection pistons of upper chambers; (**B**) upper and lower diffusion chambers with temperature and stirring control; (**C**) automated module for sampling and collection.

2. Materials and Methods

2.1. Materials

Membrane supports were purchased from Millipore® (Mixed Cellulose Esters VCWP 047000; 0.1 μm × 47 mm, white plain, New York, NY, USA). All 19 compounds for permeation studies (acyclovir, amoxicillin, atenolol, caffeine, cimetidine, diclofenac, furosemide, hydrochlorothiazide, ibuprofen, mannitol, metoprolol, naproxen, piroxicam, propranolol, ranitidine hydrochloride, trimethoprim, and verapamil hydrochloride) were of analytical grade and kindly supplied by ICF (Pharmaceutical Sciences Institute, Goiânia, Brazil). All organic solvents were of HPLC grade and solid reagents were of analytical grade.

The spin labels 5-doxyl stearic acid (5-DSA) and 16-doxyl stearic acid (16-DSA) used for electron paramagnetic resonance (EPR) spectroscopy were purchased from Sigma-Aldrich Chem Co. (St. Louis, MO, USA). The spin labels 1-palmitoyl-2-stearoyl-(5-doxyl)-sn-glycero-3-phosphocholine

(5-PC) and 1,2-dipalmitoleoyl-sn-glycero-3-phosphocholin (16-PC) were purchased from Avanti (Avanti Polar Lipids, Inc., Alabaster, AL, USA).

2.2. Methods

2.2.1. Impregnation of Membrane Support

Membranes were impregnated by immersion for 60 min (22 ± 1 °C) with a lipid solution (mixture of phospholipids), as previously reported [5]. Briefly, the lipid phase solution for impregnation was a mixture of 1.7% phospholipids (Lipoid® E 80, Ludwigshafen, Germany), 2.1% cholesterol (Sigma–Aldrich Chemical Co., Milan, Italy), and 96.2% n-octanol (Synth, Diadema, Brazil). Excess lipid was absorbed with cellulose filter paper over 30 min. Next, all impregnated membranes (N = 20) were weighed on a microanalytical scale (Mettler Toledo, mod. XPE56DR, Columbus, OH, USA) and evaluated to check for its accuracy (211.2 mg ± 6.0%). Prior to use, impregnated membranes were protected from moisture atmosphere and refrigerated (−8 °C, 24 h). It is worth mentioning that all membranes were stabilized prior to use. Stabilization was confirmed by EPR spectra which did not show any signals of physicochemical degradation: none of membranes showed any difference on ^{14}N-hyperfine coupling constant value (14.8 G) demonstrating its stability [25]. EPR signals were compared just after 24 h of refrigeration and post-run permeability studies as well as after a month of refrigerated storage time *(data not shown)*.

2.2.2. Electronic Paramagnetic Resonance (EPR)

The biomimetic membranes were impregnated, as described above. Spin labeling technique was employed to examine the conformational structure of the membrane using 5-DSA or 16-DSA. EPR was performed using a Bruker ESP 300 spectrometer (Bruker, Rheinstetten, Germany) equipped with an ER 4102 ST resonator. The instrument settings were microwave power of 2 mW; modulation frequency of 100 KHz; modulation amplitude of 1.0 G; magnetic field scan of 100 G; sweep time of 168 s; and a detector time constant of 41 ms. EPR spectral simulations were performed using the nonlinear-least-squares (NLLS) program for an isotropic model. The biomimetic membrane was introduced into flat, quartz EPR cell to perform the EPR measurements at room temperature (~25°C).

2.2.3. Permeation Studies

Permeation studies were performed using a Franz vertical diffusion cell (MicroettePlus, Hanson Research, CA, USA). Impregnated artificial membranes (Franz–PAMPA) were positioned between upper and lower part of diffusion cells and, the donor (1 mL) and receptor (7 mL) compartments holding phosphate-buffered solution (PBS) pH 7.4 (USP 32). In order to minimize the unstirred water layer (UWL), receptor compartment media was stirred (500 rpm). The temperature was kept constant (37.0 ± 0.5 °C). Each drug (n = 3) was added in the donor compartment at a fixed concentration (=10 mg/mL). One milliliter of saturated drug solutions was transferred to the donor compartments and capped to prevent evaporation. The experiments were performed under 'infinite dose' conditions [26,27], except for caffein, metoprolol, propranolol, naproxen, ranitidine, and atenolol ($D_0 \leq 0.01$). Individual drug solubility is further shown in results section. Metoprolol was used as a low/high BCS permeability class boundary reference drug for the Franz–PAMPA assay [28].

Samples from permeation studies were collected during 12 h (0.25; 0.5; 1.0; 2.0; 3.0; 4.0; 5.0; 6.0; 10.0, and 12.0 h) and analyzed by HPLC (Shimadzu Class VP; Kyoto, Japan or Agilent 1220, Santa Clara, CA, USA) according to official compendiums (USP 32 or Brazilian Pharmacopeia 4th edition). The sampling volume was immediately replaced with the same volume of fresh PBS prewarmed solution at 37° ± 0.5 °C. Calibration curves were performed at least at three concentration levels for each drug tested, in a GLP-accredited laboratory (Institute of Pharmaceutical Sciences, Goiânia, Goiás, Brazil). The validated chromatographic conditions used for the drug permeability assay are given in Table 1.

Table 1. Pharmacopeial methods applied on drug analysis and their respective limit of quantification (LOQs).

Drug	Chromatographic Conditions (Stationary and Mobile Phase; λ; Flow Rate; Injection Volume)	LOQ (µg/mL)
Acyclovir	C-18 (5 µm; 250 × 4.2 mm), acetic acid: water (1:1000); 254 nm; 3.0 mL/min; 20 µL	46.3
Amoxicillin	C18 (5 µm; 250 × 4.0 mm); acetonitrile phosphate buffer pH 5.0 (4:96); 230 nm, 1.5 mL/min, 10 µL	1.00
Atenolol	C-18 (5 µm; 300 × 3.9 mm); Dissolve 1.1 g of sodium heptane sulfonate and 0.71 g of sodium phosphate dibasic anhydrous in 700 mL of water. Add 2 mL of dibutylamine. Adjust pH 3.0. Add methanol (300 mL); 226 nm; 0.6 mL/min; 10 µL	3.4
Caffeine	C-18 (5 µm; 150 × 4.6 mm); Solution of 1.64 g anhydrous sodium acetate in 2000 mL of water. Take 1910 mL of this solution add acetonitrile (50 mL), tetrahydrofuran (40 mL). Adjust pH 4.5 with glacial acetic acid; 275 nm; 1.0 mL/min; 10 µL	19.0
Carbamazepine	CN ((250 mm × 4,.6 mm); Water, methanol, and tetrahydrofuran (85:12:3), 0.22 mL formic acid and 0.5 mL triethylamine; 230 nm, 1.5 mL/min, 20 µL	0.03
Cimetidine	C-18 (5 µm; 300 × 3.9 mm); 20% methanol in 0.3% phosphoric acid solution; 220 nm; 2.0 mL/min; 50 µL	1.0
Diclofenac sodium	C-8 (5 µm; 250 × 4.6 mm); phosphate buffer pH 2.5 and methanol (30:70); 254 nm; 1.0 mL/min; 10 µL	0.20
Furosemide	C-18 (5 µm; 250 × 4.6 mm); Water, tetrahydrofuran, and glacial acetic acid (70:30:1); 254 nm; 1.0 mL/min; 20 µL	16.6
Hydrochlor-thiazide	C-18 (5 µm; 150 × 4.6 mm); Solution A: acetonitrile and methanol (3:1). Solution B: 0.5% formic acid. Gradient: 0–3 min. Sol A: Sol B (3:97), 5–14 min. Sol A: Sol. B (3 to 36:97 to 64), 14–18 min. The Sol. A: Sol B (36 to 3:64 to 97), 18–20 min. Sol A: Sol B (3:97); 275 nm; 1.0 mL/min; 10 µL	7.8
Ibuprofen	C-18 (5 µm; 250 × 4.6 mm); 4% chloroacetic acid pH 3.0 and acetonitrile (40:60); 254 nm; 2.0 mL/min; 10 µL	13.9
Ketoprophen	C18 (3 µm; 150 × 4.6 mm); water, acetonitrile, and phosphate buffer pH13.5 (55:43:22); 233 nm, 1.0 mL/min, 20 µL	1.56
Metoprolol	C-18 (5 µm; 300 × 3.9 mm); 961 mg of pentane sulfonate, 82 mg of anhydrous sodium acetate, 550 mL of methanol, 470 mL of water and 0.57 mL of acetic acid; 254 nm; 1.0 mL/min; 30 µL	13.8
Methyldopa	C18 (5 µm; 300 × 3.9 mm); Monobasic phosphate buffer pH 3.5; 280 nm, 1.0 mL/min, 50 µL	0.12
Naproxen	C-18 (5 µm; 150 × 4.6 mm); Acetonitrile, water, and glacial acetic acid (50:49:1); 254 nm; 1.2 mL/min; 20 µL	3.6
Piroxicam	C-18 (5 µm; 250 × 4.6 mm); Buffer solution containing 7.72 g of anhydrous citric acid in 400 mL of water and 5.35 g dibasic sodium phosphate in 100 mL of water, mix the two solutions and adjust volume to 1000 mL with water.Mix buffer and methanol (55:45); 254 nm; 1.2 mL/min; 20 µL	4.0
Propranolol	C-8 (5 µm; 250 × 4.6 mm); Dissolve 0.5 g of sodium dodecyl sulfate in 18 mL of 0.15 M phosphoric acid. Add 90 mL of acetonitrile, 90 mL of methanol, dilute with water to complete 250 mL; 290 nm; 1.5 mL/min; 20 µL	8.2
Ranitidine	C-18 (3.5 µm; 10 × 4.6 mm); buffer phosphate pH 7.1: acetonitrile (80:20); 230 nm, 1.5 mL/min, 35°C, 10 µL	7.4
Trimethoprim	C-18 (5 µm; 250 × 4.2 mm); 1% glacial acetic acid: acetonitrile (21:4); 254 nm, 2 mL/min, 10 µL	0.15
Theophylline	C-18 (5 µm; 300 × 4.0 mm); 7% acetonitrile in sodium acetate buffer; 280 nm, 1 mL/min, 10 µL	0.22
Verapamil	C-18 (5 µm; 150 × 4.6 mm); 0.015 N sodium acetate in 3.3% glacial acetic acid. add acetonitrile and 2-amino-heptane (70:30:0.5); 278 nm; 0.9 mL/min; 10 µL	0.50

2.2.4. Permeability Calculations

The diffusion area (A) was calculated from the radius of the Franz cell and was 1.77 cm^2. Flux through membrane to receptor compartment (J; µg/cm^2/s) was calculated by dividing the amount of drug accumulated in the receptor compartment by A. The Fick's first law was derived to calculate flux (J) at steady state (Equation (1)):

$$J = dQ/dt * A \qquad (1)$$

where dQ is the amount of drug across the membrane (in moles), dt the permeation time (in seconds), and A the diffusion area (in cm^2). Note that J was obtained from the slope of the curve at steady state from typical mean cumulative concentration-time plots (minimum of triplicates), as further shown in results section (Figure 2). Coefficient of variation (CV) of flux for each drug was also measured.

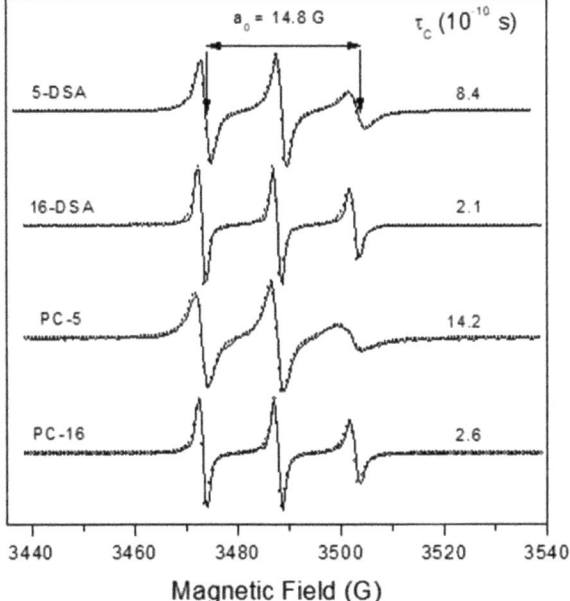

Figure 2. Experimental (solid line) and best-fit (empty circles) EPR spectra for several spin labels in BAMPA. The isotropic 14N-hyperfine coupling constant, a_0, showed equal spectra values of 14.8 G, consistent with a spin label in phospholipidic bilayer of eukaryotic cells. The rotational correlation time value, τC, is also showed. 5-DSA or 16-DSA: 5- or 16-doxylstearic acid); 5-PC or 16-PC:5-0r 16-phosphatidylcholine).

The apparent permeability ($Papp$) was calculated normalizing the flux (J) over the drug concentration in the donor compartment C_0, as described by the following Equation (2):

$$Papp = J/C_0 \qquad (2)$$

This approximation was used in all cases, even when sink conditions do not hold and donor concentrations change with time, as already described for some experiments [29]. In addition, the following equation was used to account for the fact that in most cases sink conditions were not maintained [30].

$$C_{receiver,t} = \frac{Q_{total}}{V_{receiver} + V_{donor}} + \left((C_{receiver,t-1} \cdot f) - \frac{Q_{total}}{V_{receiver} + V_{donor}} \right) \cdot e^{-P_{eff} \cdot S \cdot \left(\frac{1}{V_{receiver}} + \frac{1}{V_{donor}} \right) \cdot \Delta t} \qquad (3)$$

where $C_{receiver,t}$ is the drug concentration in the receiver chamber at time t, Q_{total} is the total amount of drug in both chambers, $V_{receiver}$ and V_{donor} are the volumes of each chamber, $C_{receiver,t-1}$ is the drug concentration in receiver chamber at previous time, f is the sample replacement dilution factor, S is the surface area of the membrane, Δt is the time interval and P_{eff} is the permeability coefficient. This equation considers a continuous change of the donor and receiver concentrations, and it is valid in either sink or non-sink conditions. The curve-fitting is performed by non-linear regression, by minimization of the sum of squared residuals (SSR), where:

$$SSR = \sum [C_{r,i,obs} - C_{r,i}(t_{end,i})]^2 \quad (4)$$

$C_{r,i,obs}$ is the observed receiver concentration at the end of interval i, and $C_{r,I}(t_{end,i})$ is the corresponding concentration at the same time calculated according to Equation (3) [29].

Classification as high permeability was established if the calculated permeability (under sink or non-sink conditions was higher than 0.8* metoprolol permeability [31].

The in vitro permeability (Papp) of each drug studied was compared to in vivo absorption in humans (Fa%), Papp in Corti artificial membrane [16], and Papp in Caco-2 cells.

3. Results

3.1. EPR Analysis and Membrane Stability

The Franz–PAMPA was characterized by EPR spectroscopy of lipid spin labels of doxyl class. The spectra showed a movement consistent with lipid bilayer (Figure 1). Two analogs of stearic acid, 5-DSA and 16-DSA, and two analogs of phosphatidylcholine, 5-PC and 16-PC, having the nitroxide radical positioned at the 5th and 16th carbon atom of the acyl chain, respectively, were used to examine the molecular dynamic at two regions into the bilayer. The EPR spectra of these four spin labels are shown in Figure 2.

The EPR parameter—isotropic ^{14}N-hyperfine coupling constant, a_0—increased with increasing dielectric constant (i.e., solvent polarity) in which the nitroxide radical is dissolved. The measured value of 14.8 G is consistent with a spin label in a membrane [32]. The spin labels 5-DSA and 5-PC with the nitroxide moiety in the region near the polar head group of the bilayer showed more restricted rotational motion relative to their positional isomers 16-DSA and 16-PC, in which the nitroxide radical is more deeply inserted in the hydrophobic core. These results indicate the existence of a gradient of flexibility along the acyl chain, with more restricted motion in the polar region. This pattern is consistent with the properties of lipid bilayers from eukaryotic cells. The rotational motion at the polar interface of the membrane was more restricted for the spin label analog of phosphatidylcholine (5-PC) with τ_C of 14.2×10^{-10} s than for the stearic acid one (5-DSA) whose τ_C was of 8.4×10^{-10} s (Figure 2).

Membrane barriers from similar models such as PAMPA and PVPA have been proven to be stable in a pH range from 2 to 8 [33]. Here, EPR spectra were also recorded before and after permeation studies to check for the integrity of biomimetic membranes. No leaching of barrier-constituents such as phosphatidylcholine and lipids into the donor compartment could be evidenced as none of membranes showed any difference on ^{14}N-hyperfine coupling constant value (14.8 G) demonstrating its stability [34]. Likewise, using the same chemical composition as Corti (2006) [5], acidic and basic drugs also showed pH-dependent permeability according to the pH partition theory [25,35]. Accordingly, close Person's correlation coefficient was seen (r = 0.7355) to our data from Franz–PAMPA *versus* PAMPA pH 7.4 data from literature.

In this regard, pHs of drug solutions were all measured to assure buffer capacity and drug stability. Some authors correlated membrane flux with the fraction absorbed in human, showing that the flux through the egg lecithin/dodecane membrane correlated better than octanol/water logD values with the fraction absorbed in humans [17]. Later, an in-depth investigation of pH impact on drug Franz–PAMPA permeability will be necessary to increase the biomimetic and absorption predictive power of this method, although the study of this factor was beyond the scope of this work.

3.2. Membrane Validation and Performance

Studies here deals with a modified PAMPA method over Franz cell apparatus. The biomimetic membrane (Franz–PAMPA) has been previously described by Corti and coworkers [5] as a modified version from Kansy et al. (1998) [36]. Mannitol and metoprolol were used as a marker for the cutoff point between low and high permeability drugs.

The apparent permeability coefficient (Papp) values found for mannitol and metoprolol, over the lipid impregnated membrane (2.27×10^{-5} and 2.55×10^{-5} cm/s, respectively) were higher when compared to the non-impregnated one across Franz–PAMPA (3.20×10^{-7} and 1.61×10^{-5} cm/s, respectively), indicating the resistivity of the lipid membrane itself.

Membrane performance was assessed using 14 representative model drugs (Table 2) cited in the FDA BCS guidance [37]. Class I model compounds were caffeine, metoprolol, propranolol and verapamil. Class II model compounds were diclofenac, ibuprofen, naproxen and, piroxicam. Class III model compounds were atenolol, cimetidine, ranitidine, and trimethoprim. Class IV model compounds were acyclovir, furosemide and hydrochlorothiazide. This classification was based in the permeability class indicated in the FDA guidance [37] and, on solubility from literature [28].

Cumulative drug transport through Franz–PAMPA was plotted over 12 h and the Papp was calculated from the slopes obtained from linear regressions (Figure 3, Table 2). Of the 21 compounds studied by Corti and coworkers and of the 14 compounds studied here, there were 11 common compounds tested in both studies: acyclovir, atenolol, caffeine, cimetidine, furosemide, hydrochlorothiazide, metoprolol tartrate, naproxen, propranolol, ranitidine, and trimethoprim. For these drugs Caco-2 Papp values were also surveyed from literature and compared here (Table 2).

For high permeability drugs (BCS I and II, Table 2), the Papp values showed to be in the range of 4.6–75.2×10^{-6} cm/s in Franz–PAMPA. For Caco-2 assay, values were narrower (15.8–52.5×10^{-6} cm/s) and, for Corti membranes they were most narrow (39.7–48.8×10^{-6} cm/s).

For low permeability drugs (BCS III and IV, Table 2), the Papp coefficient found were consistently much lower than high permeability drugs. Franz–PAMPA, Caco-2, and Corti membrane provided value ranges of 0.2–24.6×10^{-6} cm/s, 0.1–83.0×10^{-6} cm/s, and 3.2–45.5×10^{-6} cm/s, respectively. Permeability of most drugs tested here showed Papp $>1.0 \times 10^{-5}$ cm/s (Figure 4).

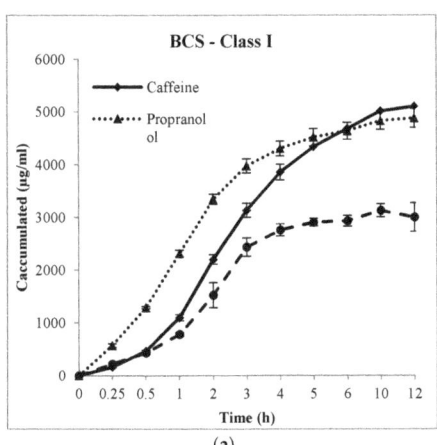
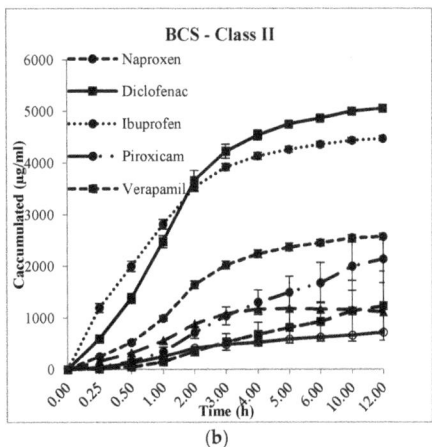

Figure 3. *Cont.*

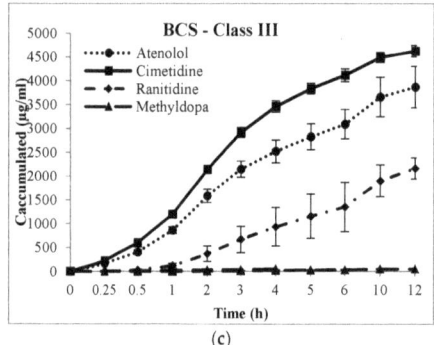
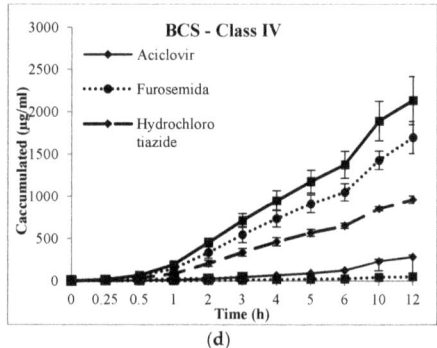

(c)   (d)

Figure 3. Cumulative transport (µg/mL, h) of drugs across Franz-PAMPA: (**a**) BCS class I; (**b**) BCS class II; (**c**) BCS class III; and (**d**) BCS class IV. Permeability was calculated from the linear portion (R^2). Data are presented as mean ± SD, n = 3

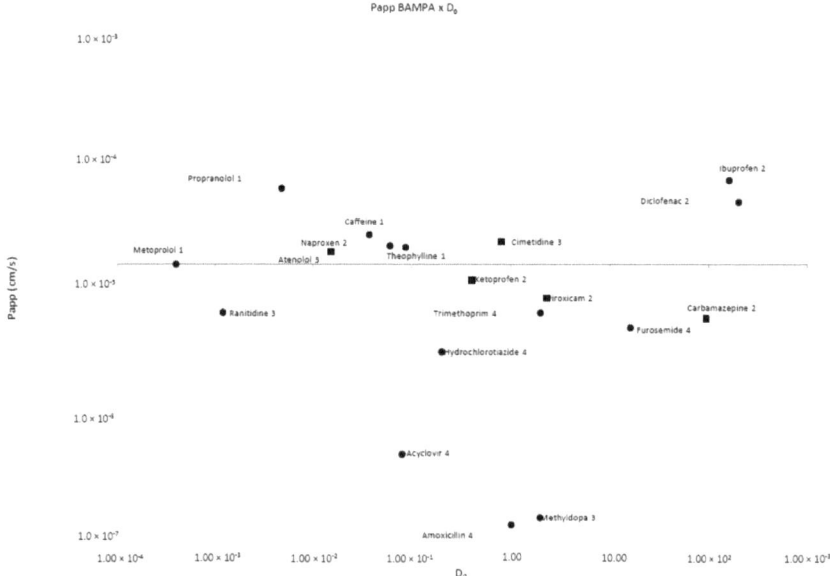

Figure 4. Permeability values for Franz-PAMPA *versus* D_0 drugs using metoprolol as reference drug. Most drugs (•; 14 out of 19) were in accordance with previous Biopharmaceutic Classification System (BCS) classification. Some of them (■; 5 out of 19) disagreed.

Table 2. Papp calculated values in Franz-PAMPA and using Non-Sink Arthursson equation. BCS classification of studied drugs and literature data to all other parameters.

Drug	[5] BCS	[1] Fa(%)	Franz–PAMPA	Non-Sink Arthurson	Papp × 10⁻⁶ cm/s [1] Caco-2	[2] Corti	[3] PAMPA pH 7.4	[3] Permeapad™	[5] LogP	[5] Log D pH 7.4	[5] pKa	[4,5] Intrinsic Solubility (mg/mL)
Metoprolol	I	95	15.8 (HP)	59.0	23.7 (HP)	48.1 (HP)	3.5	1.0	1.9	−0.2	9.6	1000.0
Caffeine		100	36.2 (HP)	53.3	30.8 (HP)	41.1	10.8	20.4	−0.1	0.02	0.6	21.17
Propranolol		93	33.1 (HP)	88.4	41.9 (HP)	39.7	23.5	nC	2.65	1.3	9.5	33.0
Theophylline		97	22.1 (HP)	—	25.0 (HP)	40.5	-	7.2	−0.25	−0.05	0.6 & 8.55	8.33
Carbamazepine	II	100	5.97	—	-	-	11.3	nC	2.5	1.8	1.0 & 13.9 15.96, −3.8	0.12
Diclofenac		100	68.1 (HP)	104.9	-	-	12.5	nC	4.4	1.2	3.99	0.001
Ibuprofen		93	57.5 (HP)	36.0	52.5 (HP)	-	6.8	16.6	3.1	0.7	4.9	0.01
Ketoprofen (AT)		100	12.1	—	20.1	42.7	16.7	nC	3.3	−1.51	4.5	0.051
Naproxen		98	2.89 (HP)	1.7	39.5 (HP)	48.8 (HP)	10.6	nC	3.2	0.2	4.2	33.0
Piroxicam		100	11.0	9.6	35.6 (HP)	-	8.2	nC	2.0	−0.07	2.33 & 5.1	0.11
Verapamil (AT)		98	5.39	5.0	15.8	41.6	7.4	9.3	3.8	2.7	8.9	0.44
Atenolol	III	52	25.8 (HP)	22.0	0.2	20.9	0.0	4.3	0.2	0.4	9.6	26.5
Cimetidine		93	35.6 (HP)	31.0	0.7	-	0.0	nC	0.4		6.8	6.0
Methyldopa		41	—	—	0.2	3.2	-	nC	0.4		1.7 & 9.9	10.0
Ranitidine (AT)		55	6.81	5.3	0.5	21.5	0.5	nC	0.3	−0.3	2.1 & 8.1	100.0
Acyclovir	IV	21	0.40	0.4	0.3	9.1	0.0	7.9	−1.7	−1.7	2.3 & 9.3	10.0
Amoxicillin		93	0.85	0.07	0.8	-	1.5	nC	0.9	—	3.2 & 11.7	4.0
Furosemide		60	4.57	4.5	0.1	27.5	0.6	nC	2.3	−0.7	3.5 & 10.6	0.01
Hydrochlorothiazide		70	2.74	2.7	0.5	31.0	0.1	nC	−0.1	−0.1	7.9	1.0
Trimethoprim (AT)		97	6.61	7.7	83.0 (HP)	45.5	5.0	nC	0.9	0.7	7.1	0.4

nC = non classified [1] Yamashita et al., 2000 (17) and Zhu et al., 2002 [38]; [2] Corti and co-workers, 2006 [5]; [3] Di Cagno et al. [22]; [4] Lindenberg et al. 2004 [39], [5] Kasim et al., 2004 [28] (AT) actively transported drugs. (HP) high permeability drug [38]—Data not available for non-sink calculations.

Typically, PAMPA methods are affected by high variability, and therefore, data can be somehow noisy for poorly permeable drugs. Variability is also an issue that impacts permeability for Caco-2 [5] and other in situ [19] and in vivo [24] models. For low permeability drugs (Fa < 80%), Avdeef and coworkers (2003) [6] measured variability for more than 200 different drugs accounting for more than 600 measurements. Papp values close to 10×10^{-6} cm/s showed variability of around 10%. Such error can increase slightly for higher Papp values but is larger for Papp $< 0.1 \times 10^{-6}$ (60%), with 0.01×10^{-6} values exhibiting variability of 100% or more. Although, currently BBB (blood brain barrier) [40] or Skin-PAMPA [41] methods can achieve higher precision and reproducibility with some other controlled protocols. Specific adjustments include setting incubation time as low as possible, increasing sensitivity of analytical methods, controlling membrane homogeneity either on the filter or among filters, besides the rationale for compounds dataset amongst others.

Likewise, permeability of small hydrophilic compounds is frequently underestimated in PAMPA since the membrane has hydrophobic nature besides being a cell-free system [42]. For the FDA-listed drugs, PAMPA Papp displayed values ranged from 0.00 to 2.35×10^{-5} cms^{-1}, indicating it was not sensitive enough to discriminate and rank poorly permeable compounds. In contrast, Franz–PAMPA showed values in a wider Papp range of $0.4–68.1 \times 10^{-6}$ cm/s. This could be tentatively explained due to the hydrophilic nature of membrane support and pH-dependent characteristics of the drugs [22,24,31]. Moreover, Franz cell stirring clearly reduces the unstirred water layer resistance in the system.

Additionally, variability of Papp values was also addressed by the calculation methods. A more sophisticated analysis is done using Artursson's equation [15] for sink and non-sink conditions as well as checking the impact of extracting a permeability coefficient from data that are not at true steady state and, thus, possibly impacted by dose depletion. Note that for both the sink and the non-sink equation, Papp values showed a particularly good correlation between them (0.8984). Similarly, Papp values obtained by us showed to be very alike to values calculated according to Artursson's non-sink equation (Table 2, Figure 5). The reason is that we used the same systematic procedure, i.e., the best fit method through the linear portion, to calculate all the slopes characterizing an accurate permeability flow, so that the impact from dose depletion is considered not above average. As a result, all drugs got the same BCS classification in both methods.

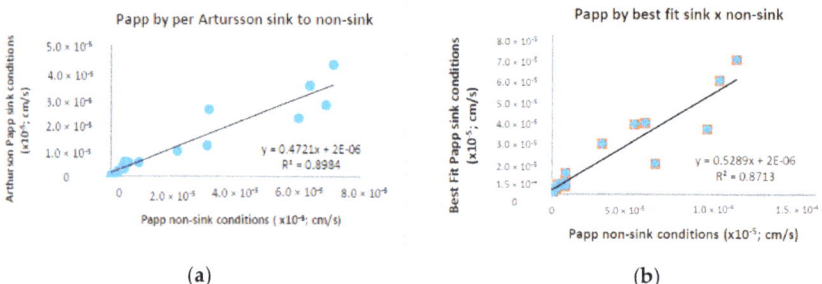

Figure 5. Papp calculations using equations by (**a**) per Artursson *non-sink versus sink* conditions and, (**b**) per Artursson *non-sink* compared to *sink* conditions best fit method of the linear portion.

In this context, Franz–PAMPA profile is mimicking biological permeation in a graphical pattern related to permeation through Caco-2 cells ($R^2 = 0.826$). Obtained Papp values *versus* fraction of dose absorbed in humans (Fa%) showed log linear correlation (Figure 6), as also described by Zhu et al. [38] when analyzing permeability performance of 93 commercial drugs as for artificial membranes. As expected, Franz–PAMPA also showed a significantly improved log linear correlation ($R^2 = 0.6982$) when actively transported compounds ranitidine, trimethoprim, and verapamil were not incorporated in the regression analysis. In contrast, the Fa% *versus*. Corti membrane correlation was linear ($R^2 = 0.904$). Such discrepancy from Franz–PAMPA and Caco-2 reveals that passive permeability of tested drugs through Corti membrane was greater and better suitable, especially for low and moderate permeability drugs, as discussed elsewhere [39]. PAMPA and Caco-2 technique would be best suited for compounds with medium and high permeabilities. For low permeability compounds, small differences in measured Papp are expected to yield large differences in Fa% values resulting in imprecise measurements.

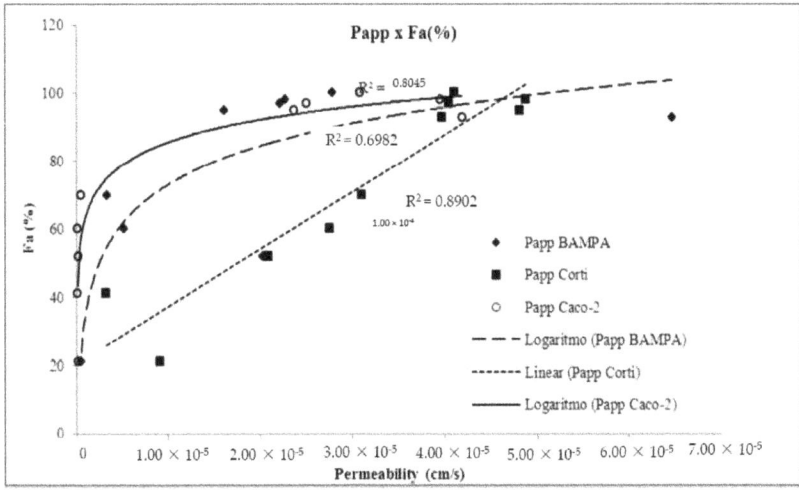

Figure 6. Demonstration of method suitability from Franz–PAMPA assay permeability and fraction of dose absorbed in humans (Fa%) compared to Caco-2 cells (○) and Corti membrane (■). Actively transported drugs were removed for R^2 calculation. Corti membrane Papp (♦) correlation to %Fa (R^2 = 0.890) was essentially unchanged.

Currently, a promising biomimetic barrier also adapted to Franz diffusion cells Permeapad™— [22] was reported for six drugs concurrent to our model (acyclovir, atenolol, caffeine, ibuprofen, and metoprolol). Even if a satisfactorily comparative analysis was not straightforward, BCS classification of most drugs (4 out of 5) showed to be identical with similar Papp rank order (Table 2).

4. Conclusions

The Franz–PAMPA method provided a permeability pattern similar to those from Caco-2. Methodologically, the advantages of Franz–PAMPA over Caco-2 are the lower costs and simplicity of membrane preparation (e.g., reagents and artificial membrane are commercially available). Furthermore, the method is very versatile and could be transformed in a high-throughput in vitro method to detect and classify compounds absorbed by passive diffusion.

Using metoprolol as a high permeability marker (Papp = 1.61×10^{-5} cm/s; Figure 1), seven drugs were classified as highly permeable (best fit method): atenolol, caffeine, cimetidine, diclofenac, ibuprofen, naproxen, and propranolol (Table 2). Only atenolol and cimetidine were misclassified as highly permeable drugs, relative to their prior literature classification as BCS 3 drugs.

Additionally, 10 out of 17 drugs were classified as low permeability drugs in Franz–PAMPA. Nevertheless, only naproxen, piroxicam, and verapamil (3 out of 10) had their permeability underestimated according to BCS, as they performed as low permeability drugs instead of BCS2 drugs.

Summing up, a potential limitation of our study is that the Papp values were calculated with an equation in which the underlying assumptions are constant donor concentration and sink conditions. In order to account for that, we also did the calculations to estimate permeability values under non-sink conditions. The obtained values are about the same compared with the true values (i.e., assuming donor concentration change and non-sink conditions). Although the relative estimation error does change across high *versus* low permeability compounds [29], the practical implications for predicting oral fraction absorbed would only be a "shift" to the left on the abscissa. In the case of a direct correlation with Caco-2 values, it would be reflected in a different slope, but it would not change the significance of the regression line. In the case of the use of the apparent permeabilities for classification of compounds, the reference value of metoprolol is also underestimated, so the classification outcome would not be changed [29].

As a final comment, the ability of Franz–PAMPA to classify drugs was good and can be potentially challenged at different pH conditions to predict intestinal permeability of drugs showing passive transport. Eventually, the Franz–PAMPA cell diffusion can be modulated in lipid composition and may be a suitable alternative for studying other biological barriers such as blood–brain barrier, skin, and mucosal barriers as buccal or nasal. The current dataset adds valuable information for future analysis of drug-molecular interactions at the lipid layer and in silico model development. Additionally, all apparatus and supplies experimentally used on Franz–PAMPA are commercially available and affordable to facilitate drug discovery method application.

Author Contributions: Conceptualization, funding acquisition, project administration, K.R.R.; T.V.C. and L.d.S.T.; methodology, formal analysis, investigation, data curation, A.A. methodology, investigation, data curation, discussion; I.G.-A., M.B.; J.P. discussion, supervision. All authors have read and agreed to the published version of the manuscript.

Funding: This research was funded by CNPq, FINEP and FAPEG.

Conflicts of Interest: The authors declare no conflict of interest.

References

1. Petereit, A.C.; Swinney, K.; Mensch, J.; Mackie, C.; Stokbroekx, S.; Brewster, M.; Dressman, J.B. Prediction of blood-brain barrier penetration of poorly soluble drug candidates using surface activity profiling. *Eur. J. Pharm. Biopharm.* **2010**, *75*, 405–410. [CrossRef]
2. Waring, M.J.; Arrowsmith, J.; Leach, A.R.; Leeson, P.D.; Mandrell, S.; Owen, R.M.; Pairaudeau, G.; Pennie, W.D.; Pickett, S.D.; Wang, J.; et al. An analysis of the attrition of drug candidates from four major pharmaceutical companies. *Nat. Rev. Drug Discov.* **2015**, *14*, 475–486. [CrossRef] [PubMed]
3. Amidon, G.L.; Lennernäs, H.; Shah, V.P.; Crison, J.R. A Theoretical Basis for a Biopharmaceutic Drug Classification: The Correlation of in vitro Drug Product Dissolution and in vivo Bioavailability. *Pharm. Res.* **1995**, *12*, 413–420. [CrossRef]
4. Wu, C.-Y.Y.; Benet, L.Z.Z. *Predicting Drug Disposition via Application of BCS: Transport/Absorption/Elimination Interplay and Development of a Biopharmaceutics Drug Disposition Classification System*; Kluwer Academic Publishers-Plenum Publishers: Amsterdam, The Netherlands, 2005; Volume 22, pp. 11–23.
5. Corti, G.; Maestrelli, F.; Cirri, M.; Furlanetto, S.; Mura, P. Development and evaluation of an in vitro method for prediction of human drug absorption I. Assessment of artificial membrane composition. *Eur. J. Pharm. Sci.* **2006**, *27*, 346–353. [CrossRef] [PubMed]
6. Ruell, J.A.; Tsinman, K.L.; Avdeef, A. PAMPA—A drug absorption in vitro model. 5. Unstirred water layer in iso-pH mapping assays and pKa(flux)—Optimized design (pOD-PAMPA). *Eur. J. Pharm. Sci.* **2003**, *20*, 393–402. [CrossRef] [PubMed]
7. Kortejärvi, H.; Urtti, A.; Yliperttula, M. Pharmacokinetic simulation of biowaiver criteria: The effects of gastric emptying, dissolution, absorption and elimination rates. *Eur. J. Pharm. Sci.* **2007**, *30*, 155–166. [CrossRef] [PubMed]
8. Matsson, P.; Doak, B.C.; Over, B.; Kihlberg, J. Cell permeability beyond the rule of 5. *Adv. Drug Deliv. Rev.* **2016**, *101*, 42–61. [CrossRef]
9. Benet, L.Z.; Hosey, C.M.; Ursu, O.; Oprea, T.I. BDDCS, the Rule of 5 and drugability. *Adv. Drug Deliv. Rev.* **2016**, *101*, 89–98. [CrossRef]
10. Bergström, C.A.S.; Holm, R.; Jørgensen, S.A.; Andersson, S.B.E.; Artursson, P.; Beato, S.; Borde, A.; Box, K.; Brewster, M.; Dressman, J.; et al. Early pharmaceutical profiling to predict oral drug absorption: Current status and unmet needs. *Eur. J. Pharm. Sci.* **2014**, *57*, 173–199. [CrossRef]

11. Lennernäs, H. Regional intestinal drug permeation: Biopharmaceutics and drug development. *Eur. J. Pharm. Sci.* **2014**, *57*, 333–341. [CrossRef]
12. Sjögren, E.; Eriksson, J.; Vedin, C.; Breitholtz, K.; Hilgendorf, C. Excised segments of rat small intestine in Ussing chamber studies: A comparison of native and stripped tissue viability and permeability to drugs. *Int. J. Pharm.* **2016**, *505*, 361–368. [CrossRef] [PubMed]
13. Miyake, M.; Toguchi, H.; Nishibayashi, T.; Higaki, K.; Sugita, A.; Koganei, K.; Kamada, N.; Kitazume, M.T.; Hisamatsu, T.; Sato, T.; et al. Establishment of Novel Prediction System of Intestinal Absorption in Humans Using Human Intestinal Tissues. *J. Pharm. Sci.* **2013**, *102*, 2564–2571. [CrossRef] [PubMed]
14. Hilgendorf, C.; Spahn-Langguth, H.; Regårdh, C.G.; Lipka, E.; Amidon, G.L.; Langguth, P. Caco-2 versus Caco-2/HT29-MTX co-cultured cell lines: Permeabilities via diffusion, inside- and outside-directed carrier-mediated transport. *J. Pharm. Sci.* **2000**, *89*, 63–75. [CrossRef]
15. Artursson, P.; Karlsson, J. Correlation between oral drug absorption in humans and apparent drug permeability coefficients in human intestinal epithelial (Caco-2) cells. *Biochem. Biophys. Res. Commun.* **1991**, *175*, 885. [CrossRef]
16. Corti, G.; Maestrelli, F.; Cirri, M.; Zerrouk, N.; Mura, P. Development and evaluation of an in vitro method for prediction of human drug absorption II. Demonstration of the method suitability. *Eur. J. Pharm. Sci.* **2006**, *27*, 354–362. [CrossRef]
17. Faller, B. Artificial membrane assays to assess permeability. *Curr. Drug Metab.* **2008**, *9*, 886–892. [CrossRef] [PubMed]
18. Mirmehrabi, M.; Rohani, S.; Perry, L. Thermodynamic modeling of activity coefficient and prediction of solubility: Part 2. Semipredictive or semiempirical models. *J. Pharm. Sci.* **2006**, *95*, 798–809. [CrossRef]
19. Lozoya-Agullo, I.; González-Álvarez, I.; González-Álvarez, M.; Merino-Sanjuán, M.; Bermejo, M. In Situ Perfusion Model in Rat Colon for Drug Absorption Studies: Comparison with Small Intestine and Caco-2 Cell Model. *J. Pharm. Sci.* **2015**, *104*, 3136–3145. [CrossRef]
20. Yamashita, S.; Furubayashi, T.; Kataoka, M.; Sakane, T.; Sezaki, H.; Tokuda, H. Optimized conditions for prediction of intestinal drug permeability using Caco-2 cells. *Eur. J. Pharm. Sci.* **2000**, *10*, 195–204. [CrossRef]
21. Oltra-Noguera, D.; Mangas-Sanjuan, V.; Centelles-Sangüesa, A.; Gonzalez-Garcia, I.; Sanchez-Castaño, G.; Gonzalez-Alvarez, M.; Casabo, V.-G.; Merino, V.; Gonzalez-Alvarez, I.; Bermejo, M. Variability of permeability estimation from different protocols of subculture and transport experiments in cell monolayers. *J. Pharmacol. Toxicol. Methods* **2015**, *71*, 21–32. [CrossRef]
22. Di Cagno, M.; Bibi, H.A.; Bauer-Brandl, A. New biomimetic barrier Permeapad™ for efficient investigation of passive permeability of drugs. *Eur. J. Pharm. Sci.* **2015**, *73*, 29–34. [CrossRef] [PubMed]
23. Berben, P.; Bauer-Brandl, A.; Brandl, M.; Faller, B.; Flaten, G.E.; Jacobsen, A.-C.; Brouwers, J.; Augustijns, P. Drug permeability profiling using cell-free permeation tools: Overview and applications. *Eur. J. Pharm. Sci.* **2018**, *119*, 219–233. [CrossRef] [PubMed]
24. Billat, P.-A.; Roger, E.; Faure, S.; Lagarce, F. Models for drug absorption from the small intestine: Where are we and where are we going? *Drug Discov. Today* **2017**, *22*, 761–775. [CrossRef] [PubMed]
25. Flaten, G.E.; Bunjes, H.; Luthman, K.; Brandl, M. Drug permeability across a phospholipid vesicle-based barrier 2. Characterization of barrier structure, storage stability and stability towards pH changes. *Eur. J. Pharm. Sci.* **2006**, *28*, 336–343. [CrossRef]
26. OECD. Joint Meeting of the Chemicals Committee and the Working Party on Chemicals, Pesticides and Biotechnology. *Ser. Chem. Accid.* **2017**, *33*, 1–117.
27. Selzer, D.; Abdel-Mottaleb, M.M.A.; Hahn, T.; Schaefer, U.F.; Neumann, D. Finite and infinite dosing: Difficulties in measurements, evaluations and predictions. *Adv. Drug Deliv. Rev.* **2013**, *65*, 278–294. [CrossRef]
28. Kasim, N.A.; Whitehouse, M.; Ramachandran, C.; Bermejo, M.; Lennernäs, H.; Hussain, A.S.; Junginger, H.E.; Stavchansky, S.A.; Midha, K.K.; Shah, V.P.; et al. Molecular Properties of WHO Essential Drugs and Provisional Biopharmaceutical Classification. *Mol. Pharm.* **2004**, *1*, 85–96. [CrossRef]
29. Tavelin, S.; Gråsjö, J.; Taipalensuu, J.; Ocklind, G.; Artursson, P. Applications of epithelial cell culture in studies of drug transport. *Methods Mol. Biol.* **2002**, *188*, 233–272. [CrossRef]
30. Mangas-Sanjuan, V.; González-Álvarez, I.; González-Álvarez, M.; Casabó, V.G.; Bermejo, M. Modified nonsink equation for permeability estimation in cell monolayers: Comparison with standard methods. *Mol. Pharm.* **2014**, *11*, 1403–1414. [CrossRef]

31. Kim, J.-S.; Mitchell, S.; Kijek, P.; Tsume, Y.; Hilfinger, J.; Amidon, G.L. The suitability of an in situ perfusion model for permeability determinations: Utility for BCS class I biowaiver requests. *Mol. Pharm.* **2006**, *3*, 686–694. [CrossRef]
32. Collado, M.I.; Goñi, F.M.; Alonso, A.; Marsh, D. Domain Formation in Sphingomyelin/Cholesterol Mixed Membranes Studied by Spin-Label Electron Spin Resonance Spectroscopy. *Biochemistry* **2005**, *44*, 4911–4918. [CrossRef] [PubMed]
33. Bermejo, M.; Avdeef, A.; Ruiz, A.; Nalda, R.; Ruell, J.A.; Tsinman, O.; González, I.; Fernández, C.; Sánchez, G.; Garrigues, T.M.; et al. PAMPA—A drug absorption in vitro model 7. Comparing rat in situ, Caco-2, and PAMPA permeability of fluoroquinolones. *Eur. J. Pharm. Sci.* **2004**, *21*, 429–441. [CrossRef] [PubMed]
34. Flaten, G.E.; Luthman, K.; Vasskog, T.; Brandl, M. Drug permeability across a phospholipid vesicle-based barrier 4. The effect of tensides, co-solvents and pH changes on barrier integrity and on drug permeability. *Eur. J. Pharm. Sci.* **2008**, *34*, 173–180. [CrossRef]
35. Naderkhani, E.; Isaksson, J.; Ryzhakov, A.; Flaten, G.E. Development of a biomimetic phospholipid vesicle-based permeation assay for the estimation of intestinal drug permeability. *J. Pharm. Sci.* **2014**, *103*, 1882–1890. [CrossRef]
36. Kansy, M.; Senner, F.; Gubernator, K. Physicochemical high throughput screening: Parallel artificial membrane permeation assay in the description of passive absorption processes. *J. Med. Chem.* **1998**, *41*, 1007–1010. [CrossRef] [PubMed]
37. Food and Drug Administration Guidance for Industry: Waiver of In vivo Bioavailability and Bioequivalence Studies for Immediate-Release Solid Oral Dosage Forms Based on a Biopharmaceutics Classification System. Available online: https://www.fda.gov/media/70963/download (accessed on 20 December 2017).
38. Plöger, G.F.; Hofsäss, M.A.; Dressman, J.B. Solubility Determination of Active Pharmaceutical Ingredients Which Have Been Recently Added to the List of Essential Medicines in the Context of the Biopharmaceutics Classification System–Biowaiver. *J. Pharm. Sci.* **2018**, *107*, 1478–1488. [CrossRef]
39. Mensch, J.; Melis, A.; Mackie, C.; Verreck, G.; Brewster, M.E.; Augustijns, P. Evaluation of various PAMPA models to identify the most discriminating method for the prediction of BBB permeability. *Eur. J. Pharm. Biopharm.* **2010**, *74*, 495–502. [CrossRef]
40. Sinkó, B.; Garrigues, T.M.; Balogh, G.T.; Nagy, Z.K.; Tsinman, O.; Avdeef, A.; Takács-Novák, K. Skin-PAMPA: A new method for fast prediction of skin penetration. *Eur. J. Pharm. Sci.* **2012**, *45*, 698–707. [CrossRef]
41. Zhu, C.; Jiang, L.; Chen, T.M.; Hwang, K.K. A comparative study of artificial membrane permeability assay for high throughput profiling of drug absorption potential. *Eur. J. Med. Chem.* **2002**, *37*, 399–407. [CrossRef]
42. Lindenberg, M.; Kopp, S.; Dressman, J.B. Classification of orally administered drugs on the World Health Organization Model list of Essential Medicines according to the biopharmaceutics classification system. *Eur. J. Pharm. Biopharm.* **2004**, *58*, 265–278. [CrossRef]

Publisher's Note: MDPI stays neutral with regard to jurisdictional claims in published maps and institutional affiliations.

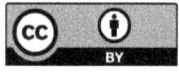

© 2020 by the authors. Licensee MDPI, Basel, Switzerland. This article is an open access article distributed under the terms and conditions of the Creative Commons Attribution (CC BY) license (http://creativecommons.org/licenses/by/4.0/).

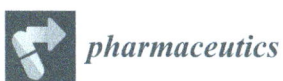

Article

Development of a Hierarchical Support Vector Regression-Based In Silico Model for Caco-2 Permeability

Giang Huong Ta [1], Cin-Syong Jhang [1], Ching-Feng Weng [2] and Max K. Leong [1,*]

[1] Department of Chemistry, National Dong Hwa University, Shoufeng, Hualien 974301, Taiwan; 810812203@gms.ndhu.edu.tw (G.H.T.); 610512002@gms.ndhu.edu.tw (C.-S.J.)
[2] Department of Physiology, School of Basic Medical Science, Xiamen Medical College, Xiamen 361023, China; cfweng@gms.ndhu.edu.tw
* Correspondence: leong@gms.ndhu.edu.tw; Tel.: +886-3-890-3609

Abstract: Drug absorption is one of the critical factors that should be taken into account in the process of drug discovery and development. The human colon carcinoma cell layer (Caco-2) model has been frequently used as a surrogate to preliminarily investigate the intestinal absorption. In this study, a quantitative structure–activity relationship (QSAR) model was generated using the innovative machine learning-based hierarchical support vector regression (HSVR) scheme to depict the exceedingly confounding passive diffusion and transporter-mediated active transport. The HSVR model displayed good agreement with the experimental values of the training samples, test samples, and outlier samples. The predictivity of HSVR was further validated by a mock test and verified by various stringent statistical criteria. Consequently, this HSVR model can be employed to forecast the Caco-2 permeability to assist drug discovery and development.

Keywords: intestinal absorption; intestinal permeability; human colon carcinoma cell layer (Caco-2); hierarchical support vector regression (HSVR)

Citation: Ta, G.H.; Jhang, C.-S.; Weng, C.-F.; Leong, M.K Development of a Hierarchical Support Vector Regression-Based In Silico Model for Caco-2 Permeability. *Pharmaceutics* 2021, *13*, 174. https://doi.org/10.3390/pharmaceutics13020174

Academic Editor: Maria Isabel Gonzalez-Alvarez
Received: 27 December 2020
Accepted: 21 January 2021
Published: 28 January 2021

Publisher's Note: MDPI stays neutral with regard to jurisdictional claims in published maps and institutional affiliations.

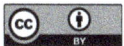

Copyright: © 2021 by the authors. Licensee MDPI, Basel, Switzerland. This article is an open access article distributed under the terms and conditions of the Creative Commons Attribution (CC BY) license (https://creativecommons.org/licenses/by/4.0/).

1. Introduction

Clinically, the majority of drugs are orally administered [1]. Prior to reaching the blood circulation system, the administered pharmaceutical agents have to pass through the intestinal barrier via passive diffusion, active uptake, and/or efflux transport processes [2–4], as illustrated by Figure 10.2 of Proctor et al. [2]. In passive diffusion, drug molecules can permeate the epithelial cell layers through the transcellular pathway, in which they penetrate through the cell membrane, or the paracellular pathway, in which they can cross the epithelial cell layer through the tight junction between cells [5]. The significance of active transporters on intestinal absorption has been detailed elsewhere [6]. Principally, active transport can be modulated by the efflux transporters of the ATP-binding cassette (ABC) family as well the influx transporters of the solute carrier (SLC) family [6], of which the efflux transporters can pump the administrated drugs out of enterocytes, leading to the reduction of the accumulated concentration, whereas the influx can enhance the intestinal uptake, resulting in the increased drug accumulation [7]. Of various active influx and efflux transporters, P-glycoprotein (P-gp), also termed multidrug resistance 1 protein (MDR1/encoded by *ABCB1* gene), breast cancer resistance protein (BCRP/*ABCG2*), organic anion transporting polypeptide 2B1 (OATP2B1/*SLCO2B1*), and peptide transporter 1 (PEPT1/*SLC15A1*) play predominant roles in intestinal absorption [8].

Passive diffusion depends on a number of physicochemical properties, whereas active transport relies on the characteristics of specific binding sites on the transport proteins [9]. The uncharged and modest hydrophobic drugs such as testosterone [10] can permeate through the membrane. Conversely, it is very difficult for highly hydrophobic molecules to get across cells, since they can be adhered to the membrane [5]. On the other hand, hydrophilic drugs such as mannitol predominantly pass through the paracellular pathway [10].

Of various drug absorption, distribution, metabolism, elimination, and toxicity (ADME/Tox) properties, drug absorption plays a pivotal role in drug discovery, since they substantially contribute to the earlier preclinical go/no-go decisions for the drug candidates [10,11] to achieve the "fail fast, fail early" paradigm [12]. As such, numerous in vivo and in situ assays have been developed to evaluate the intestinal absorption [13,14]. For instance, the in situ single-pass intestinal perfusion (SPIP) model measures the appearance of the drug in plasma after intravenous and intraintestinal drug administration [13,15]. The drug is orally administered or directly given into the intestine or stomach in some animal species in in vivo assay [13,14,16].

In addition to in vivo and in situ assays, various in vitro assays have been devised, since they have more advantages such as low cost and time efficiency as compared with their in situ and in vivo counterparts [15]. Of various in vitro assays to evaluate intestinal absorption, human colon carcinoma monolayer cells (Caco-2) [3], parallel artificial membrane permeability (PAMPA) [17,18], and Madin–Darby canine kidney cells (MDCK) [19] are most frequently used. In fact, a comprehensive drug absorption profile should include the Caco-2, MDCK, and PAMPA permeability data to explore drug solubility and bioavailability [20]. Moreover, Caco-2, which can be adopted to evaluate the drug permeability through the cytoplasm (transcellular uptake) or between cells (paracellular uptake) and active transport [6], has become the golden standard for predicting intestinal drug permeability and absorption because of its similarity in morphology and function with human enterocytes [21–23]. The Caco-2 protocol has been clearly described in detail by Hubatsch et al. As compared with the biological membrane, the Caco-2 system still suffers from a range of disadvantages such as high technical complexity, the limitations related to the differences between cell monolayers and intestinal membrane structurally and functionally [24], in addition to its long culture periods (21-24 days) with the significantly extensive costs, contributing to the major concerns in practical applications [21,25].

The Caco-2 permeability is normally expressed by the apparent permeability coefficient (P_{app}), in which the drug solution is added to the apical side, viz. the donor compartment, and the P_{app} value in the basolateral side, viz. the receiver compartment, is measured [23]

$$P_{app} = \frac{dQ}{dt} \times \frac{1}{(A \times C_0)} \qquad (1)$$

where dQ/dt is the linear appearance rate of mass in the receiver solution transported during sink conditions, A is the membrane surface area, and C_0 is the initial concentration at the donor compartment [26]. However, it is not uncommon to observe in vitro permeability variations among different from research groups, because the cultured cells can vary based on culture conditions, passage number, monolayer age, seeding density, and stage of differentiation [27,28], as exemplified by those compounds listed in Table 3 of Lee et al. [29]. Furthermore, Yamashita et al. have found that the different pH values of apical medium and the different solvents can produce different drug absorption values [30]. For instance, the P_{app} values of alprenolol are $(6.06 \pm 0.18) \times 10^{-6}$ cm/s and $(30.0 \pm 1.8) \times 10^{-6}$ cm/s at pH 6.0 and pH 7.4, respectively. More examples of P_{app} variations at different pH values can be found in Table 1 of Yamashita et al. [30].

In silico technologies have become an essential component in drug discovery and development according to the fact that they can provide guidance in the early stages in the drug discovery process such as the activity classification (high/moderate/poor) or quantitative predictions [31,32]. As such, a great number of in silico models have been established to predict the ADME/Tox properties [33]. The relationship between biological activity and chemical characteristics can be established by quantitative structure–activity or structure–property relationships (QSAR and QSPR) [34]. Numerous QSAR models have been generated to predict Caco-2 permeability based on a variety of physicochemical and physiological descriptors [35–51]. Nevertheless, the difficulties in developing sound in silico models to predict the intestinal permeability still remain unanswered mainly due to the fact that Caco-2 permeability is a dramatically perplexing process that can take place through numerous non-linear routes (vide supra).

More specifically, the ABC transporters, which are efflux transporters, can reduce the drug absorption, whereas the SLC transporters, which are influx transporters, can enhance the drug uptake, leading to the decrease and/or increase of drug absorption, respectively. In fact, such controversy can establish a paramount barrier in model development. For instance, the number of aromatic rings (n_{Ar}) can enhance the compound hydrophobicity [52] and facilitate the passive diffusion consequently. Conversely, n_{Ar} is also an important feature for P-gp substrate recognition and modulates the compound efflux correspondingly [53]. Thus, n_{Ar} can simultaneously affect the active efflux and passive diffusion.

It is exceedingly difficult, if not nearly impossible, to derive a robust in silico model, which can properly render the complex relationships between the selected descriptors and Caco-2 permeability. However, the hierarchical support vector regression (HSVR) scheme, which is an innovative machine learning-based scheme initially developed by Leong et al. [54], can properly address the complicated and varied dependencies of descriptors that, in turn, can be greatly contributed to its advantageous features of both a local model and a global model, namely wider coverage of applicability domain (AD) and a higher capability of prediction, respectively. When comparing with most theoretical models, which are vulnerable to the outliers that represent mathematic extrapolations, HSVR can still show consistent performance, as demonstrated elsewhere [1,54–57]. Herein, the objective of this study was to develop an in silico model based on the HSVR scheme to predict Caco-2 permeability in conjunction with previously published PAMPA permeability, intestinal absorption, and MDCK efflux in silico models [1,55,57] to facilitate drug discovery and development, since medicinal chemists can employ these models to predict the drug absorption of (virtual) hit compounds as well as drug metabolism and pharmacokinetics (DM/PK) scientists can adopt these models to prioritize the lead compounds.

2. Materials and Methods

2.1. Data Collection

The P_{app} values were collected from the various sources after a comprehensive literature search [22,23,58–66]. Assay systems were carefully scrutinized to ensure data consistency, since various assay conditions such as pH value and solvent system, for example, can affect the Caco-2 permeability [30]. Only P_{app} values, which were measured in the Hank's balanced salt solution (HBSS) buffer and 4-(2-hydroxyethyl)-1-piperazineethanesulfonic acid (HEPES) including ca. 1% dimethylsulfoxide (DMSO) at pH 7.4 were chosen in this study. The average P_{app} value was selected to warrant better consistency in case there was more than one P_{app} value for a given compound within a near range. Finally, 144 compounds were chosen in this study and their corresponding logarithm P_{app} values, simplified molecular input line entry system (SMILES) strings, Chemical Abstracts Service (CAS) registry numbers, and references to the literature are listed in Table S1.

2.2. Molecular Descriptors

The density functional theory (DFT), Becke 3-parameter Lee–Yang–Parr (B3LYP) method was employed to do full geometry optimization by the Gaussian package (Gaussian, Wallingford, CT, USA) for all recruited samples with the selection of basis set 6-31G (d,p). The solvent system was taken into consideration by the polarizable continuum model (PCM) [67,68]. The atomic charges, upon which the dipole moments depend, were calculated by the molecular electrostatic potential (MEP) [69]. The frontier orbitals energies, namely the highest occupied molecular orbital energy (E_{HOMO}) and the lowest unoccupied molecular orbital energy (E_{LUMO}), molecular dipole (μ), as well as the maximum absolute component of μ ($|\mu|_{max}$) were also recovered from the optimization calculations.

In total, more than 100 descriptors, which feature one-, two-, and three-dimensional ones and can be categorized into a variety of classes consisting of topological descriptors, electronic descriptors, thermodynamic descriptors, structure descriptors, spatial descriptors, and E-state indices, were enumerated by Discovery Studio (BIOVIA, San Diego, CA, USA) and E-Dragon (available at the website http://www.vcclab.org/lab/edragon/). The logarithm of the n-octanol–water partition coefficient at pH 7.4 (log P) was calculated by XLOGP3 of SwissADME (available at the website http://www.swissadme.ch/index.php). Furthermore, the cross-sectional area (CSA), which has been implicated in membrane permeability [70,71], was calculated using the method modified by Muehlbacher et al. [72]. The collected compounds were divided into 4 ion classes [73], namely zwitterion, base, acid, and neutral ions according to their pK_a values. The neutral ions only have one pK_a value, the zwitterion ions are those whose strongest acidic pK_a values are larger than 7 and the strongest basic ones are smaller than 7, the acidic ions have all their pK_a values smaller than 7, whereas the basic ions have all their pK_a values larger than 7.

2.3. Descriptor Selection

Descriptor selection was initially executed by removing those descriptors missing more than one molecule or displaying little or no distinction among all molecules. Furthermore, the Spearman's matrix between calculated descriptors was constructed to minimize the chance of spurious correlations, and those descriptors with intercorrelation values of $r^2 > 0.80$ were discarded, since the threshold was proposed by Topliss and Edwards [74]. In this study, a more conservative value of $r^2 \geq 0.64$ was taken to further ensure the quality of derived models.

Descriptor values can span a wide range due to their diverse nature (vide supra). It is of necessity to transfer descriptors into a more consistent range to decrease the chance of descriptors with broader ranges overriding those with narrower ranges [75]. Accordingly, descriptors were subjected to normalization by centering and scaling

$$\hat{x}_{ij} = \frac{x_{ij} - \langle x_j \rangle}{\sqrt{\sum_{i=1}^{n}(x_{ij} - \langle x_j \rangle)^2 / (n-1)}} \quad (2)$$

where x_{ij} and $\hat{x}_{ij}$ symbolize the jth original and normalized descriptors of the ith molecule, respectively; $\langle x_j \rangle$ is the average value of the original jth descriptor; and n is the number of molecules.

The descriptor selection is of pivotal importance in the performance of QSAR models [76]. Thus, genetic function approximation (GFA) bundled in the QSAR module of Discovery Studio was used for the initial descriptor because of its effectiveness and efficiency [77]. The recursive feature elimination (RFE) scheme was adopted for additional selection, in which the model was repeatedly generated by all but one descriptor. The descriptor, which had the less contribution in predictive performance, was removed after ranking their contributions [78].

2.4. Dataset Selection

It is not uncommon to identify the outliers and remove them from data collection for model development [79]. As such, outliers were recognized by inspecting molecular distribution in the chemical space [80], which was created by principal components (PCs) using the Diverse Molecules/Principal Component Analysis embedded in Discovery Studio, followed by discovering the outliers.

The remaining molecules were arbitrarily allocated into the training set and test set with an about 4:1 portion as recommended [81] to generate and verify the built model, respectively, using the Diverse Molecules/Library Analysis function within Discovery Studio. Golbraikh et al. have postulated that a sound model can be resulted only when both samples in the training set and test set can show high levels of chemical and biological similarity [82]. Thus, the data distributions in the training and test set were carefully checked to ensure the high similarity degrees biologically and chemically in both datasets.

2.5. Hierarchical Support Vector Regression

Leong et al. originally invented HSVR [54] which was evolved from support vector machine (SVM) proposed by Vapnik et al. [83]. Initially, SVM was designed for classification only and the regression function, termed as support vector regression (SVR), was introduced later [84]. HSVR has a higher level of predictivity and broader applicability domain (AD) as compared with SVR, since it can seamlessly combine the advantages of the local model and global model [56]. More significantly, the superiority of HSVR has been revealed by some studies [1,54–57].

The theory and fulfillment of HSVR have been delineated in detail elsewhere, and the schematic presentation of HSVR can be depicted by Figure 1 of Leong et al. [54]. Basically, an SVR ensemble (SVRE) is used to build an HSVR model, and SVR models in the ensemble are generated from different descriptor combinations and function as local models with their own ADs. Briefly, the svm-train module in *LIBSVM* (software available at http://www.csie.ntu.edu.tw/~cjlin/libsvm/) was employed to build various SVR models using those samples in the training set with different descriptor combinations and SVR run conditions. The module svm-predict in *LIBSVM* was adopted to validate the produced SVR models using the samples in the test set. Radial basis function (RBF) was the designated kernel function due to its simplicity and better functionality [85]. Both ε-SVR and ν-SVR regression functions were tested. The SVR runtime conditions including ε-SVR and ν-SVR, their associated ε and ν, the kernel width γ, and cost C were tuned by the grid-search technique.

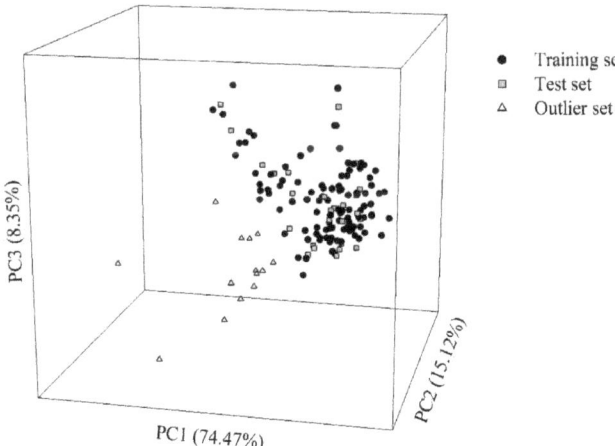

Figure 1. The chemical space spanned by three principle components (PCs) displays the distribution of the data samples in the training set (solid circle), test set (gray square), and outlier set (open triangle).

According to the principle of Occam's razor, i.e., the principle of parsimony, the number of descriptors selected to build SVR models should be minimized as much as possible. This principle was also applied to the construction of SVRE, which demanded the minimum number of ensemble members [86]. Initially, the combinations of two SVR models were adopted to generate the HSVR model; this process was repeated until the production of a predictive HSVR. Otherwise, the combinations of three- or even four-member SVRE were used to develop the HSVR models if the two-SVR ensembles failed to perform well.

2.6. Predictive Evaluation

The residual yielded by the difference between the observed value (y_i) and the predicted value ($\hat{y}_i$) for the ith molecule was computed based on the following equation:

$$\Delta_i = y_i - \hat{y}_i \tag{3}$$

In addition, standard deviation (s), maximum residual (Δ_{Max}), root mean square error (RMSE), and mean absolute error (MAE) in a dataset with n samples were evaluated.

$$\text{RMSE} = \sqrt{\sum_{i=1}^{n} \Delta_i^2 / n} \tag{4}$$

$$\text{MAE} = \frac{1}{n}\sum_{i=1}^{n} |\Delta_i| \tag{5}$$

Various statistic metrics were adopted to evaluate the produced models. The squared correlation coefficients including r^2 and q^2 in the training set and external set, respectively, were computed by the following equation.

$$r^2, q^2 = 1 - \sum_{i=1}^{n}(\hat{y}_i - y_i)^2 / \sum_{i=1}^{n}(y_i - \langle\hat{y}\rangle)^2 \tag{6}$$

where $\langle \hat{y}_i \rangle$ represents the average predicted value, and n is the number of samples in the dataset. The derived models were subjected to the 10-fold cross-validation using the function embedded in *LIBSVM* to give rise to the squared correlation coefficient of 10-fold cross-validation q_{CV}^2. Another internal validation was carried out by the Y-scrambling test [87], in which the log P_{app} values were randomly permuted and then reapplied to the previous developed model without altering the descriptors. This process was repeated 25 times as suggested [87] to generate the average squared correlation coefficient $\langle r_s^2 \rangle$.

The external dataset was evaluated predictivity by the squared correlation coefficients q_{F1}^2, q_{F2}^2, and q_{F3}^2, and the concordance correlation coefficient (CCC) [88–93] using *QSARINS* [94,95].

$$q_{F1}^2 = 1 - \sum_{i=1}^{n_{EXT}}(y_i - \hat{y}_i)^2 / \sum_{i=1}^{n_{EXT}}(y_i - \langle y_{TR} \rangle)^2 \tag{7}$$

$$q_{F2}^2 = 1 - \sum_{i=1}^{n_{EXT}}(y_i - \hat{y}_i)^2 / \sum_{i=1}^{n_{EXT}}(y_i - \langle y_{EXT} \rangle)^2 \tag{8}$$

$$q_{F3}^2 = 1 - \left[\sum_{i=1}^{n_{EXT}}(y_i - \hat{y}_i)^2 / n_{EXT}\right] / \left[\sum_{i=1}^{n_{EXT}}(y_i - \langle y_{TR} \rangle)^2 / n_{TR}\right] \tag{9}$$

$$\text{CCC} = \frac{2\sum_{i=1}^{n_{EXT}}(y_i - \langle y_{EXT} \rangle)(\hat{y}_i - \langle \hat{y}_{EXT} \rangle)}{\sum_{i=1}^{n_{EXT}}(y_i - \langle y_{EXT} \rangle)^2 + \sum_{i=1}^{n_{EXT}}(\hat{y}_i - \langle \hat{y}_{EXT} \rangle)^2 + n_{EXT}(\langle y_{EXT} \rangle - \langle \hat{y}_{EXT} \rangle)^2} \tag{10}$$

where $\langle y_{TR} \rangle$ is the averaged observed values in the training set, $\langle y_{EXT} \rangle$ and $\langle \hat{y}_{EXT} \rangle$ are the averaged observed and predicted values in the external set, respectively; n_{TR} and n_{EXT} stand for the numbers of samples in the training set and external set, respectively.

In addition, some modified squared correlation coefficients r^2 were estimated [96,97]

$$r_m^2 = r^2\left(1 - \sqrt{|r^2 - r_0^2|}\right) \tag{11}$$

$$r_m'^2 = r^2\left(1 - \sqrt{|r^2 - r_0'^2|}\right) \tag{12}$$

$$\left\langle r_m^2 \right\rangle = \left(r_m^2 + r'^2_m \right)/2 \tag{13}$$

$$\Delta r_m^2 = \left| r_m^2 - r'^2_m \right| \tag{14}$$

$$\left(r^2 - r_0^2 \right)/r^2 < 0.10 \text{ and } 0.85 \leq k \leq 1.15. \tag{15}$$

To externally evaluate the predictivity of the generated models, the most stringent criteria validation values jointly proposed by Golbraikh et al. [82], Ojha et al. [96], Roy et al. [98], and Chirico and Gramatica [89] were adopted

$$r^2, q_{CV}^2, q^2, q_{Fn}^2 \geq 0.70 \tag{16}$$

$$\left| r^2 - q_{CV}^2 \right| < 0.10 \tag{17}$$

$$\left| r_0^2 - r'^2_0 \right| < 0.30 \tag{18}$$

$$r_m^2 \geq 0.65 \tag{19}$$

$$\left\langle r_m^2 \right\rangle \geq 0.65 \text{ and } \Delta r_m^2 < 0.20 \tag{20}$$

$$CCC \geq 0.85 \tag{21}$$

where r^2 in Equations (15) and (18)-(20) symbolize r^2 and q^2 in the training set and external set, respectively. The q_{Fn}^2 in Equation (16) stands for q_{F1}^2, q_{F2}^2, and q_{F3}^2.

3. Results

3.1. Dataset Selection

Of all the molecules enrolled in this study, 104 and 26 molecules were randomly selected as the training set and test set, respectively, giving rise to a ca. 4:1 ratio as suggested [81]. The chemical space with the projection of all molecules is displayed in Figure 1. Three principle components (PCs), which accounted for 97.94% of the variance in the original data, were used to create the chemical space. This figure shows that samples in the training set and test set had similar distribution in the chemical space. The high levels of the biological and chemical similarity between both datasets can be illustrated by the histograms of log P_{app}, molecular weight (MW), surface area (SA), polar surface area (PSA), number of hydrogen bond acceptor (HBA), number of hydrogen bond donor (HBD), and n-octanol-water partition coefficient (log P) in the density form (Figure S1). Thus, it is plausible to assert that the substantial bias did not appear in the data partition.

It is of great significance to characterize the AD of the predictive model and to exclude the outliers from data collection [94]. Various methods to detect outliers have been proposed [99]. The scheme based on the chemical similarity/dissimilarity using principle component analysis (PCA) was adopted in this study [94]. Accordingly, 14 molecules were specified as outliers, which are substantially dissimilar to those ones in both the training and test sets, as shown in the chemical space (Figure 1), from which it can be observed that they are located far from the others. The distinction between the outliers and the others can be actually recognized by the fact that they contain more than nine rings or more than 12 HBAs as compared with the other molecules.

3.2. SVR Models

Numerous SVR models were generated using different descriptor combinations and runtime conditions. Three SVR models, coined as SVR A, SVR B, and SVR C, were assembled to establish the SVR ensemble, which was successively utilized to generate the HSVR model by another SVR. The optimal runtime conditions of SVR A, SVR B, SVR C, and HSVR are listed in Table S2.

SVR A, SVR B, and SVR C adopted five, five, and seven descriptors, respectively, with different combinations (Table 1). These SVR models in the ensemble were assembled according to their performances on the molecules and statistical assessments in the training set and test set. Their runtime conditions and their predicted log P_{app} values are listed in Tables S1 and S2, respectively. Tables 2 and 3 record their associated statistical evaluations in the training set and test set, respectively.

Table 1. The list of ensemble support vector regression (SVR) models and their descriptors, the correlation coefficient (r) with P_{app}, and their descriptions.

Descriptor	SVR A	SVR B	SVR C	r	Description
log P	X [†]	X		0.15	Logarithm of the n-octanol-water partition coefficient
n_{Ar}		X		−0.07	Number of aromatic rings
PSA	X	X		−0.56	Polar surface area
μ		X		−0.27	Dipole moment
$|\mu|_{max}$	X		X	−0.08	The maximum dipole component
α	X			−0.34	Sum of atomic polarizabilities over all the molecule atoms
n_{Ring}			X	−0.31	Number of rings
V_m			X	−0.35	Molecular volume
n_{Rot}			X	−0.21	Number of rotatable bonds in a molecule
HBD		X	X	−0.40	Number of hydrogen-bond donors
$pK_{a(Max)}$	X		X	−0.13	The maximum pK_a for a molecule
ion class			X	N/A [‡]	Four classes are separated by the pK_a of molecules

[†] Selected. [‡] Not applicable.

Table 2. Statistic metrics including r^2, Δ_{Max}, mean absolute error (MEA), s, root mean square error (RMSE), q^2_{CV}, and $\langle r^2_s \rangle$ assessed by support vector regression (SVR) A, SVR B, SVR C, and hierarchical support vector regression (HSVR) in the training set.

Statistic Metrics	SVR A	SVR B	SVR C	HSVR
r^2	0.69	0.77	0.76	0.91
Δ_{Max}	1.31	1.19	1.66	0.98
MAE	0.28	0.17	0.17	0.1
s	0.25	0.28	0.29	0.18
RMSE	0.38	0.32	0.33	0.2
q^2_{CV}	0.16	0.19	0.21	0.81
$\langle r^2_s \rangle$	0.05	0.03	0.03	0.03

Table 3. Statistic metrics including q^2, q^2_{F1}, q^2_{F2}, q^2_{F3} CCC, Δ_{Max}, MAE, s, and RMSE assessed by SVR A, SVR B, SVR C, and HSVE in the test set.

Statistic Metrics	SVR A	SVR B	SVR C	HSVR
q^2	0.50	0.58	0.60	0.75
q^2_{F1}	0.42	0.58	0.59	0.71
q^2_{F2}	0.41	0.57	0.59	0.71
q^2_{F3}	0.30	0.50	0.50	0.70
CCC	0.62	0.74	0.77	0.85
Δ_{Max}	1.27	1.06	0.88	0.72
MAE	0.42	0.35	0.39	0.33
s	0.35	0.31	0.23	0.20
RMSE	0.54	0.46	0.45	0.38

The observed versus the predicted log P_{app} values by SVR A, SVR B, SVR C, and HSVR are displayed by the scatter plot in Figure 2, from which it can be observed that SVR A, SVR B, and SVR C predicted the observed values well for the majority of the molecules in the training set, producing small MAE and s values consequently (Table 2). Moreover, it can be found from Figure 2 that the points predicted by SVR B are generally closer to the regression line than SVR A and SVR C. SVR B, consequently, gave rise to the lowest

Δ_{Max} (1.19), MAE (0.17), and RMSE (0.32), and the largest r^2 (0.77), suggesting that SVR B performed marginally better than SVR A and SVR C in the training set.

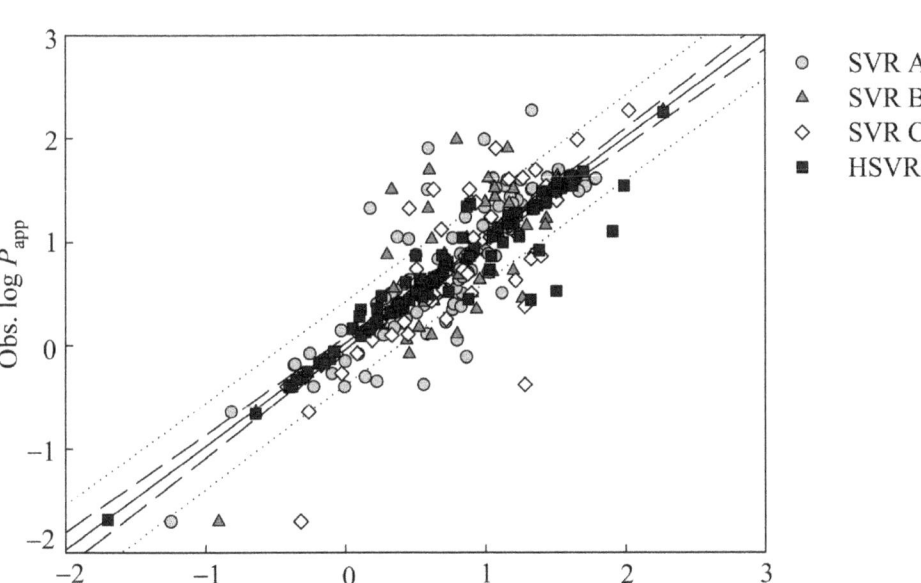

Figure 2. Observed log P_{app} versus the log P_{app} predicted by SVR A (gray circle), SVR B (gray triangle), SVR C (open diamond), and HSVR (solid square) for the training samples. The solid, dashed, and dotted lines represent to the HSVR regression of the data, 95% confidence intervals for the HSVR regression, and 95% confidence intervals for the prediction, respectively.

Furthermore, the difference between r^2 and q^2_{CV} evaluated by SVR B was 0.58 when subjected to the leave-one-out cross-validation, indicating that SVR B was over-trained which, in turn, can severely limit its application. Over-training was also associated with SVR A and SVR C as manifested by their extremely low q^2_{CV} values. The $\langle r_s^2 \rangle$ values produced by SVR A, SVR B, and SVR C were 0.05, 0.03, and 0.03 (Table 2), respectively, when subjected in Y-scrambling. These near zero values suggest that there is an almost zero chance correlation associated with those SVR models [87].

The predicted values by SVR A, SVR B, and SVR C are in moderate agreement with the observed values for those test molecules depicted by Figure 3, which shows the scatter plot of observed versus the log P_{app} predictions by SVR A, SVR B, SVR C, and HSVR for those samples in the test set. The MAE values generated by SVR A, SVR B, and SVR C increase from 0.28, 0.17, and 0.17 in the training set to 0.42, 0.35, and 0.39 in the test set, respectively (Table 3). RMSE along with the other statistic values also reveal deteriorating performances of these models in SVRE from the training set to the test set (Tables 2 and 3). Moreover, the q^2 values produced by SVR A, SVR B, and SVR C were 0.50, 0.58, and 0.60 in the test set, respectively, which are much less than their r^2 counterparts in the training set.

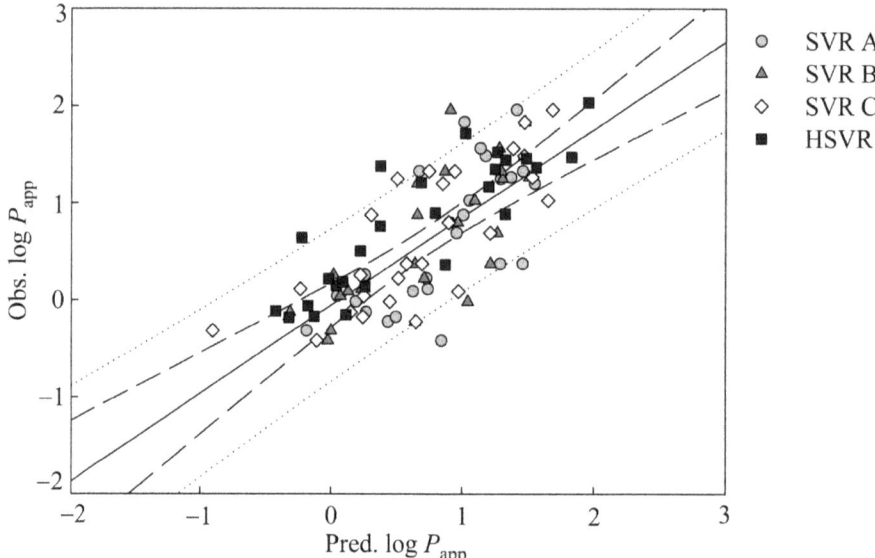

Figure 3. Observed log P_{app} versus the log P_{app} predicted by SVR A (gray circle), SVR B (gray triangle), SVR C (open diamond), and HSVR (solid square) for the test samples. The solid, dashed, and dotted lines represent the HSVR regression of the data, 95% confidence intervals for the HSVR regression, and 95% confidence intervals for the prediction, respectively.

The prediction performances of those SVR models in the SVRE were significantly decreased when applied to those samples in the outlier set as suggested by the statistical metrics listed in Table 4. For example, SVR A, SVR B, and SVR C yielded the q_{F2}^2 values of −0.18, −0.41, and 0.16, respectively, which are substantially smaller than the r^2 values in the training set and the q_{F2}^2 values in the test set (Tables 2 and 3). Furthermore, the distances between the points and the regression line in the outlier set were much greater than those in the training set shown in Figure 4. As such, it can be asserted that those three models in the SVRE are vulnerable to the outliers that, actually, are not uncommon for most predictive models [100].

Table 4. Statistic metrics including q^2, q_{F1}^2, q_{F2}^2, q_{F3}^2, CCC, Δ_{Max}, MAE, s, and RMSE assessed by SVR A, SVR B, SVR C, and HSVE in the outlier set.

Statistic Metrics	SVR A	SVR B	SVR C	HSVR
q^2	0.45	0.36	0.40	0.76
q_{F1}^2	0.75	0.70	0.82	0.95
q_{F2}^2	−0.18	−0.41	0.16	0.76
q_{F3}^2	0.39	0.27	0.56	0.87
CCC	0.49	0.56	0.58	0.87
Δ_{Max}	1.58	0.91	0.82	0.49
MAE	0.35	0.47	0.16	0.17
s	0.41	0.34	0.56	0.17
RMSE	0.52	0.57	0.58	0.24

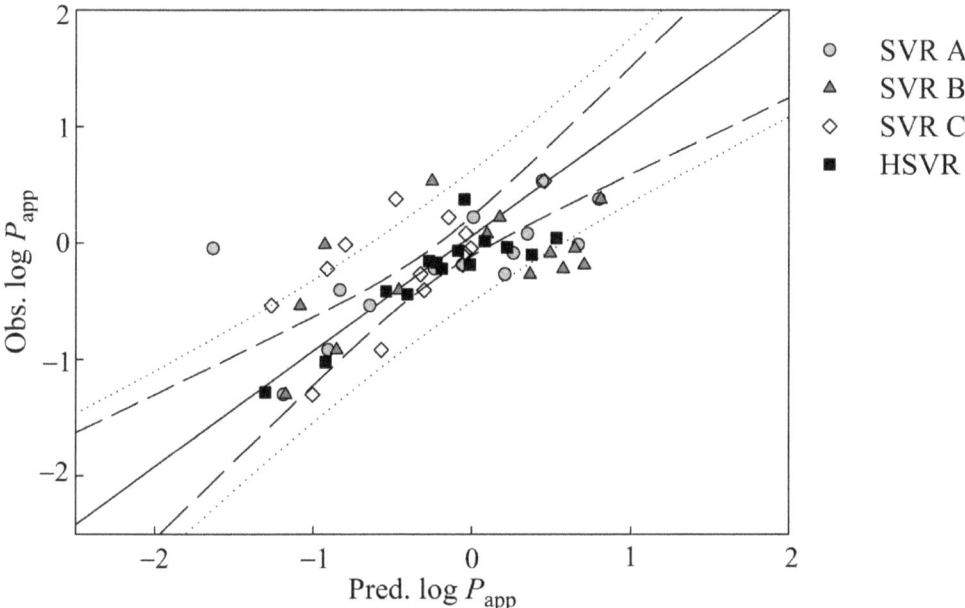

Figure 4. Observed log P_{app} versus the log P_{app} predicted by SVR A (gray circle), SVR B (gray triangle), SVR C (open diamond), and HSVR (solid square) for the outlier samples. The solid, dashed, and dotted lines represent the HSVR regression of the data, 95% confidence intervals for the HSVR regression, and 95% confidence intervals for the prediction, respectively.

3.3. HSVR Model

The HSVR model was generated by the regression of SVRE according to the predictions of all molecules and statistical assessments in the training set (Table S1 and Table 2), and its runtime parameters are recorded in Table S2. HSVR commonly predicted better than SVR A, SVR B, and SVR C for the samples in the training set, as demonstrated by Figure 2, from which it can be noticed that most of predictions by HSVR lie in the range between the largest and the smallest ones predicted by those models in the SVRE. HSVR can improve the predictions in some cases. For instance, the prediction of compound **101** (omeprazole) by HSVR yielded an absolute residual of 0.02, whereas SVR A, SVR B, and SVR C produced the absolute errors of 0.34, 1.10, and 0.18, respectively (Table S1). In addition, HSVR produced the highest r^2 (0.91) and q^2_{CV} (0.81) and the lowest Δ_{Max} (0.98), MAE (0.10), s (MAE), and RMSE (0.20) values when compared with those models in the SVRE, suggesting that HSVR statistically performed better SVR A, SVR B, and SVR C in the training set. Furthermore, HSVR gave rise to a $\langle r_s^2 \rangle$ value of 0.03, indicating that it is least possible that HSVR was created by chance correlation [87].

When applied to the test molecules, marginal performance deteriorations can be found for HSVR. For example, s increased from 0.18 in the training set to 0.20 in the test set (Tables 2 and 3). However, Δ_{Max} dropped from 0.98 in the training set to 0.72 in the test set. HSVR still executed better than SVR A, SVR B, and SVR C in the test set as shown in Figure 3. The other statistical parameters listed in Table 3 also assert the performance dominance of HSVR. For instance, the q^2 values were 0.50, 0.58, 0.60, and 0.75 generated by SVR A, SVR B, SVR C, and HSVR, respectively. Similarly, HSVR also produced smaller absolute deviations than its counterparts in the SVRE in the test set. For example, the absolute residuals of compound 36 (clozapine) were 0.35, 0.54, 0.35, and 0.03 yielded by SVR A, SVR B, SVR C, and HSVR, respectively (Table S1). HSVR generally produced consistent and small deviations in both training and test sets as asserted by those parameters listed in Tables 2 and 3 in comparison with its counterparts in the SVRE. More importantly, the HSVR model generated the largest q^2 (0.75) in the test set and the smallest difference between r^2 and q^2_{CV} (0.10), suggesting that it is less likely that HSVR model was over-trained or over-fitted.

HSVR even displayed better performance than the SVR models in the ensemble in the outlier set as depicted by those statistical assessments listed in Table 4. The HSVR model generated the largest q^2 value (0.76) and yet SVR A, SVR B, and SVR C yielded 0.45, 0.36, and 0.40, respectively. The superiority of HSVR in the outlier set can also be assured by the other statistical parameters, which is mainly due to the broader application domain of HSVR when compared with its counterparts in the ensemble. That robust HSVR feature makes it more utilizable in practical applications [101].

3.4. Predictive Evaluations

The scatter plot of residual versus the log P_{app} prediction by HSVR for the training, test, and outlier samples is shown in Figure 5, from which it can be found that the residuals are commonly situated on both sides of x-axis along with the prediction range in those three datasets, suggesting that it is least likely that systematic error is associated with HSVR. Additionally, the training set, test set, and outlier set had the average residuals of 0.02, −0.13, and 0.06, respectively (Table S1), denoting that there is no biased prediction by HSVR.

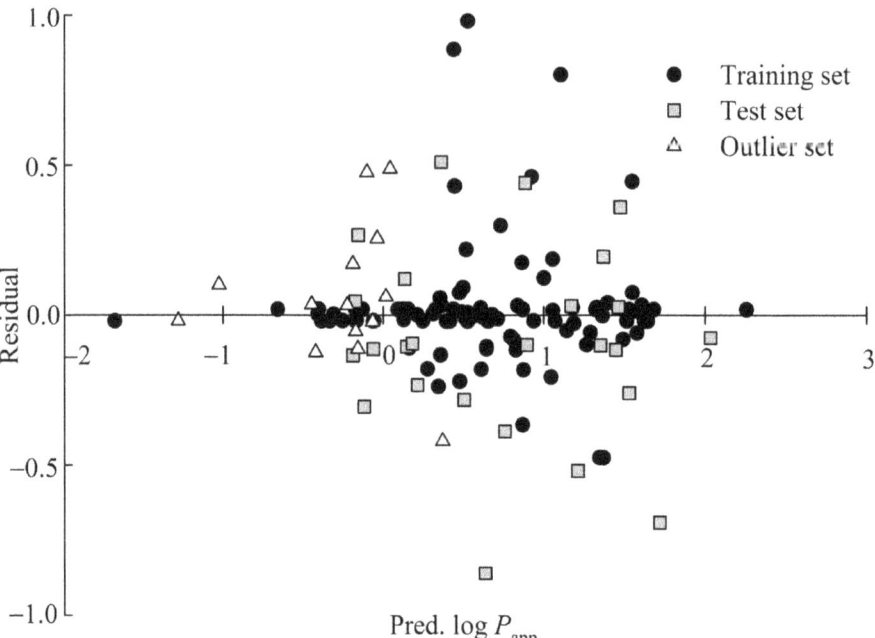

Figure 5. Residual versus the log P_{app} prediction by HSVR in the training set (solid circle), test set (gray square), and outlier set (open triangle).

Table 5 lists the results when the developed HSVR model was further subjected to the most stringent validation criteria collectively recommended by Golbraikh et al. [82], Ojha et al. [96], Roy et al. [98], and Chirico and Gramatica [89] in the three datasets (Equations (15)–(21)). It can be observed that HSVR completely met those proposed validation requirements in addition to the fact that HSVR exhibited a similar degrees of performance in the training set, test set, and outlier set. As such, it can be asserted that HSVR is an extremely accurate and predictive theoretical model.

Table 5. Validation verification of HSVR based on prediction performance of the training, test, and outlier samples.

Validation Verification	Training Set	Test Set	Outlier Set
r_0^2	0.91	0.75	0.75
k	1.01	0.86	0.93
r'^2_0	0.91	0.68	0.71
r_m^2	0.84	0.71	0.68
r'^2_m	0.91	0.75	0.76
$\langle r_m^2 \rangle$	0.87	0.73	0.72
Δr_m^2	0.06	0.04	0.08
$r^2 \geq 0.70$	X [†]	X	X
Equation (15)	X	X	X
Equation (16)	X	N/A	N/A
Equation (17)	X	X	X
Equation (18)	X	X	X
Equation (19)	X	X	X
Equation (20)	X	X	X
Equation (21)	N/A [‡]	X	X

[†] Fulfilled; [‡] Not applicable.

3.5. Mock test

To verify the practical applicability of the generated HSVR model, this model was applied to those drugs measured by Yamashita et al. [30]. There were eight compounds commonly adopted by this study and Yamashita et al., furnishing a sound way to calibrate the challenging system. However, Yamashita et al. assayed the P_{app} values at pH 6.0, instead of pH 7.4 used by those compounds collected in this study, suggesting that some P_{app} variations can be resulted from both systems (vide supra). These discrepancies make those drugs assayed by Yamashita et al. not appropriate as the second external dataset or the test set because those validation criteria listed in Table 5 cannot be applied to those drugs. The relationship between both different experimental conditions was initially constructed for those eight common compounds, and the resulting scatter plot is exhibited in Figure 6, from which it can be found that both assay systems were reasonably correlated with each other with an r value of 0.86), suggesting that this HSVR can be adopted to predict those novel compounds measured by Yamashita et al.

Figure 7 shows the predicted results of seven novel drugs in the mock test. The correlation coefficient r value between the predicted log P_{app} (pH 7.4) and observed log P_{app} (pH 6.0) was 0.86, suggesting that the HSVR model can nearly reproduce the experimental results. In addition, the produced p-value was <0.05. This mock test ensured the predictive ability of generated HSVR when applied to the novel compounds with different experimental conditions.

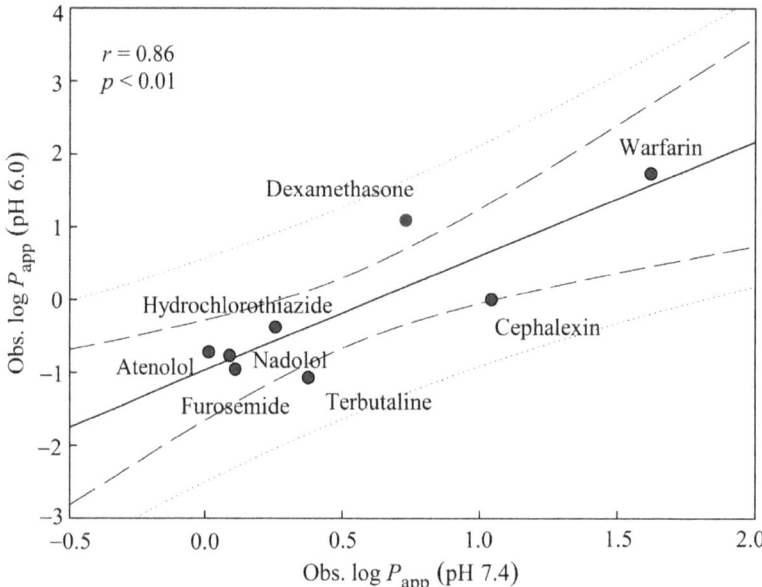

Figure 6. Observed log P_{app} at pH 7.4 versus observed log P_{app} at pH 6.0 for the common drugs in the mock test. The solid, dashed, and dotted lines represent the mock test regression of the observed data, 95% confidence interval for the mock test regression, and 95% confidence interval for the observation, respectively.

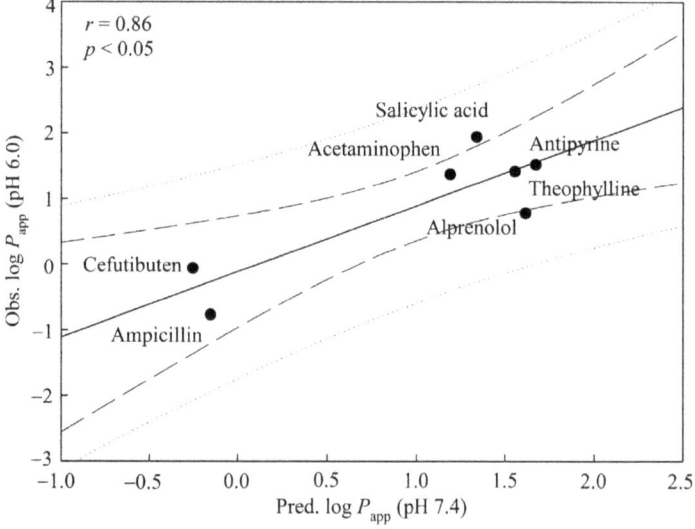

Figure 7. Predicted log P_{app} at pH 7.4 versus observed log P_{app} at pH 6.0 by the HSVR model for the drugs in the mock test. The solid, dashed, and dotted lines represent the HSVR regression data, 95% confidence interval for the HSVR regression, and 95% confidence interval for prediction, respectively.

3.6. Classification

It is of interest to verify the qualitative predictivity of HSVR, since a number of qualitative models have been published [25,102]. Accordingly, compounds enlisted in this study were classified as Caco-2 permeable (Caco-2$^+$) and Caco-2 impermeable (Caco-2$^-$) based on the threshold value of P_{app} (8×10^{-6} cm/s) as suggested [25,102]. Initially, the confusion matrix was constructed (Table S3), and the Cooper statistics and Kubat's G-mean [103] (Table S4) were employed to qualitatively evaluate the predictivity of HSVR. The results were also compared with predictions made by *admetSAR* [104] (available at website: http://lmmd.ecust.edu.cn/admetsar2/), since *admetSAR* has been adopted by DrugBank (available at: https://go.drugbank.com/) to qualitatively predict Caco-2 permeability. The results are listed in Table 6, from which it can be asserted that HSVR outperformed *admetSAR* in every aspect. For instance, the parameter accuracy was 93.1% produced by HSVR, which is substantially higher than that generated by *admetSAR* (50.7%). The metric MCC is the most distinction between HSVR and *admetSAR* (85.0% vs. −8.0%). Thus, it can be asserted that HSVR is also an accurate and predictive qualitative predictive model.

Table 6. Statistical parameters of qualitative predictions by HSVR and *admetSAR*.

Statistical Parameters	HSVR	admetSAR
Se	90.0%	32.0%
Sp	94.7%	60.6%
Acc	93.1%	50.7%
PP	90.0%	30.2%
NP	94.7%	62.6%
MCC	85.0%	−8.0%
G-mean	92.3%	44.1%
F-measure	90.0%	31.1%
κ	85.0%	−8.0%

4. Discussion

Caco-2 has been commonly adopted to predict the intestinal permeability in the process of drug discovery because of its morphological and functional similarity with human enterocytes [105]. The mechanism of Caco-2 permeation is rather complex, since it can take place through passive diffusion, which can go through the paracellular and transcellular routes and active transport. The passive diffusion is predominately governed by the concentration gradient, and most hydrophilic drugs prefer to penetrate between cells in a paracellular fashion, whereas hydrophobic drugs are inclined to get across the cells via the transcellular route. Drugs that can permeate the Caco-2 cells by the active transport can interact with the influx and/or efflux transporters expressed on the cell surface [106]. As such, Caco-2 permeability is affected by some physicochemical and physiological properties [106].

Hydrophobicity or lipophilicity plays an important role in passive diffusion through membranes as well as the drug–receptor interactions [17,107,108]. In addition, hydrophobicity, which can represent by the *n*-octanol-water partition coefficient, *viz*. log *P*, is also an important factor affecting the interaction between the molecules and the target protein, since more lipophilic molecules tend to have stronger interactions with both target protein and biological membrane. Therefore, the very lipophilic molecules have poor oral absorption from the stomach [107,109]. Polar and hydrophobic drug must penetrate through the Caco-2 cell membrane [17,110]. In addition, it has been observed that log *P*, hydrogen bond propensity, weight, and volume are closely related with P_{app} [43]. As such, log *P* was adopted in this study (Table 1), which is consistent with the fact that numerous published in silico models to predict intestinal absorption, PAMPA permeability [1,111], and Caco-2 permeability also have employed this descriptor [40,112–114]. It can be observed from Figure 8, which displays the average log P_{app} for each histogram bin of log *P* for all molecules included in this investigation, that log P_{app} increased with log *P* value initially and then decreased afterward, leading to a seemingly bilinear relationship between log P_{app} and log *P*. This perplexing dependency can be realized by the fact that the more hydrophobic solutes can easier approach the lipid bilayer to penetrate the membrane. The opposite relationship between hydrophobicity and permeability will be resulted when the solutes are too hydrophobic due to stronger attractions between solutes and the membrane as well as stronger repulsive forces from the solvent molecules upon the entrance to the solvent environment that can be illustrated by the PAMPA permeability [1,115,116]. Complexity can be even profound when taking into account the fact that P-gp and BCRP, which are efflux transporters in Caco-2 (vide supra), can interact with substrates by hydrophobicity [117], subsequently leading to a low correlation between log P_{app} and log P (r = 0.15).

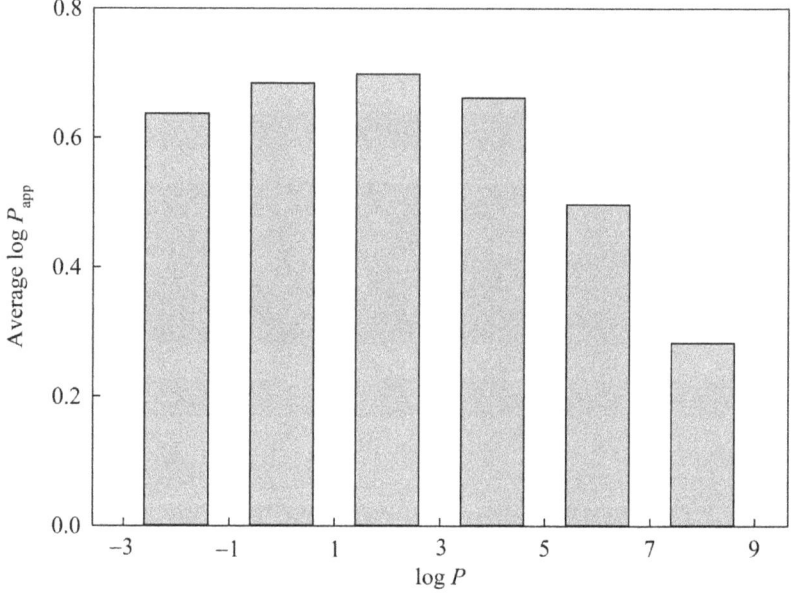

Figure 8. Histogram of average log P_{app} versus the distribution of log P.

It has been observed that the number of aromatic rings (n_{Ar}) has a positive correlation with log P with an r value of 0.67 [118], suggesting that a predictive model can be overtrained once both log P and n_{Ar} are adopted simultaneously. However, this issue was not concerned in this study, since only SVR C adopted this descriptor, whereas SVR A and SVR B included log P (Table 1). In addition, the aromatic ring is a non-polar group, which can enhance the hydrophobicity [52] and increase the passive diffusion [119,120]. In addition, aromatic ring moieties have been implicated in P-gp substrate recognition and efflux modulation [53], leading to the fact that n_{Ar} can be an important factor in P-gp modulation action [121] and BCRP-substrate interactions [122]. As such, n_{Ar} plays a complex role in both passive diffusion and active transport in Caco-2 permeability.

It has been recognized that both PSA and μ are associated with passive diffusion [37,123–125]. In addition, these descriptors have been adopted by published in silico Caco-2 permeability models [37,45–49,126–128]. It has been reported in the PAMPA permeability study that larger PSA, μ, and polarity can enhance the solute-solute and solute-solvent interactions, which, in turn, require more desolvation energy when the solutes penetrate through the lipophilic membrane to the donor compartment [123,129–132], and conversely decrease the passive diffusion [1], consequently, making permeability less favorable. Therefore, it has been shown that PSA has a negative impact in the permeation rate [133,134]. In addition, Joung et al. have indicated that PSA shows an important role in distinguishing the P-gp substrate from the non-substrates [135]. Accordingly, PSA and μ were adopted in this study due to their pivotal roles in Caco-2 permeability.

It is seemingly unusual to include the descriptor $|\mu|_{max}$, which is the absolute maximum component of the molecular dipole, in this study, since it has never been employed by any published model before. This inconsistency actually can be manifested by Figure 9, which displays the average $|\mu|_{max}$ for each histogram bin of μ, that the larger μ, the larger $|\mu|_{max}$, suggesting that they were positively correlated with each other. In addition, μ was recruited by SVR A and SVR C, whereas $|\mu|_{max}$ was enlisted by SVR B only, suggesting that it is less likely to produce an over-trained HSVR, since no single model adopted both two descriptors simultaneously. More importantly, the empirical observation has revealed that HSVR including these selections executed better than the others (data not shown) plausibly because of the descriptor-descriptor interaction [1]. Any other traditional linear or machine learning-based QSAR schemes, conversely, cannot properly render such contradictory descriptor selections.

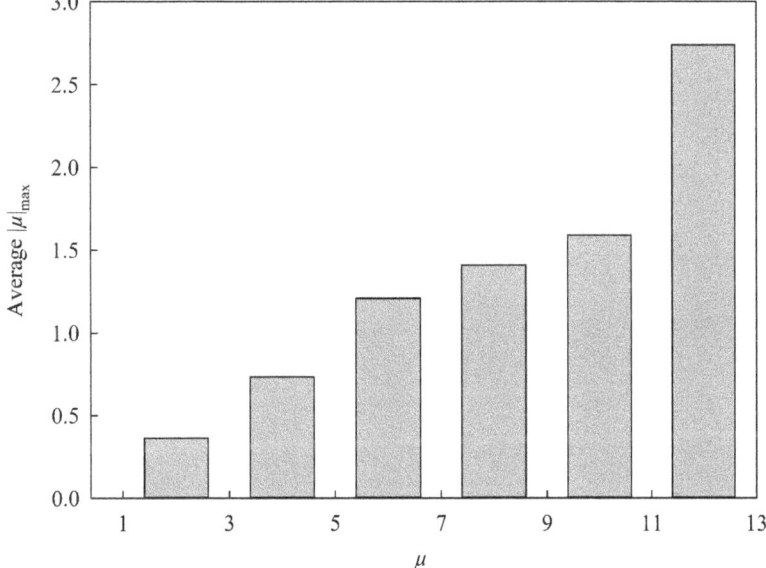

Figure 9. Histogram of average $|\mu|_{max}$ versus the distribution of μ.

It has been reported that the molecular size of the solute molecule is of critical importance in the diffusivity of the biological membrane [37,125,136], and the intestinal absorption can decrease with the increase of molecular size [137]. Furthermore, the molecular size also affects passive diffusion through membranes [138,139] and active transport through the P-gp-substrate interactions [121,138]. Molecular size can be represented by a number of descriptors such α, n_{Ring}, V_m, and n_{rot} [140–142], which were adopted in the investigation and negatively associated with log P_{app} (Table 1). Conversely, Fujiwara et al. adopted the descriptor molecule weight (MW) to develop a theoretical Caco-2 permeability model [37], whereas MW was not included in this study. This discrepancy can be realized by the fact that α was highly correlated with MW with an r value of 0.98 for all molecules enlisted in this study, suggesting that it is plausible to replace MW by α in order not to produce an over-trained model. In addition, it has been observed that α is positively correlated to log P [143] and is highly associated with absorption [50].

The descriptor n_{Ring}, which is reportedly related to molecular size [136,141], has never been adopted by any published Caco-2 permeability predictive model and yet was selected by SVR C (Table 1). This disagreement can be recognized by the fact that n_{Ring} was greatly correlated with α with an r value of 0.78 for all molecules recruited in this study. As such, it is plausible to expect that both n_{Ring} and α play similar roles in Caco-2 permeability. The relationship among log P_{app}, n_{Ring}, and log P can be further perplexing as illustrated by Figure 10, which shows the 3D plot of log P_{app}, n_{Ring}, and log P. The relationship between n_{Ring} and log P has been detailed by Pham-The et al. [125].

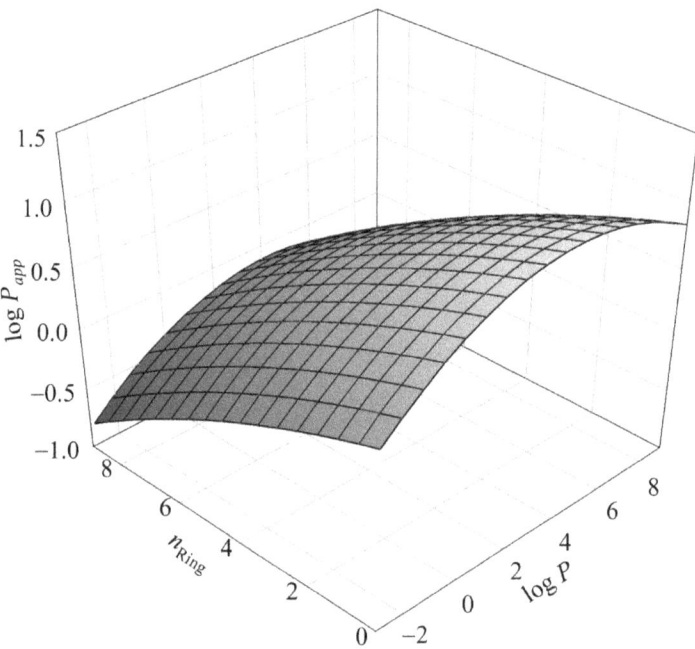

Figure 10. The relationship among log P_{app}, n_{Ring}, and log P in 3D presentation.

It has been observed that V_m plays an important role in passive absorption [9,144,145] and it is adopted by a published Caco-2 permeability model [146] as well as in this study. It has been observed in the rat that fewer rotatable bonds, viz. smaller n_{rot}, can lead to better oral bioavailability, and n_{rot} can also exert a positive effect on the permeation rate [133,143], since more rigid molecules will have smaller n_{rot} values that, in turn, can enhance permeability [125]. Furthermore, n_{rot} is of importance in intestinal absorption [147], since increased n_{rot} can reduce the permeability [133]. Furthermore, a number of published membrane permeability models have also employed the descriptor CSA, which is another feature associated with molecular size and also plays a pivotal role in membrane permeability [70,71]. However, n_{rot} was greatly associated with CSA with an r value of 0.80 for all molecules enrolled in this investigation, suggesting that using n_{rot} in lieu of CSA without producing the over-trained model is plausible. Li et al. also have found that n_{rot} is another feature to discriminate P-gp substrates from non-substrates [148]. As such, it is of necessity to recruit n_{rot} in model development to properly render Caco-2 permeability as suggested [71,72].

Hydrogen bonding potential, which can be expressed by HBD and HBA, is another important factor in determining the solute–solvent interactions [37], and it is the main contributor for the passive diffusion [143]. It has been observed that Caco-2 permeability is a function of HBD and/or HBA, since more permeable solutes tend to have smaller HBD and/or HBA [130,131,149]. Between HBD and HBA, HBD seemingly shows a more profound effect on Caco-2 permeability as compared with HBA [150] as manifested by the fact that several published in silico models have selected HBD to predict Caco-2 permeability instead of HBA [35,42]. Mechanistically, HBD is one of the features associated with P-gp-substrate interactions [148,151]. In addition to efflux transport, HDB is one of the features linked to substrate binding with OATP2B1 [7] as well as PepT1 [152]. Thus, it is of necessity to include in Caco-2 predictive models to take into consideration the passive diffusion as well as the active influx/efflux transport.

The descriptor $pK_{a(Max)}$ was selected in this study due to the fact that higher $pK_{a(Max)}$ can lead to the lower ionized form of drugs in the donor compartment, which, in turn, can increase the penetration through hydrophobic membrane [153]. Furthermore, it has been recognized that neutral compounds can have higher membrane permeability than the other ion classes [154]. Accordingly, all molecules included in this investigation were categorized into different ion classes based on their pK_a values. In addition, ABC and/or SLC substrates were also identified based on the drug information retrieved from DrugBank to understand if the dependence of ion class can be varied by their ion classes. It can be found from Figure 11, which displays the histograms of median log P_{app} versus all molecules, ABC substrates, SLC substrates, as well as ABC and SLC substrates for four different ion classes, that the median log P_{app} values of neutral compounds are substantially larger than the others, suggesting that neutral compounds exhibit higher Caco-2 permeability regardless of active transporter substrate classes, viz. influx transporter or efflux transporter. This observation actually is very similar to the PAMPA permeability, since the ionized compounds will demand larger desolvation energies, which, in turn, can hinder their penetration [134].

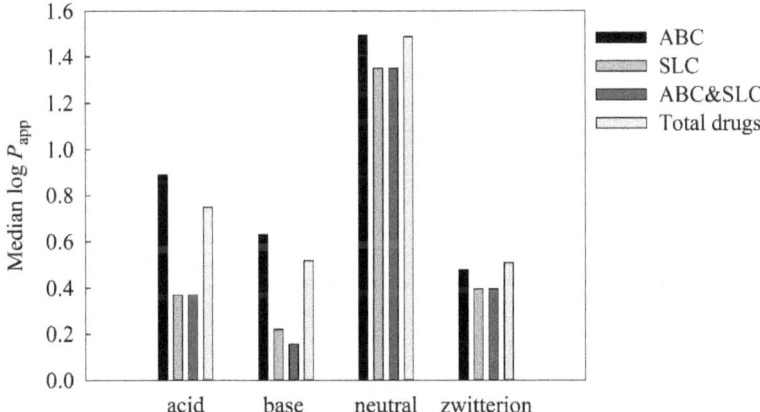

Figure 11. The histogram represents the log P_{app} versus the molecules belong to ATP-binding cassette (ABC) substrate, solute carrier (SLC) substrate, both ABC and SLC substrate, and total drugs in the acid class, base class, neutral class, and zwitterion class, respectively.

Initially, numerous efforts were made in attempting to build assorted 2-QSAR models by employing the partial least square (PLS) scheme, and yet no productive models were produced (data not shown) [1]. This challenge can be realized by the fact that the correlations between the designated descriptors and log P_{app} for all molecules included in this investigation were small, and the largest absolute maximum r was only 0.56 between PSA and log P_{app} (Table 1), signifying the high non-linearity between them. More significantly, the substantial difference in 2-QSAR development between the passive diffusion, viz. the PAMPA system, and Caco-2 permeability can be greatly attributed to the complex active (influx and efflux) transport. Thus, it is extremely difficult, if not absolutely impossible, to derive a linear Cacao-2 permeability QSAR model. Conversely, the accurate and predictive HSVR model can properly render such non-linear dependence of log P_{app} on descriptors.

5. Conclusions

Intestinal permeability is one of the important ADME/Tox metrics that should be addressed in the process of drug discovery and development. The Caco-2 system has been frequently used as a surrogate to preliminarily investigate the intestinal absorption. An in silico model can be a useful approach to predict Caco-2 permeability in assisting drug discovery and development. However, Caco-2 permeability can occur through passive diffusion and active transport, leading to a complex process. Therefore, it is of necessity to include different descriptor combinations and diverse relationships to address these variations in distinct mechanisms. The innovative machine learning-based HSVR scheme, which possesses the superior features of a local model (greater predictivity) and a global model (larger coverage of the application domain), was employed in this study to construct a theoretical model to predict the Caco-2 permeability. The generated HSVR models unveiled great prediction accuracy for the training, test, and outlier samples. When challenged by a group of drugs assayed at different experimental conditions, the developed HSVR model also executed equivalently well. In addition, HSVR showed excellent qualitative performance in recognizing Caco-2 permeable and impermeable compounds, and the selected descriptors can completely justify the diverse mechanisms related to the passive diffusion and active transport. Thus, it can be assured that this HSVR model can be useful to accurately and swiftly predict the Caco-2 permeability of novel compounds in order to assist drug discovery and development.

Supplementary Materials: The following are available online at https://www.mdpi.com/1999-4923/13/2/174/s1, Table S1. Selected compounds for this study; their names, SMILES strings, CAS numbers, and observed log P_{app} values; their predicted values by SVR A, SVR B, SVR C, and HSVR; data partitions; and references; Table S2. Optimal runtime parameters for the SVR models; Table S3. Confusion matrix for the qualitative predictive model; Table S4. The Cooper statistics and Kubat's G-mean calculated from the confusion matrix. Optimal runtime parameters for the SVR models; Figure S1. Histograms of: (A) log P_{app}, (B) molecular weight (MW), (C) surface area (SA), (D) polar surface area (PSA), (E) number of hydrogen bond acceptor (HBA), (F) number of hydrogen bond donor (HBD), (G) and the n-octanol-water partition coefficient (log P) in the training set, test set, and outlier set.

Author Contributions: G.H.T., C.-F.W., and M.K.L. conceived and designed the study; G.H.T., C.-S.J., and M.K.L. performed the experiments and analyzed the data; and G.H.T., C.-F.W., and M.K.L. wrote the paper. The final version of manuscript is reviewed and approved by all authors. All authors have read and agreed to the published version of the manuscript.

Funding: This work was supported by the Ministry of Science and Technology, Taiwan.

Institutional Review Board Statement: Not applicable.

Informed Consent Statement: Not applicable.

Data Availability Statement: Not applicable.

Acknowledgments: Parts of calculations were performed at the National Center for High-Performance Computing, Taiwan. The authors are grateful to Paola Gramatica for providing the free license of *QSARINS*.

Conflicts of Interest: The authors declare no conflict of interest.

References

1. Chi, C.-T.; Lee, M.-H.; Weng, C.-F.; Leong, M.K. In Silico Prediction of PAMPA Effective Permeability Using a Two-QSAR Approach. *Int. J. Mol. Sci.* **2019**, *20*, 3170. [CrossRef] [PubMed]
2. Proctor, W.R.; Ming, X.; Thakker, D.R. In Vitro Techniques to Study Drug–Drug Interactions Involving Transport: Caco-2 Model for Study of P-Glycoprotein and Other Transporters. In *Enzyme- and Transporter-Based Drug-Drug Interactions: Progress and Future Challenges*; Pang, S.K., Rodrigues, D.A., Peter, M.R., Eds.; Springer: New York, NY, USA, 2010; pp. 257–282.
3. Volpe, D.A. Advances in cell-based permeability assays to screen drugs for intestinal absorption. *Expert. Opin. Drug Discov.* **2020**, *15*, 539–549. [CrossRef] [PubMed]

4. Dobson, P.D.; Kell, D.B. Carrier-mediated cellular uptake of pharmaceutical drugs: An exception or the rule? *Nat. Rev. Drug Discov.* **2008**, *7*, 205–220. [CrossRef]
5. Artursson, P.; Bergström, C.A.S. Intestinal Absorption: The Role of Polar Surface Area. In *Drug Bioavailability: Estimation of Solubility, Permeability, Absorption and Bioavailability*; van de Waterbeemd, H., Lennernäs, H., Artursson, P., Eds.; WILEY-VCH Verlag GmbH & Co. KGaA: Weinheim, Germany, 2004; Volume 18, pp. 339–357.
6. Müller, J.; Keiser, M.; Drozdzik, M.; Oswald, S. Expression, regulation and function of intestinal drug transporters: An update. *Biol. Chem.* **2017**, *398*, 175–192. [CrossRef] [PubMed]
7. Varma, M.V.; Ambler, C.M.; Ullah, M.; Rotter, C.J.; Sun, H.; Litchfield, J.; Fenner, K.S.; El-Kattan, A.F. Targeting Intestinal Transporters for Optimizing Oral Drug Absorption. *Curr. Drug Metab.* **2010**, *11*, 730–742. [CrossRef]
8. Seithel, A.; Karlsson, J.; Hilgendorf, C.; Björquist, A.; Ungell, A.L. Variability in mRNA expression of ABC- and SLC-transporters in human intestinal cells: Comparison between human segments and Caco-2 cells. *Eur. J. Pharm. Sci.* **2006**, *28*, 291–299. [CrossRef]
9. Agatonovic-Kustrin, S.; Beresford, R.; Yusof, A.P.M. Theoretically-derived molecular descriptors important in human intestinal absorption. *J. Pharm. Biomed. Anal.* **2001**, *25*, 227–237. [CrossRef]
10. Li, A.P. Screening for human ADME/Tox drug properties in drug discovery. *Drug Discov. Today* **2001**, *6*, 357–366. [CrossRef]
11. Caldwell, G.W.; Yan, Z.; Tang, W.; Dasgupta, M.; Hasting, B. ADME optimization and toxicity assessment in early- and late-phase drug discovery. *Curr. Top. Med. Chem.* **2009**, *9*, 965–980. [CrossRef]
12. Wishart, D.S. Improving early drug discovery through ADME modelling: An overview. *Drugs R D* **2007**, *8*, 349–362. [CrossRef]
13. Dahlgren, D.; Lennernäs, H. Intestinal Permeability and Drug Absorption: Predictive Experimental, Computational and In Vivo Approaches. *Pharmaceutics* **2019**, *11*, 411. [CrossRef] [PubMed]
14. Petri, N.; Lennernäs, H. In Vivo Permeability Studies in the Gastrointestinal Tract of Humans. In *Drug Bioavailability: Estimation of Solubility, Permeability, Absorption and Bioavailability*; van de Waterbeemd, H., Lennernäs, H., Artursson, P., Eds.; WILEY-VCH Verlag GmbH & Co. KGaA: Weinheim, Germany, 2004; Volume 18, pp. 155–188.
15. Dezani, T.M.; Dezani, A.B.; Junior, J.B.; Serra, C.H. Single-Pass Intestinal Perfusion (SPIP) and prediction of fraction absorbed and permeability in humans: A study with antiretroviral drugs. *Eur. J. Pharm. Biopharm.* **2016**, *104*, 131–139. [CrossRef]
16. Lennernäs, H. Human in Vivo Regional Intestinal Permeability: Importance for Pharmaceutical Drug Development. *Mol. Pharm.* **2014**, *11*, 12–23. [CrossRef] [PubMed]
17. Chmiel, T.; Mieszkowska, A.; Kempińska-Kupczyk, D.; Kot-Wasik, A.; Namieśnik, J.; Mazerska, Z. The impact of lipophilicity on environmental processes, drug delivery and bioavailability of food components. *Microchem. J.* **2019**, *146*, 393–406. [CrossRef]
18. Kansy, M.; Fischer, H.; Kratzat, K.; Senner, F.; Wagner, B.; Parrilla, I. High-Throughput Artificial Membrane Permeability Studies in Early Lead Discovery and Development. In *Pharmacokinetic Optimization in Drug Research*; Testa, B., Van de Waterbeend, H., Folkers, G., Guy, R., Eds.; Verlag Helvetica Chimica Acta/Wiley/VCH: Zurich, Switzerland; Weinheim, Germany, 2001; pp. 447–464.
19. Irvine, J.D.; Takahashi, L.; Lockhart, K.; Cheong, J.; Tolan, J.W.; Selick, H.E.; Grove, J.R. MDCK (Madin–Darby canine kidney) cells: A tool for membrane permeability screening. *J. Pharm. Sci.* **1999**, *88*, 28–33. [CrossRef] [PubMed]
20. Avdeef, A.; Nielsen, P.E.; Tsinman, O. PAMPA—a drug absorption in vitro model: 11. Matching the in vivo unstirred water layer thickness by individual-well stirring in microtitre plates. *Eur. J. Pharm. Sci.* **2004**, *22*, 365–374. [CrossRef]
21. Wang, N.-N.; Dong, J.; Deng, Y.-H.; Zhu, M.-F.; Wen, M.; Yao, Z.-J.; Lu, A.-P.; Wang, J.-B.; Cao, D.-S. ADME Properties Evaluation in Drug Discovery: Prediction of Caco-2 Cell Permeability Using a Combination of NSGA-II and Boosting. *J. Chem. Inf. Model.* **2016**, *56*, 763–773. [CrossRef]
22. Uchida, R.; Okamoto, H.; Ikuta, N.; Terao, K.; Hirota, T. Investigation of Enantioselective Membrane Permeability of α-Lipoic Acid in Caco-2 and MDCKII Cell. *Int. J. Mol. Sci.* **2016**, *17*, 155. [CrossRef]
23. Zeng, Z.; Shen, Z.L.; Zhai, S.; Xu, J.L.; Liang, H.; Shen, Q.; Li, Q.Y. Transport of curcumin derivatives in Caco-2 cell monolayers. *Eur. J. Pharm. Biopharm.* **2017**, *117*, 123–131. [CrossRef]
24. Sánchez, A.B.; Calpena, A.C.; Mallandrich, M.; Clares, B. Validation of an Ex Vivo Permeation Method for the Intestinal Permeability of Different BCS Drugs and Its Correlation with Caco-2 In Vitro Experiments. *Pharmaceutics* **2019**, *11*, 638. [CrossRef]
25. Ponce, Y.M.; Pérez, M.A.C.; Zaldivar, V.R.; Sanz, M.B.; Mota, D.S.; Torrens, F. Prediction of Intestinal Epithelial Transport of Drug in (Caco-2) Cell Culture from Molecular Structure using *in silico* Approaches During Early Drug Discovery. *Internet Electron. J. Mol. Des.* **2005**, *4*, 124–150.
26. Petri, N.; Tannergren, C.; Rungstad, D.; Lennernäs, H. Transport Characteristics of Fexofenadine in the Caco-2 Cell Model. *Pharm. Res.* **2004**, *21*, 1398–1404. [CrossRef] [PubMed]
27. Volpe, D.A. Variability in Caco-2 and MDCK cell-based intestinal permeability assays. *J. Pharm. Sci.* **2008**, *97*, 712–725. [CrossRef] [PubMed]
28. Hosey, C.M.; Benet, L.Z. Predicting the Extent of Metabolism Using *in Vitro* Permeability Rate Measurements and *in Silico* Permeability Rate Predictions. *Mol. Pharm.* **2015**, *12*, 1456–1466. [CrossRef] [PubMed]
29. Lee, J.B.; Zgair, A.; Taha, D.A.; Zang, X.; Kagan, L.; Kim, T.H.; Kim, M.G.; Yun, H.-y.; Fischer, P.M.; Gershkovich, P. Quantitative analysis of lab-to-lab variability in Caco-2 permeability assays. *Eur. J. Pharm. Biopharm.* **2017**, *114*, 38–42. [CrossRef]
30. Yamashita, S.; Furubayashi, T.; Kataoka, M.; Sakane, T.; Sezaki, H.; Tokuda, H. Optimized conditions for prediction of intestinal drug permeability using Caco-2 cells. *Eur. J. Pharm. Sci.* **2000**, *10*, 195–204. [CrossRef]

31. Bergström, C.A. In silico predictions of drug solubility and permeability: Two rate-limiting barriers to oral drug absorption. *Basic Clin. Pharmacol. Toxicol.* **2005**, *96*, 156–161. [CrossRef]
32. Parrott, N.; Lavé, T. Prediction of intestinal absorption: Comparative assessment of gastroplus™ and idea™. *Eur. J. Pharm. Sci.* **2002**, *17*, 51–61. [CrossRef]
33. Pelkonen, O.; Turpeinen, M.; Raunio, H. In vivo-in vitro-in silico pharmacokinetic modelling in drug development: Current status and future directions. *Clin. Pharm.* **2011**, *50*, 483–491. [CrossRef]
34. Cherkasov, A.; Muratov, E.N.; Fourches, D.; Varnek, A.; Baskin, I.I.; Cronin, M.; Dearden, J.; Gramatica, P.; Martin, Y.C.; Todeschini, R.; et al. QSAR modeling: Where have you been? Where are you going to? *J. Med. Chem* **2014**, *57*, 4977–5010. [CrossRef]
35. Subramanian, G.; Kitchen, D.B. Computational approaches for modeling human intestinal absorption and permeability. *J. Mol. Model.* **2006**, *12*, 577–589. [CrossRef] [PubMed]
36. Karelson, M.; Karelson, G.; Tamm, T.; Indrek, T.; Jänes, J.; Tämm, K.; Lomaka, A.; Savchenko, D.; Dobcheva, D. QSAR study of pharmacological permeabilities. *Arkivoc* **2009**, *2*, 218–238. [CrossRef]
37. Fujiwara, S.-I.; Yamashita, F.; Hashida, M. Prediction of Caco-2 cell permeability using a combination of MO-calculation and neural network. *Int. J. Pharm.* **2002**, *237*, 95–105. [CrossRef]
38. Van de Waterbeemd, H.; Camenisch, G.; Folkers, G.; Raevsky, O.A. Estimation of Caco-2 Cell Permeability using Calculated Molecular Descriptors. *Quant. Struct. Act. Relat.* **1996**, *15*, 480–490. [CrossRef]
39. Refsgaard, H.H.F.; Jensen, B.F.; Brockhoff, P.B.; Guldbrandt, M.; Christensen, M.S. In Silico Prediction of Membrane Permeability from Calculated Molecular Parameters. *J. Med. Chem.* **2005**, *48*, 805–811. [CrossRef]
40. Paixão, P.; Gouveia, L.F.; Morais, J.A.G. Prediction of the *in vitro* permeability determined in Caco-2 cells by using artificial neural networks. *Eur. J. Pharm. Sci.* **2010**, *41*, 107–117. [CrossRef]
41. Nordqvist, A.; Nilsson, J.; Lindmark, T.; Eriksson, A.; Garberg, P.; Kihlén, M. A General Model for Prediction of Caco-2 Cell Permeability. *QSAR Comb. Sci.* **2004**, *23*, 303–310. [CrossRef]
42. Ma, G.; Cheng, Y. Predicting Caco-2 Permeability Using Support Vector Machine and Chemistry Development Kit. *J. Pharm. Pharm. Sci.* **2006**, *9*, 210–221.
43. Di Fenza, A.; Alagona, G.; Ghio, C.; Leonardi, R.; Giolitti, A.; Madami, A. Caco-2 cell permeability modelling: A neural network coupled genetic algorithm approach. *J. Comput. Aided Mol. Des.* **2007**, *21*, 207–221. [CrossRef]
44. Chan, E.C.Y.; Tan, W.L.; Ho, P.C.; Fang, L.J. Modeling Caco-2 permeability of drugs using immobilized artificial membrane chromatography and physicochemical descriptors. *J. Chromatogr. A* **2005**, *1072*, 159–168. [CrossRef]
45. Santos-Filho, O.A.; Hopfinger, A.J. Combined 4D-Fingerprint and Clustering Based Membrane-Interaction QSAR Analyses for Constructing Consensus Caco-2 Cell Permeation Virtual Screens. *J. Pharm. Sci.* **2008**, *97*, 566–583. [CrossRef] [PubMed]
46. Tantishaiyakul, V. Prediction of Caco-2 cell permeability using partial least squares multivariate analysis. *Pharmazie* **2001**, *56*, 407–411.
47. Welling, S.H.; Clemmensen, L.K.H.; Buckley, S.T.; Hovgaard, L.; Brockhoff, P.B.; Refsgaard, H.H.F. In silico modelling of permeation enhancement potency in Caco-2 monolayers based on molecular descriptors and random forest. *Eur. J. Pharm. Biopharm.* **2015**, *94*, 152–159. [CrossRef]
48. Yamashita, F.; Wanchana, S.; Hashida, M. Quantitative structure/property relationship analysis of Caco-2 permeability using a genetic algorithm-based partial least squares method. *J. Pharm. Sci.* **2002**, *91*, 2230–2239. [CrossRef] [PubMed]
49. Yamashita, F.; Fujiwara, S.-i.; Hashida, M. The "Latent Membrane Permeability" Concept: QSPR Analysis of Inter/Intralaboratorically Variable Caco-2 Permeability. *J. Chem. Inf. Comput. Sci.* **2002**, *42*, 408–413. [CrossRef]
50. Norinder, U.; Osterberg, T.; Artursson, P. Theoretical calculation and prediction of intestinal absorption of drugs using Molsurf parametrization and PLS statistics. *Eur. J. Pharm. Sci.* **1999**, *8*, 49–56. [CrossRef]
51. Pham The, H.; González-Álvarez, I.; Bermejo, M.; Mangas Sanjuan, V.; Centelles, I.; Garrigues, T.M.; Cabrera-Pérez, M. In Silico Prediction of Caco-2 Cell Permeability by a Classification QSAR Approach. *Mol. Inform.* **2011**, *30*, 376–385. [CrossRef] [PubMed]
52. Shinde, R.N.; Srikanth, K.; Sobhia, M.E. Insights into the permeability of drugs and drug-likemolecules from MI-QSAR and HQSAR studies. *J. Mol. Model.* **2012**, *18*, 947–962. [CrossRef] [PubMed]
53. Wang, B.; Ma, L.-Y.; Wang, J.-Q.; Lei, Z.-N.; Gupta, P.; Zhao, Y.-D.; Li, Z.-H.; Liu, Y.; Zhang, X.-H.; Li, Y.-N.; et al. Discovery of 5-Cyano-6-phenylpyrimidin Derivatives Containing an Acylurea Moiety as Orally Bioavailable Reversal Agents against P-Glycoprotein-Mediated Mutidrug Resistance. *J. Med. Chem.* **2018**, *61*, 5988–6001. [CrossRef]
54. Leong, M.K.; Chen, Y.-M.; Chen, T.-H. Prediction of human cytochrome P450 2B6-substrate interactions using hierarchical support vector regression approach. *J. Comput. Chem.* **2009**, *30*, 1899–1909. [CrossRef] [PubMed]
55. Lee, M.-H.; Ta, G.H.; Weng, C.-F.; Leong, M.K. In Silico Prediction of Intestinal Permeability by Hierarchical Support Vector Regression. *Int. J. Mol. Sci.* **2020**, *21*, 3582. [CrossRef] [PubMed]
56. Leong, M.K.; Lin, S.-W.; Chen, H.-B.; Tsai, F.-Y. Predicting Mutagenicity of Aromatic Amines by Various Machine Learning Approaches. *Toxicol. Sci.* **2010**, *116*, 498–513. [CrossRef] [PubMed]
57. Chen, C.; Lee, M.H.; Weng, C.F.; Leong, M.K. Theoretical Prediction of the Complex P-Glycoprotein Substrate Efflux Based on the Novel Hierarchical Support Vector Regression Scheme. *Molecules* **2018**, *23*, 1820. [CrossRef] [PubMed]
58. Bergström, C.A.S.; Bolin, S.; Artursson, P.; Rönn, R.; Sandström, A. Hepatitis C virus NS3 protease inhibitors: Large, flexible molecules of peptide origin show satisfactory permeability across Caco-2 cells. *Eur. J. Pharm. Sci.* **2009**, *38*, 556–563. [CrossRef] [PubMed]

59. Skolnik, S.; Lin, X.; Wang, J.; Chen, X.-H.; He, T.; Zhang, B. Towards prediction of *in vivo* intestinal absorption using a 96-well Caco-2 assay. *J. Pharm. Sci.* **2010**, *99*, 3246–3265. [CrossRef] [PubMed]
60. Lazorova, L.; Hubatsch, I.; Ekegren, J.K.; Gising, J.; Nakai, D.; Zaki, N.M.; Bergström, C.A.S.; Norinder, U.; Larhed, M.; Artursson, P. Structural features determining the intestinal epithelial permeability and efflux of novel HIV-1 protease inhibitors. *J. Pharm. Sci.* **2011**, *100*, 3763–3772. [CrossRef]
61. Nti-Addae, K.W.; Guarino, V.R.; Dalwadi, G.; Stella, V.J. Determination of the permeability characteristics of two sulfenamide prodrugs of linezolid across Caco-2 cells. *J. Pharm. Sci.* **2012**, *101*, 3134–3141. [CrossRef]
62. Deng, X.; Zhang, G.; Shen, C.; Yin, J.; Meng, Q. Hollow fiber culture accelerates differentiation of Caco-2 cells. *Appl. Microbiol. Biotechnol.* **2013**, *97*, 6943–6955. [CrossRef]
63. Yang, Y.; Bai, L.; Li, X.; Xiong, J.; Xu, P.; Guo, C.; Xue, M. Transport of active flavonoids, based on cytotoxicity and lipophilicity: An evaluation using the blood–brain barrier cell and Caco-2 cell models. *Toxicol. Vitro* **2014**, *28*, 388–396. [CrossRef]
64. Wu, S.; Xu, W.; Wang, F.-R.; Yang, X.-W. Study of the Biotransformation of Tongmai Formula by Human Intestinal Flora and Its Intestinal Permeability across the Caco-2 Cell Monolayer. *Molecules* **2015**, *20*, 18704. [CrossRef]
65. Zhou, L.; Lee, K.; Thakker, D.R.; Boykin, D.W.; Tidwell, R.R.; Hall, J.E. Enhanced Permeability of the Antimicrobial Agent 2,5-Bis(4-Amidinophenyl)Furan Across Caco-2 Cell Monolayers Via Its Methylamidoxime Prodrug. *Pharm. Res.* **2002**, *19*, 1689–1695. [CrossRef]
66. Troutman, M.D.; Thakker, D.R. Efflux Ratio Cannot Assess P-Glycoprotein-Mediated Attenuation of Absorptive Transport: Asymmetric Effect of P-Glycoprotein on Absorptive and Secretory Transport Across Caco-2 Cell Monolayers. *Pharm. Res.* **2003**, *20*, 1200–1209. [CrossRef] [PubMed]
67. Miertuš, S.; Scrocco, E.; Tomasi, J. Electrostatic interaction of a solute with a continuum. A direct utilizaion of AB initio molecular potentials for the prevision of solvent effects. *Chem. Phys.* **1981**, *55*, 117–129. [CrossRef]
68. Cammi, R.; Tomasi, J. Remarks on the use of the apparent surface charges (ASC) methods in solvation problems: Iterative versus matrix-inversion procedures and the renormalization of the apparent charges. *J. Comput. Chem.* **1995**, *16*, 1449–1458. [CrossRef]
69. Besler, B.H.; Merz, K.M., Jr.; Kollman, P.A. Atomic charges derived from semiempirical methods. *J. Comput. Chem.* **1990**, *11*, 431–439. [CrossRef]
70. Gerebtzoff, G.; Seelig, A. *In Silico* Prediction of Blood–Brain Barrier Permeation Using the Calculated Molecular Cross-Sectional Area as Main Parameter. *J. Chem. Inf. Model.* **2006**, *46*, 2638–2650. [CrossRef]
71. Leung, S.S.F.; Sindhikara, D.; Jacobson, M.P. Simple Predictive Models of Passive Membrane Permeability Incorporating Size-Dependent Membrane-Water Partition. *J. Chem. Inf. Model.* **2016**, *56*, 924–929. [CrossRef]
72. Muehlbacher, M.; Spitzer, G.M.; Liedl, K.R.; Kornhuber, J. Qualitative prediction of blood–brain barrier permeability on a large and refined dataset. *J. Comput. Aided Mol. Des.* **2011**, *25*, 1095–1106. [CrossRef]
73. Fridén, M.; Winiwarter, S.; Jerndal, G.; Bengtsson, O.; Wan, H.; Bredberg, U.; Hammarlund-Udenaes, M.; Antonsson, M. Structure–Brain Exposure Relationships in Rat and Human Using a Novel Data Set of Unbound Drug Concentrations in Brain Interstitial and Cerebrospinal Fluids. *J. Med. Chem.* **2009**, *52*, 6233–6243. [CrossRef]
74. Topliss, J.G.; Edwards, R.P. Chance factors in studies of quantitative structure-activity relationships. *J. Med. Chem.* **1979**, *22*, 1238–1244. [CrossRef]
75. Kettaneh, N.; Berglund, A.; Wold, S. PCA and PLS with very large data sets. *Comput. Stat. Data Anal.* **2005**, *48*, 69–85. [CrossRef]
76. Tseng, Y.J.; Hopfinger, A.J.; Esposito, E.X. The great descriptor melting pot: Mixing descriptors for the common good of QSAR models. *J. Comput. Aided Mol. Des.* **2012**, *26*, 39–43. [CrossRef] [PubMed]
77. Rogers, D. Application of genetic function approximation to quantitative structure-activity relationships and quantitative structure-property relationships. *J. Chem. Inf. Comput. Sci.* **1994**, *34*, 854–866. [CrossRef]
78. Guyon, I.; Weston, J.; Barnhill, S.; Vapnik, V. Gene Selection for Cancer Classification using Support Vector Machines. *Mach. Learn.* **2002**, *46*, 389–422. [CrossRef]
79. Yimin, A.; Jun, X. A New Support Vector Machine Model for Outlier Detection. In Proceedings of the International Conference on Graphic and Image Processing (ICGIP 2012), Hong Kong, China, 26–27 October 2013; p. 87680E.
80. Hubert, M.; Engelen, S. Robust PCA and classification in biosciences. *Bioinformatics* **2004**, *20*, 1728–1736. [CrossRef]
81. Tropsha, A.; Gramatica, P.; Gombar, V.K. The Importance of Being Earnest: Validation is the Absolute Essential for Successful Application and Interpretation of QSPR Models. *QSAR Comb. Sci.* **2003**, *22*, 69–77. [CrossRef]
82. Golbraikh, A.; Shen, M.; Xiao, Z.; Xiao, Y.-D.; Lee, K.-H.; Tropsha, A. Rational selection of training and test sets for the development of validated QSAR models. *J. Comput. Aided Mol. Des.* **2003**, *17*, 241–253. [CrossRef]
83. Cortes, C.; Vapnik, V. Support-vector networks. *Mach. Learn.* **1995**, *20*, 273–297. [CrossRef]
84. Vapnik, V.; Golowich, S.E.; Smola, A. Support vector method for function approximation, regression estimation and signal processing. In Proceedings of the 9th International Conference on Neural Information Processing Systems; MIT Press: Denver, Colorado, 1996; pp. 281–287.
85. Kecman, V. *Learning and Soft Computing: Support. Vector Machines, Neural Networks, and Fuzzy Logic. Models*; MIT Press: Cambridge, MA, USA, 2001; p. 608.
86. Dearden, J.C.; Cronin, M.T.; Kaiser, K.L. How not to develop a quantitative structure-activity or structure-property relationship (QSAR/QSPR). *SAR QSAR Environ. Res.* **2009**, *20*, 241–266. [CrossRef]

87. Rücker, C.; Rücker, G.; Meringer, M. y-Randomization and Its Variants in QSPR/QSAR. *J. Chem. Inf. Model.* **2007**, *47*, 2345–2357. [CrossRef]
88. Chirico, N.; Gramatica, P. Real External Predictivity of QSAR Models: How To Evaluate It? Comparison of Different Validation Criteria and Proposal of Using the Concordance Correlation Coefficient. *J. Chem. Inf. Model.* **2011**, *51*, 2320–2335. [CrossRef] [PubMed]
89. Chirico, N.; Gramatica, P. Real External Predictivity of QSAR Models. Part 2. New Intercomparable Thresholds for Different Validation Criteria and the Need for Scatter Plot Inspection. *J. Chem. Inf. Model.* **2012**, *52*, 2044–2058. [CrossRef] [PubMed]
90. Consonni, V.; Ballabio, D.; Todeschini, R. Comments on the Definition of the Q2 Parameter for QSAR Validation. *J. Chem. Inf. Model.* **2009**, *49*, 1669–1678. [CrossRef] [PubMed]
91. Lin, L.I. A concordance correlation coefficient to evaluate reproducibility. *Biometrics* **1989**, *45*, 255–268. [CrossRef]
92. Lin, L.I.K. Assay Validation Using the Concordance Correlation Coefficient. *Biometrics* **1992**, *48*, 599–604. [CrossRef]
93. Schüürmann, G.; Ebert, R.-U.; Chen, J.; Wang, B.; Kühne, R. External Validation and Prediction Employing the Predictive Squared Correlation Coefficient—Test Set Activity Mean vs Training Set Activity Mean. *J. Chem. Inf. Model.* **2008**, *48*, 2140–2145. [CrossRef]
94. Gramatica, P.; Cassani, S.; Chirico, N. QSARINS-chem: Insubria datasets and new QSAR/QSPR models for environmental pollutants in QSARINS. *J. Comput. Chem.* **2014**, *35*, 1036–1044. [CrossRef]
95. Gramatica, P.; Chirico, N.; Papa, E.; Cassani, S.; Kovarich, S. QSARINS: A new software for the development, analysis, and validation of QSAR MLR models. *J. Comput. Chem.* **2013**, *34*, 2121–2132. [CrossRef]
96. Ojha, P.K.; Mitra, I.; Das, R.N.; Roy, K. Further exploring rm2 metrics for validation of QSPR models. *Chemom. Intell. Lab. Syst.* **2011**, *107*, 194–205. [CrossRef]
97. Roy, P.P.; Roy, K. On Some Aspects of Variable Selection for Partial Least Squares Regression Models. *QSAR Comb. Sci.* **2008**, *27*, 302–313. [CrossRef]
98. Roy, K.; Mitra, I.; Kar, S.; Ojha, P.K.; Das, R.N.; Kabir, H. Comparative Studies on Some Metrics for External Validation of QSPR Models. *J. Chem. Inf. Model.* **2012**, *52*, 396–408. [CrossRef] [PubMed]
99. Gajewicz, A. How to judge whether QSAR/read-across predictions can be trusted: A novel approach for establishing a model's applicability domain. *Environ. Sci. Nano* **2018**, *5*, 408–421. [CrossRef]
100. Caudill, M. Using neural networks: Hybrid expert networks. *AI Expert* **1990**, *5*, 49–54.
101. Gnanadesikan, R.; Kettenring, J.R. Robust Estimates, Residuals, and Outlier Detection with Multiresponse Data. *Biometrics* **1972**, *28*, 81–124. [CrossRef]
102. Shin, M.; Jang, D.; Nam, H.; Lee, K.H.; Lee, D. Predicting the Absorption Potential of Chemical Compounds Through a Deep Learning Approach. *IEEE/ACM Trans. Comput Biol. Bioinform.* **2018**, *15*, 432–440. [CrossRef]
103. Ma, L.; Fan, S. CURE-SMOTE algorithm and hybrid algorithm for feature selection and parameter optimization based on random forests. *BMC Bioinform.* **2017**, *18*, 169. [CrossRef]
104. Cheng, F.; Li, W.; Zhou, Y.; Shen, J.; Wu, Z.; Liu, G.; Lee, P.W.; Tang, Y. admetSAR: A Comprehensive Source and Free Tool for Assessment of Chemical ADMET Properties. *J. Chem. Inf. Model.* **2012**, *52*, 3099–3105. [CrossRef]
105. Grandvuinet, A.S.; Gustavsson, L.; Steffansen, B. New Insights into the Carrier-Mediated Transport of Estrone-3-sulfate in the Caco-2 Cell Model. *Mol. Pharm.* **2013**, *10*, 3285–3295. [CrossRef]
106. Volpe, D.A. Drug-permeability and transporter assays in Caco-2 and MDCK cell lines. *Future Med. Chem.* **2011**, *3*, 2063–2077. [CrossRef]
107. Valkó, K.L. Lipophilicity and biomimetic properties measured by HPLC to support drug discovery. *J. Pharm. Biomed. Anal.* **2016**, *130*, 35–54. [CrossRef]
108. Lipinski, C.A.; Lombardo, F.; Dominy, B.W.; Feeney, P.J. Experimental and computational approaches to estimate solubility and permeability in drug discovery and development settings. *Adv. Drug Deliv. Rev.* **2001**, *46*, 3–26. [CrossRef]
109. Liu, X.; Testa, B.; Fahr, A. Lipophilicity and its relationship with passive drug permeation. *Pharm. Res.* **2011**, *28*, 962–977. [CrossRef]
110. Volpe, D.A. Drug Permeability Studies in Regulatory Biowaiver Applications. In *Drug Absorption Studies: In Situ, In Vitro and In Silico Models*; Ehrhardt, C., Kim, K.-J., Eds.; Springer US: Boston, MA, USA, 2008; pp. 665–680.
111. Akamatsu, M.; Fujikawa, M.; Nakao, K.; Shimizu, R. In silico prediction of human oral absorption based on QSAR analyses of PAMPA permeability. *Chem. Biodivers* **2009**, *6*, 1845–1866. [CrossRef] [PubMed]
112. Pham-The, H.; Cabrera-Pérez, M.Á.; Nam, N.-H.; Castillo-Garit, J.A.; Rasulev, B.; Le-Thi-Thu, H.; Casañola-Martin, G.M. In silico assessment of ADME properties: Advances in Caco-2 cell monolayer permeability modeling. *Curr. Top. Med. Chem.* **2018**, *18*, 2209–2229. [CrossRef] [PubMed]
113. Faassen, F.; Vogel, G.; Spanings, H.; Vromans, H. Caco-2 permeability, P-glycoprotein transport ratios and brain penetration of heterocyclic drugs. *Int. J. Pharm.* **2003**, *263*, 113–122. [CrossRef]
114. Faassen, F.; Kelder, J.; Lenders, J.; Onderwater, R.; Vromans, H. Physicochemical Properties and Transport of Steroids Across Caco-2 Cells. *Pharm. Res.* **2003**, *20*, 177–186. [CrossRef] [PubMed]
115. Verma, R.P.; Hansch, C.; Selassie, C.D. Comparative QSAR studies on PAMPA/modified PAMPA for high throughput profiling of drug absorption potential with respect to Caco-2 cells and human intestinal absorption. *J. Comput. Aided Mol. Des.* **2007**, *21*, 3–22. [CrossRef]

116. Fujikawa, M.; Nakao, K.; Shimizu, R.; Akamatsu, M. QSAR study on permeability of hydrophobic compounds with artificial membranes. *Bioorg. Med. Chem.* **2007**, *15*, 3756–3767. [CrossRef]
117. Billat, P.-A.; Roger, E.; Faure, S.; Lagarce, F. Models for drug absorption from the small intestine: Where are we and where are we going? *Drug Discov. Today* **2017**, *22*, 761–775. [CrossRef]
118. Ward, S.E.; Beswick, P. What does the aromatic ring number mean for drug design? *Expert. Opin. Drug Discov.* **2014**, *9*, 995–1003. [CrossRef]
119. Camenisch, G.; Alsenz, J.; van de Waterbeemd, H.; Folkers, G. Estimation of permeability by passive diffusion through Caco-2 cell monolayers using the drugs' lipophilicity and molecular weight. *Eur. J. Pharm. Sci.* **1998**, *6*, 317–324. [CrossRef]
120. Yang, N.J.; Hinner, M.J. Getting across the cell membrane: An overview for small molecules, peptides, and proteins. *Methods Mol. Biol.* **2015**, *1266*, 29–53. [PubMed]
121. Beck, W.T.; Qian, X.-d. Photoaffinity substrates for P-glycoprotein. *Biochem. Pharmacol.* **1992**, *43*, 89–93. [CrossRef]
122. Ebert, B.; Seidel, A.; Lampen, A. Identification of BCRP as transporter of benzo[a]pyrene conjugates metabolically formed in Caco-2 cells and its induction by Ah-receptor agonists. *Carcinogenesis* **2005**, *26*, 1754–1763. [CrossRef]
123. Clark, D.E. Rapid calculation of polar molecular surface area and its application to the prediction of transport phenomena. 1. Prediction of intestinal absorption. *J. Pharm. Sci.* **1999**, *88*, 807–814. [CrossRef]
124. Palm, K.; Luthman, K.; Ungell, A.-L.; Strandlund, G.; Artursson, P. Correlation of drug absorption with molecular surface properties. *J. Pharm. Sci.* **1996**, *85*, 32–39. [CrossRef]
125. Pham-The, H.; González-Álvarez, I.; Bermejo, M.; Garrigues, T.; Le-Thi-Thu, H.; Cabrera-Pérez, M.Á. The Use of Rule-Based and QSPR Approaches in ADME Profiling: A Case Study on Caco-2 Permeability. *Mol. Inf.* **2013**, *32*, 459–479. [CrossRef]
126. Değim, Z. Prediction of Permeability Coefficients of Compounds Through Caco-2 Cell Monolayer Using Artificial Neural Network Analysis. *Drug Dev. Ind. Pharm.* **2005**, *31*, 935–942. [CrossRef]
127. Hou, T.J.; Zhang, W.; Xia, K.; Qiao, X.B.; Xu, X.J. ADME Evaluation in Drug Discovery. 5. Correlation of Caco-2 Permeation with Simple Molecular Properties. *J. Chem. Inf. Comput. Sci.* **2004**, *44*, 1585–1600. [CrossRef]
128. Palm, K.; Luthman, K.; Ungell, A.-L.; Strandlund, G.; Beigi, F.; Lundahl, P.; Artursson, P. Evaluation of Dynamic Polar Molecular Surface Area as Predictor of Drug Absorption: Comparison with Other Computational and Experimental Predictors. *J. Med. Chem.* **1998**, *41*, 5382–5392. [CrossRef]
129. Bergström, C.A.S.; Strafford, M.; Lazorova, L.; Avdeef, A.; Luthman, K.; Artursson, P. Absorption Classification of Oral Drugs Based on Molecular Surface Properties. *J. Med. Chem.* **2003**, *46*, 558–570. [CrossRef] [PubMed]
130. Burton, P.S.; Conradi, R.A.; Hilgers, A.R.; Ho, N.F.H.; Maggiora, L.L. The relationship between peptide structure and transport across epithelial cell monolayers. *J. Control. Release* **1992**, *19*, 87–97. [CrossRef]
131. Kulkarni, A.; Han, Y.; Hopfinger, A.J. Predicting Caco-2 Cell Permeation Coefficients of Organic Molecules Using Membrane-Interaction QSAR Analysis. *J. Chem. Inf. Comput. Sci.* **2002**, *42*, 331–342. [CrossRef]
132. Rossi Sebastiano, M.; Doak, B.C.; Backlund, M.; Poongavanam, V.; Over, B.; Ermondi, G.; Caron, G.; Matsson, P.; Kihlberg, J. Impact of Dynamically Exposed Polarity on Permeability and Solubility of Chameleonic Drugs Beyond the Rule of 5. *J. Med. Chem.* **2018**, *61*, 4189–4202. [CrossRef] [PubMed]
133. Veber, D.F.; Johnson, S.R.; Cheng, H.-Y.; Smith, B.R.; Ward, K.W.; Kopple, K.D. Molecular Properties That Influence the Oral Bioavailability of Drug Candidates. *J. Med. Chem.* **2002**, *45*, 2615–2623. [CrossRef]
134. Yang, Y.; Engkvist, O.; Llinàs, A.; Chen, H. Beyond Size, Ionization State, and Lipophilicity: Influence of Molecular Topology on Absorption, Distribution, Metabolism, Excretion, and Toxicity for Druglike Compounds. *J. Med. Chem.* **2012**, *55*, 3667–3677. [CrossRef]
135. Joung, J.Y.; Kim, H.; Kim, H.M.; Ahn, S.K.; Nam, K.-Y.; No, K.T. Prediction Models of P-Glycoprotein Substrates Using Simple 2D and 3D Descriptors by a Recursive Partitioning Approach. *Bull. Korean Chem. Soc.* **2012**, *33*, 1123–1127. [CrossRef]
136. Newby, D.A. *Data Mining Methods for the Prediction of Intestinal Absorption Using QSAR*; University of Kent: Kent, UK, 2014.
137. Helen Chan, O.; Stewart, B.H. Physicochemical and drug-delivery considerations for oral drug bioavailability. *Drug Discov. Today* **1996**, *1*, 461–473. [CrossRef]
138. Ferté, J. Analysis of the tangled relationships between P-glycoprotein-mediated multidrug resistance and the lipid phase of the cell membrane. *Eur. J. Biochem.* **2000**, *267*, 277–294. [CrossRef]
139. Litman, T.; Zeuthen, T.; Skovsgaard, T.; Stein, W.D. Structure-activity relationships of P-glycoprotein interacting drugs: Kinetic characterization of their effects on ATPase activity. *Biochim. Biophys. Acta Mol. Basis Dis.* **1997**, *1361*, 159–168. [CrossRef]
140. Kaliszan, R. QSRR: Quantitative Structure-(Chromatographic) Retention Relationships. *Chem. Rev.* **2007**, *107*, 3212–3246. [CrossRef] [PubMed]
141. Kouskoura, M.G.; Kachrimanis, K.G.; Markopoulou, C.K. Modeling the drugs' passive transfer in the body based on their chromatographic behavior. *J. Pharm. Biomed. Anal.* **2014**, *100*, 94–102. [CrossRef] [PubMed]
142. Winiwarter, S.; Ridderström, M.; Ungell, A.L.; Andersson, T.B.; Zamora, I. Use of Molecular Descriptors for Absorption, Distribution, Metabolism, and Excretion Predictions. In *Comprehensive Medicinal Chemistry II*; John, B.T., David, J.T., Eds.; Elsevier: Oxford, UK, 2007; pp. 531–554.
143. Raevsky, O.A. Physicochemical Descriptors in Property-Based Drug Design. *Mini Rev. Med. Chem.* **2004**, *4*, 1041–1052. [CrossRef] [PubMed]

consequently their bioavailabilities in rate and extent must be similar if excipients do not alter the drug absorptions. In vitro BE or biowaivers based on the BCS are now included in the main regulatory guidances around the world, with some slight discrepancies on classification boundaries summarized and discussed by Lenic et al. [1], Zheng et al. [2], and Hoffsäss and Dressman [3].

Two recent reports estimated the probability of proving BE (or the risk of obtaining non-bioequivalent (NBE) or bio-inequivalent (BI) results) for products containing drugs from all BCS classes, and whether the quality control (QC) in vitro dissolution test could predict the in vivo bioequivalence outcome [4,5].

Ramirez et al. published in 2010 a survey of 124 bioequivalence studies of drugs that were classified according to the BCS in order to explore the probability of passing the BE standard for the different BCS classes and the predictive ability of the quality control dissolution test of the BE outcome [5]. In the survey, they found several drug products (including pravastatin) that failed the BE demonstration, in spite of the adequate power of the BE study design (>80%) and the fact that the drug products passed the QC dissolution test. In other words, even if the study had enough power to correctly conclude bioequivalence (H1 alternative hypothesis), the products were found to be inequivalent, and the null hypothesis (H0) of inequivalence could not be rejected [6,7]. The authors concluded that the usually employed QC dissolution tests were not adequate to allow a biowaiver of in vivo bioequivalence studies.

In the Cristofoletti et al. report [4], the authors surveyed a random sample of 500 BE studies from a database from the Brazilian medicines agency (ANVISA). In this study, the drugs were classified according to the BCS and Biopharmaceutical Drug Disposition and Classification System (BDDCS) to evaluate the outcome of bioequivalence studies. For Cristofoletti et al., the failure in pravastatin (a class III compound), in spite of the adequate power of the studies (>80%), remains unexplained.

In both surveys, the probability of obtaining a BE result when the dissolution profiles were similar was around 90% for class I and III drug products (post-test probability or positive predictive value), whereas for class II drug products, the post-test BE probability after a similar dissolution profile was 61%. On the other hand, the probability of false positive results (i.e., similar dissolution but NBE results) was almost 90% for class II drugs. These results point out the lack of an in vivo predictive value of the pharmacopeia dissolution tests [4,5].

The purpose of this work is to explore the predictive ability of BCS biowaiver-based dissolution methods for two test pravastatin products versus the innovator reference product, where one of the test products corresponds to the failing product from Ramirez et al. survey [5], and to explore the reasons for the BE failure. In addition, we have investigated the influence of the product excipients on intestinal permeability to assess the need of additional in vitro tests (apart from dissolution) to ensure the in vitro predictability of the in vivo bioequivalence outcome.

2. Materials and Methods

2.1. Compounds

Pravastatin (MW = 446.52 g/mol) was obtained from Sigma-Aldrich (Barcelona, Spain), and Acetonitrile (ACN) was obtained from VWR International (West Chester, PA, USA). Methanol (MeOH), hydrogen chloride (HCl), and trifluoroacetic acid (TFA) were purchased from Fisher Scientific (Pittsburgh, PA, USA). Sodium hydroxide (NaOH), sodium chloride (NaCl), and sodium dihydrogen phosphate monohydrate ($NaH_2PO_4 \cdot H_2O$) were received from Sigma-Aldrich (Barcelona, Spain). Pravastatin is a weak acid with a pK_a = 4.21 and log P = 1.65 [8]. For oral administration, it is used in the form of sodium salt. Pravastatin sodium is a white hygroscopic powder, easily soluble in water and methanol, and acetonitrile, and practically insoluble in chloroform [9].

Metoprolol, n-octanol, acetonitrile, and methanol were purchased from Sigma (Barcelona, Spain).

2.2. Pravastatin Formulations

Lipemol 40 mg tablets (Bristol-Myers, Squibb, S.A., London, UK) were used as reference products. Their excipients are croscarmellose sodium, magnesium stearate, magnesium oxide, microcrystalline cellulose, yellow iron oxide, anhydrous lactose, and povidone K30.

Pravastatin bioequivalent (BE) and non-bioequivalent (NBE) formulations were donated by a Spanish pharmaceutical company. The excipients in the NBE formulations are croscarmellose sodium, magnesium stearate, microcrystalline cellulose, yellow iron oxide, colloidal silica, magnesium carbonate, and anhydrous lactose.

In the BE formulation, the excipients are magnesium stearate, microcrystalline cellulose, yellow iron oxide, povidone K30, calcium phosphate monobasic anhydrous, sodium starch glycolate, trometamol, and sodium phosphate dibasic dehydrate.

The company provided samples from the batches used in the BE study for tests and reference products.

The results obtained in their corresponding 2 × 2 crossover BE studies are reported in Table 1. The NBE formulation failed to show bioequivalence in C_{max}.

Table 1. In vivo bioequivalence results of the test formulations.

Pharmacokinetic Parameter	Point Estimate and 90% Confidence Interval (%)	
	NBE Formulation	BE Formulation
C_{max}	112.50 (100.20–126.30)	105.36 (95.66–116.04)
$AUC_{0-\infty}$	100.10 (92.50–107.50)	99.15 (92.90–105.82)

(n = 36 patients).

2.3. Experimental Techniques

2.3.1. Solubility Assays: Saturation Shake-Flask Method

To estimate pravastatin solubility, an excess of solid drug was added in buffer solutions pH 1.2, 4.5, and 6.8 at 37 °C. The solubility assays were performed according to the World Health Organization (WHO) guidelines protocols [10]. The equilibrium was reached in 8 h. A sample concentration was determined using high-performance liquid chromatography (HPLC) with ultraviolet (UV) detection.

2.3.2. Lipophilicity Indexes: Partition Coefficients

Bulk phase partition coefficients (P) between n-octanol (analytical grade, Sigma-Aldrich, Barcelona, Spain) and phosphate buffer pH 6.80, 50 mM were determined for metoprolol and pravastatin.

The partition coefficient was calculated as the ratio between octanol concentration and the aqueous concentration. Three replicates were done to determine the average value.

Partition coefficients can be used as an index to provisionally classify compounds in terms of permeability [11]. Metoprolol was chosen as the reference compound for high permeability because its oral fraction absorbed is higher than 95%. Thus, drugs that exhibit partition coefficients and human intestinal permeability values lower than the value for metoprolol are considered low-permeability drugs.

2.3.3. Permeability Assays: Cell Culture and Transport Studies

Caco-2 cells were grown in a polycarbonate membrane. To reach the confluence, 250,000 cells/cm^2 were seeded in six Transwell plates and fasted for 19–22 days with Dubelcco's Modified Eagle's Media, with 1% L-glutamine, 10% fetal bovine serum, and 1% penicillin/streptomycin, at 37 °C temperature, 90% relative humidity, and 5% CO_2.

The confluence of the cells was tested by measuring the transepithelial electrical resistance (TEER). Permeability studies were conducted with an orbital shaking (50 rpm) and with pH 7.0 in both chambers. Standard protocols were described and validated previously in our laboratory [12–16]. Four samples of 200 µL were taken and replaced with a fresh buffer from the receiver side at 15, 30, 45, and 90 min.

Pravastatin transport was studied in the solution at five concentrations (50, 100, 358 (highest single dose per tablet), 500, and 1000 µM). Permeability studies were performed in both directions: apical-to-basal (A-to-B) and basal-to-apical (B-to-A). The permeability value of pravastatin was compared with metoprolol, the high permeability reference compound.

The apparent permeability coefficient was calculated according the following equation:

$$C_{receiver,t} = \frac{Q_{total}}{V_{receiver} + V_{donor}} + \left((C_{receiver,t-1} \cdot f) - \frac{Q_{total}}{V_{receiver} + V_{donor}} \right) \cdot e^{-P_{eff}\, 0.1 \cdot S \cdot \left(\frac{1}{V_{receiver}} + \frac{1}{V_{donor}} \right) \cdot \Delta t} \quad (1)$$

where $C_{receiver,t}$ is the drug concentration in the receiver chamber at time t, Q_{total} is the total amount of drug in both chambers, $V_{receiver}$ and V_{donor} are the volumes of each chamber, $C_{receiver,t-1}$ is the drug concentration in the receiver chamber at the previous time, f is the sample replacement dilution factor, S is the surface area of the monolayer, Δt is the time interval, and P_{eff} is the permeability coefficient as was described by Mangas-Sanjuan et al. [14].

The permeability value of pravastatin 358 µM (highest single dose per tablet) was compared with the permeability value of the reference and test formulations at the same concentration of pravastatin. Experiments in the presence of the formulation excipients were done by dissolving a formulation tablet in 250 mL of buffer and filtrating the obtained dispersion to eliminate nonsoluble excipients.

2.3.4. Disintegration

These assays were performed using a tablet disintegration tester (Hanson Research, Chatsworth, CA., USA) to measure the tablet disintegration time. According to the United States Pharmacopeia (USP) and European Pharmacopeia (Ph. Eur.) guidelines, the experiments were carried out in 800 mL of the media at 37 °C ($n = 3$).

The disintegration studies were performed in different media, simulating pH in the gastrointestinal human tract at pH 1.2, 4.5, and 6.8, and unbuffered water.

2.3.5. Dissolution Assays

Drug release experiments were performed in 900 mL and 500 mL of pharmacopeia media (hydrochloric acid buffer/acetate buffer/phosphate buffer) at pH 1.2, 4.5, and 6.8, respectively, at 37 ± 0.5 °C and 50 rpm with USP 2 (Pharma-Test PT-DT70) [17]. Samples were taken at 5, 10, 15, 20, 30, 45, and 60 min, and the sample volume was replaced by a fresh preheated medium. Samples were immediately centrifuged (at 10,000 rpm for 10 min) and diluted (1:1) in methanol.

The dissolution profiles were compared by f_2 (similarity factor) [18,19]. The f_2 calculations were performed in Microsoft Excel (2016) [20].

2.4. Analysis of the Samples

The samples were analyzed by HPLC (Alliance-Waters 2695, Barcelona, Spain) using a Nova-Pak C18 column (4 µM, 3.9 × 150 mm) and UV detector (Waters 2487, Barcelona, Spain) at wavelengths of 238 nm. The flow-rate was 1.0 mL/min, and the mobile phase contained 50:40:10 methanol, water with 0.1% trifluoroacetic, and acetonitrile. The retention time of pravastatin was 3.2 min, and the limit of quantification was 0.02 µM. The analysis method fulfilled the linearity ($r > 0.99$), accuracy, and precision criteria (<5%).

The metoprolol HPLC method was published previously by our group [13,21].

2.5. Statistical Analysis

Results are shown as mean ± standard deviations. Statistical analysis of permeability values were two-tailed student t-tests, or analysis of variance (ANOVA) and Scheffé post hoc. The significance level was 0.05, and the software used was statistical package SPSS, V.20.00.

3. Results

The solubility pH profile for pravastatin at pH 1.2, 4.5, and 6.8 was 439.80 ± 17.42, 503.87 ± 24.20, and 479.58 ± 17.39 mg/mL (Figure 1). As expected considering its acidic nature, the lowest solubility was obtained at the lowest pH. The highest strength/dose of pravastatin (40 mg) would be soluble in 0.09 mL of water at pH 1.2. Dose number (Do) is 3.20×10^{-4}. Therefore, pravastatin is a highly soluble drug. ANOVA test and Scheffé post hoc comparison detected differences in the solubility values at pH 1.2 versus the higher pHs, while no differences were detected between solubility values at pH 4.5 versus 6.8.

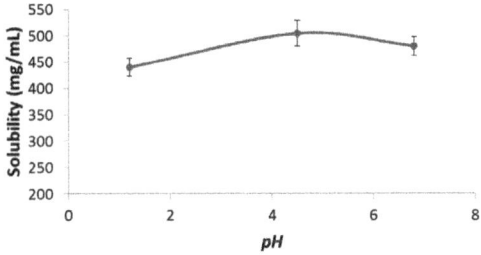

Figure 1. The pH solubility profile of pravastatin determined by the shake-flask method.

The n-Octanol partition coefficient was $P = 0.70 \pm 0.07$ for pravastatin. This value was obtained with relation to a 65:35 n-octanol/phosphate buffer, with a pH 6.80, 50 mM. For metoprolol, the partition coefficient was $P = 0.23 \pm 0.05$. According to these results, pravastatin could be provisionally classified as a high-permeability compound, but as Takagi, et al. [11] described previously, the existence of an active transport mechanism (absorptive or secretive) would bias the classification based purely on lipophilicity.

The permeability value of pravastatin was compared with a metoprolol (reference compound) value in order to classify pravastatin as a high- or low-permeability compound. Different concentrations of pravastatin were studied in order to characterize the transport mechanism of the drug across the intestinal membrane (Figure 2).

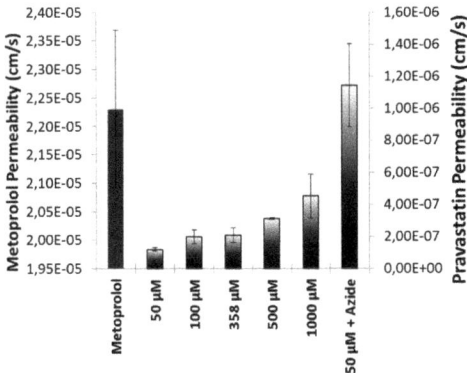

Figure 2. In vitro permeability values of pravastatin in Caco-2 cell monolayers at different drug concentrations. The highest clinical dose of pravastatin is equal to 358 μM (358 μM = 0.152 mg/mL, 100 μM = 0.04 mg/mL, 500 μM = 0.21 mg/mL, and 1000 μM = 0.42 mg/mL).

The analysis of variance (ANOVA) detected statistically significant differences among the permeability values obtained at different pravastatin concentrations ($p = 0.0003$).

Permeability values in the different formulations of pravastatin were also compared. The results are shown in Figure 3. The ANOVA and post hoc test showed statistically significant differences between the reference and NBE formulation ($p < 0.05$).

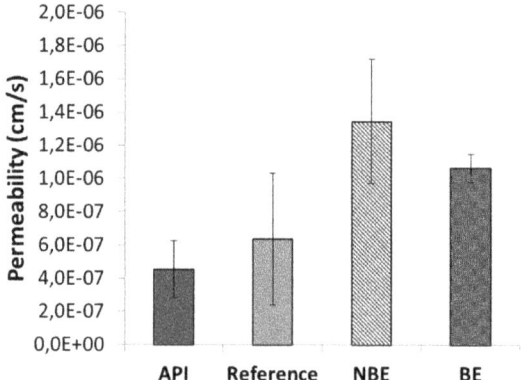

Figure 3. Pravastatin permeability values of the application programming interface (API) (358 µM), reference, non-bioequivalent (NBE), and bioequivalent (BE) formulations. Error bars represent the standard deviation.

In Figure 4, disintegration times of pravastatin products are depicted with statistical differences between formulations. The disintegration endpoint of each sample is recorded as per the United States Pharmacopeia (USP) definition, in which no palpable form or outline of the sample is observed on the screen of the test apparatus or adhering to the lower surface of the disk.

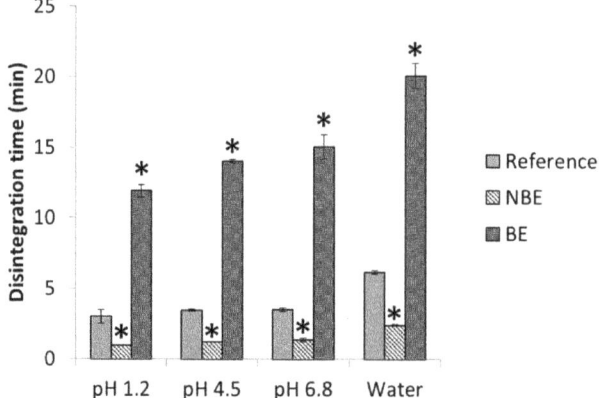

Figure 4. Disintegration times of various pravastatin products in different disintegration media. * Significant difference ($p < 0.05$).

Results of the dissolution tests in different buffers and volumes are summarized in Figure 5.

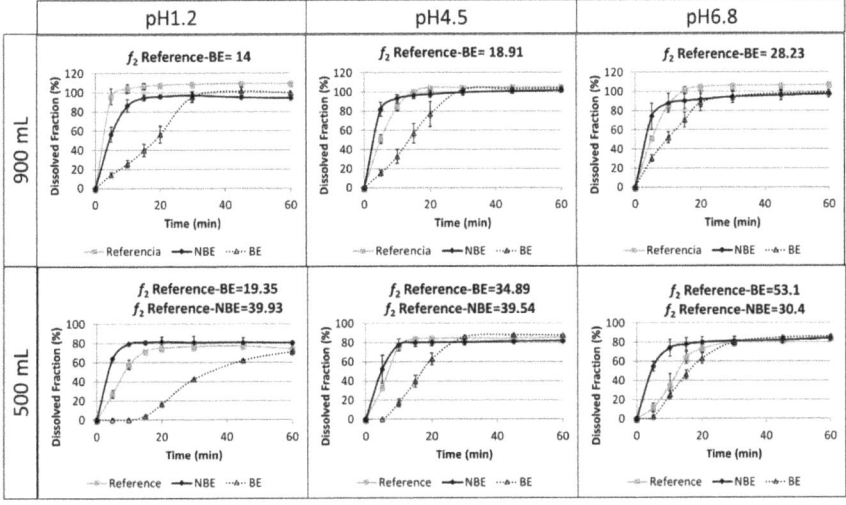

Figure 5. Dissolution profiles of three pravastatin formulations (reference product, non-bioequivalent formulation (NBE) and bioequivalent formulation (BE)) in the paddle apparatus at 50 rpm in buffered media at pH 1.2, 4.5, and 6.8 ($n = 6$).

The reference and NBE products showed complete dissolution (>85%) in 15 min in the USP 2 at 50 rpm in 900 mL of buffered media at pH 1.2, 4.5, and 6.8. However, the BE product showed complete dissolution at 30 min. The same tests were conducted at 500 mL to verify whether a volume lower than 900 mL could detect differences in BCS class III formulations. However, the amount dissolved in these reduced volumes did not reach complete dissolution. Therefore, these dissolution tests are difficult to interpret.

4. Discussion

Based on the experimental results of solubility and permeability determinations, pravastatin is classified as a class III drug according with BCS, as its Dose number (Do) is less than 1 ($\leq 3.20 \times 10^{-4}$) at all the relevant pHs, and the permeability value of pravastatin was lower than that of metoprolol. Pravastatin is classified as a low-permeability drug, which is consistent with an oral bioavailability of 17% due to a low intestinal absorption (34% of dose administered) and a first-pass hepatic effect of 66% of the absorbed drug [22]. On the other hand, our experimental results are consistent with the existence of a secretion mechanism, as permeability increased at higher concentrations. The permeability value obtained in the presence of sodium azide that corresponded with the passive diffusion permeability confirms that not even at the highest pravastatin concentration tested was the efflux mechanism saturated. In addition, the permeability obtained in the presence of sodium azide, when any potential transporter contribution was nullified, was as high as metoprolol permeability, which is consistent with the experimentally estimated partition coefficient.

The observed changes in pravastatin permeability values in different formulations demonstrated that, in spite of the assumption of excipients being inert, actually some of them affect drug bioavailability, in particular for drugs with a carrier-mediated transport mechanism like pravastatin. Many excipients have shown its ability to inhibit the secretion activity of P-glycoprotein or MRP-2 transporters, increasing the permeability of the substrate drug [23–26]. Other authors have demonstrated that changes in paracellular route permeability are also affected by the presence of excipients [27–29]. The formulation with the largest permeability is the NBE formulation, which is consistent with the failed C_{max} due to supra-bioavailability.

Disintegration differences in pravastatin products were in line with the in vivo outcome for the NBE formulation, but there was no rank order correlation in the cases of the reference and the BE formulation, which showed marked differences in disintegration times that are not reflected in vivo. This might be attributed to the differences in permeability that are compensated for by the differences in disintegration/dissolution, since the BE formulation also exhibited higher permeability than the reference formulation, but this difference was compensated for by its slower disintegration/dissolution. In 500 mL of pH 6.8 buffer, the dissolution of the formulations showed the same trend as the observed in the in vivo results, and the f_2 similarity factor indicated differences between the reference and NBE formulation. This may be because these dissolution conditions are predictive or simply a coincidence, since in these conditions complete dissolution was not achieved and the results are difficult to rely on.

Dissolution assays in the paddle apparatus at 50 rpm in 900 mL cannot detect differences in dissolution profiles of the reference and NBE formulations using classical buffers at pH 1.2, 4.5, and 6.8, because complete dissolution (>85%) was achieved in 15 min. However, in buffers of pH 1.2 and 6.8, it is evident that the dissolution was more rapid for the NBE formulation. This small difference, together with the large difference in permeability, seems to be the cause of the C_{max} failure, which was borderline, but the point estimate of the ratio test/reference was slightly >10% different, and the confidence interval did not include the 100% value. This difference in permeability highlights the relevance of requiring similar excipients for BCS class III drugs, as the high solubility could allow a similar in vitro dissolution, and even a similar in vivo dissolution, while still other factors may affect their oral fraction from being absorbed. For the BE product, the BCS-based biowaiver dissolution test in 900 mL would have led to a false negative result [3], i.e., differences observed in vitro while BE was observed in vivo. This possibility is not a problem from a regulatory point of view, since the companies always have the possibility to conduct an in vivo BE study, whereas the regulatory problem is to approve the NBE formulation based on in vitro dissolution profiles when the C_{max} is notably different and not able to show equivalence.

On the other hand, our dissolution results show that for these pravastatin products reduced volumes (500 mL) seem to be more discriminatory, i.e., both products are detected as nonsimilar at pH 1.2 and 4.5, and differences parallel or follow the same rank order correlation of the in vivo outcome at pH 6.8. However, these dissolution studies are difficult to interpret because complete dissolution is not reached and, therefore, the f_2 similarity factor lacks any meaning. In fact, at pH 1.2 and 4.5, the amounts dissolved at 15 min, which is an approximation of the median gastric emptying time in the reference and the NBE formulations, can be considered similar. Therefore, with the simplistic assumption of gastric emptying after 15 min of residence in the stomach, the same amount would be released to the duodenum. The amounts dissolved at 15 min at pH 6.8 are different, but that pH is not the expected pH when the drug is emptied from the stomach. Therefore, if the C_{max} differences are due not only to the differences in permeability but also to differences in dissolution, it is evident that the usual volume of 900 mL is not adequate. Dissolution tests in 500 mL of buffer at 50 rpm were conducted to explore if volumes closer to the fluid volume in the gastrointestinal tract offer different results. However, the predictive power at pH 6.8 was not confirmed. For example, at pH 1.2 and 6.8, the f_2 similarity factor was not able to conclude similarity because dissolution did not reach 100% at the end of the study but an asymptote. However, in relative terms, the NBE formulation and the reference exhibit similar amounts dissolved at 15 min (less than 10%). At pH 4.5, even the f_2 similarity factors concludes with the NBE formulation and the reference.

5. Conclusions

The BCS-based biowaiver dissolution tests with the paddle apparatus at 50 rpm in pH 1.2, 4.5, and 6.8 in 900 mL media were not able to detect the in vivo C_{max} differences for pravastatin products. The different C_{max} seems to be the result of the combined effect of a higher permeability of the NBE formulation due to the excipients inhibition of the efflux transporters and a more rapid disintegration and dissolution. Those combined effects could not be detected with the current dissolution conditions in a volume of 900 mL and the criteria of similarity at 15 min, but the difference of the NBE formulation was observed at earlier sampling times (e.g., 5 min) and/or when the dissolution tests were conducted in 500 mL of dissolution media. Nevertheless, at 500 mL volume and pH 1.2 and 4.5, the BE formulation was also detected as nonsimilar.

Author Contributions: Methodology, validation, and investigation, A.R.-P., S.C.-U. and B.P.-A.; formal analysis, M.G.-A. and I.M.-M.; conceptualization, writing—review and editing, A.G.-A.; writing—original draft preparation, visualization, supervision, I.G.-A.; project administration and funding acquisition M.B.

Funding: This research was funded by Agencia Estatal Investigación and European Union through FEDER (Fondo Europeo de Desarrollo Regional) by the project "Modelos in vitro de evaluacion biofarmaceutica", grant number SAF2016-78756(AEI/FEDER, EU). The author S.C.-U. APC was funded by DAP, University of Los Andes, Venezuela.

Conflicts of Interest: The authors declare no conflict of interest. Spanish Agency for Medicines and Health Care Products had no role in the design of the study; in the collection, analyses, or interpretation of data; in the writing of the manuscript; and in the decision to publish the results. This article represents the personal opinions of the authors, and does not necessarily represent the views or policies of their corresponding Regulatory Authorities.

References

1. Lenić, I.; Blake, K.; Garcia-Arieta, A.; Potthast, H.; Welink, J. Overview of the European Medicines Agency's Experience with Biowaivers in Centralized Applications. *Clin. Transl. Sci.* **2019**, *12*, 490–496. [CrossRef] [PubMed]
2. Zhang, X.; Zheng, N.; Lionberger, R.A.; Yu, L.X. Innovative approaches for demonstration of bioequivalence: The US FDA perspective. *Ther. Deliv.* **2013**, *4*, 725–740. [CrossRef] [PubMed]
3. Hofsäss, M.A.; Dressman, J.B. The Discriminatory Power of the BCS-Based Biowaiver: A Retrospective with Focus on Essential Medicines. *J. Pharm. Sci.* **2019**, *108*, 2824–2837. [CrossRef] [PubMed]
4. Cristofoletti, R.; Chiann, C.; Dressman, J.B.; Storpirtis, S. A comparative analysis of biopharmaceutics classification system and biopharmaceutics drug disposition classification system: A cross-sectional survey with 500 bioequivalence studies. *J. Pharm. Sci.* **2013**, *102*, 3136–3144. [CrossRef]
5. Ramirez, E.; Laosa, O.; Guerra, P.; Duque, B.; Mosquera, B.; Borobia, A.M.; Lei, S.H.; Carcas, A.J.; Frias, J. Acceptability and characteristics of 124 human bioequivalence studies with active substances classified according to the Biopharmaceutic Classification System. *Br. J. Clin. Pharmacol.* **2010**, *70*, 694–702. [CrossRef]
6. Walker, E.; Nowacki, A.S. Understanding equivalence and noninferiority testing. *J. Gen. Intern. Med.* **2011**, *26*, 192–196. [CrossRef]
7. Chow, S.C. Bioavailability and Bioequivalence in Drug Development. *Wiley Interdiscip. Rev. Comput. Stat.* **2014**, *6*, 304–312. [CrossRef]
8. PubChem. Available online: https://pubchem.ncbi.nlm.nih.gov/ (accessed on 25 September 2019).
9. Colon-Useche, S. Caracterización Biofarmacéutica de Zolpidem, Cloperastina y Pravastatina. Ph.D. Thesis, Universidad Completense de Madrid, Madrid, Spain.
10. World Health Organization. Protocol to Conduct Equilibrium Solubility Experiments for the Purpose of Biopharmaceutics Classification System-Based Classification of Active Pharmaceutical Ingredients for Biowaiver. Available online: http://apps.who.int/phint/en/p/docf/ (accessed on 23 May 2018).
11. Takagi, T.; Ramachandran, C.; Bermejo, M.; Yamashita, S.; Yu, L.X.; Amidon, G.L. A provisional biopharmaceutical classification of the top 200 oral drug products in the United States, Great Britain, Spain, and Japan. *Mol. Pharm.* **2006**, *3*, 631–643. [CrossRef]
12. Ruiz-García, A.; Lin, H.; Plá-Delfina, J.M.; Hu, M. Kinetic characterization of secretory transport of a new ciprofloxacin derivative (CNV97100) across Caco-2 cell monolayers. *J. Pharm. Sci.* **2002**, *91*, 2511–2519. [CrossRef]
13. Oltra-Noguera, D.; Mangas-Sanjuan, V.; Centelles-Sangüesa, A.; Gonzalez-Garcia, I.; Sanchez-Castaño, G.; Gonzalez-Alvarez, M.; Casabo, V.G.; Merino, V.; Gonzalez-Alvarez, I.; Bermejo, M. Variability of permeability estimation from different protocols of subculture and transport experiments in cell monolayers. *J. Pharmacol. Toxicol. Methods* **2015**, *71*, 21–32. [CrossRef]
14. Mangas-Sanjuan, V.; González-Álvarez, I.; González-Álvarez, M.; Casabó, V.G.; Bermejo, M. Modified nonsink equation for permeability estimation in cell monolayers: Comparison with standard methods. *Mol. Pharm.* **2014**, *11*, 1403–1414. [CrossRef] [PubMed]

15. Gundogdu, E.; Mangas-Sanjuan, V.; Gonzalez-Alvarez, I.; Bermejo, M.; Karasulu, E. In vitro-in situ permeability and dissolution of fexofenadine with kinetic modeling in the presence of sodium dodecyl sulfate. *Eur. J. Drug Metab. Pharmacokinet.* **2012**, *37*, 65–75. [CrossRef] [PubMed]
16. González-Alvarez, I.; Fernández-Teruel, C.; Garrigues, T.M.; Casabo, V.G.; Ruiz-García, A.; Bermejo, M. Kinetic modelling of passive transport and active efflux of a fluoroquinolone across Caco-2 cells using a compartmental approach in NONMEM. *Xenobiotica* **2005**, *35*, 1067–1088. [CrossRef] [PubMed]
17. Ruiz Picazo, A.; Martinez-Martinez, M.T.; Colón-Useche, S.; Iriarte, R.; Sánchez-Dengra, B.; González-Álvarez, M.; García-Arieta, A.; González-Álvarez, I.; Bermejo, M. In Vitro Dissolution as a Tool for Formulation Selection: Telmisartan Two-Step IVIVC. *Mol. Pharm.* **2018**, *15*, 2307–2315. [CrossRef]
18. Ewp. Committee for Medical Products for Human Use (CHMP) Guideline on the Investigation of Bioequivalence Discussion in the Joint Efficacy and Quality Working Group Adoption Rev.1. Available online: https://www.ema.europa.eu/en/documents/scientific-guideline/guideline-investigation-bioequivalence-rev1_en.pdf (accessed on 23 May 2018).
19. FDA. Dissolution Testing of Immediate Release Solid Oral Dosage Forms. Available online: https://www.fda.gov/regulatory-information/search-fda-guidance-documents/dissolution-testing-immediate-release-solid-oral-dosage-forms (accessed on 30 May 2018).
20. Al-Tabakha, M.M.; Fahelelbom, K.M.S.; Obaid, D.E.E.; Sayed, S. Quality Attributes and In Vitro Bioequivalence of Different Brands of Amoxicillin Trihydrate Tablets. *Pharmaceutics* **2017**, *9*, 18. [CrossRef]
21. Rodríguez-Berna, G.; Mangas-Sanjuán, V.; Gonzalez-Alvarez, M.; Gonzalez-Alvarez, I.; García-Giménez, J.L.; Cabañas, M.J.D.; Bermejo, M.; Corma, A. A promising camptothecin derivative: Semisynthesis, antitumor activity and intestinal permeability. *Eur. J. Med. Chem.* **2014**, *83*, 366–373. [CrossRef]
22. AEMPS. Available online: https://cima.aemps.es/cima/pdfs/es/ft/59028/59028_ft.pdf (accessed on 25 September 2019).
23. Shen, Q.; Lin, Y.; Handa, T.; Doi, M.; Sugie, M.; Wakayama, K.; Okada, N.; Fujita, T.; Yamamoto, A. Modulation of intestinal P-glycoprotein function by polyethylene glycols and their derivatives by in vitro transport and in situ absorption studies. *Int. J. Pharm.* **2006**, *313*, 49–56. [CrossRef]
24. Batrakova, E.V.; Li, S.; Li, Y.; Alakhov, V.Y.; Kabanov, A.V. Effect of Pluronic P85 on ATPase Activity of Drug Efflux Transporters. *Pharm. Res.* **2004**, *21*, 2226–2233. [CrossRef]
25. Tayrouz, Y.; Ding, R.; Burhenne, J.; Riedel, K.D.; Weiss, J.; Hoppe-Tichy, T.; Haefeli, W.E.; Mikus, G. Pharmacokinetic and pharmaceutic interaction between digoxin and Cremophor RH40. *Clin. Pharmacol. Ther.* **2003**, *73*, 397–405. [CrossRef]
26. Arima, H.; Yunomae, K.; Morikawa, T.; Hirayama, F.; Uekama, K. Contribution of cholesterol and phospholipids to inhibitory effect of dimethyl-beta-cyclodextrin on efflux function of P-glycoprotein and multidrug resistance-associated protein 2 in vinblastine-resistant Caco-2 cell monolayers. *Pharm. Res.* **2004**, *21*, 625–634. [CrossRef]
27. Rege, B.D.; Yu, L.X.; Hussain, A.S.; Polli, J.E. Effect of Common Excipients on Caco-2 Transport of Low-Permeability Drugs. *J. Pharm. Sci.* **2001**, *90*, 1776–1786. [CrossRef]
28. Goole, J.; Lindley, D.J.; Roth, W.; Carl, S.M.; Amighi, K.; Kauffmann, J.M.; Knipp, G.T. The effects of excipients on transporter mediated absorption. *Int. J. Pharm.* **2010**, *393*, 17–31. [CrossRef]
29. Takizawa, Y.; Kishimoto, H.; Nakagawa, M.; Sakamoto, N.; Tobe, Y.; Furuya, T.; Tomita, M.; Hayashi, M. Effects of pharmaceutical excipients on membrane permeability in rat small intestine. *Int. J. Pharm.* **2013**, *453*, 363–370. [CrossRef] [PubMed]

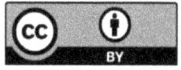

© 2019 by the authors. Licensee MDPI, Basel, Switzerland. This article is an open access article distributed under the terms and conditions of the Creative Commons Attribution (CC BY) license (http://creativecommons.org/licenses/by/4.0/).

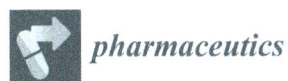

Article

A Mechanistic Physiologically-Based Biopharmaceutics Modeling (PBBM) Approach to Assess the In Vivo Performance of an Orally Administered Drug Product: From IVIVC to IVIVP

Marival Bermejo [1,2,†], Bart Hens [1,3,†], Joseph Dickens [4], Deanna Mudie [1,5], Paulo Paixão [1,6], Yasuhiro Tsume [1,7], Kerby Shedden [4] and Gordon L. Amidon [1,*]

1. Department of Pharmaceutical Sciences, College of Pharmacy, University of Michigan, 428 Church Street, Ann Arbor, MI 48109-1065, USA; mbermejo@goumh.umh.es (M.B.); bart.hens@kuleuven.be (B.H.); deanna.mudie@lonza.com (D.M.); ppaixao@ff.ulisboa.pt (P.P.); yasuhiro.tsume@merck.com (Y.T.)
2. Department of Engineering, Pharmacy Section, Miguel Hernandez University, San Juan de Alicante, 03550 Alicante, Spain
3. Department of Pharmaceutical & Pharmacological Sciences, KU Leuven, Herestraat 49, 3000 Leuven, Belgium
4. Department of Statistics, University of Michigan, Ann Arbor, MI 48109, USA; josephdi@umich.edu (J.D.); kshedden@umich.edu (K.S.)
5. Global Research and Development, Lonza, Bend, OR 97703, USA
6. Research Institute for Medicines (iMed.ULisboa), Faculty of Pharmacy, Universidade de Lisboa, Avenida Professor Gama Pinto, 1649-003 Lisboa, Portugal
7. Merck & Co., Inc., 126 E Lincoln Ave, Rahway, NJ 07065, USA
* Correspondence: glamidon@umich.edu; Tel.: +1-734-764-2464.; Fax: +1-734-764-6282
† These authors contributed equally to this work.

Received: 14 December 2019; Accepted: 15 January 2020; Published: 17 January 2020

Abstract: The application of in silico modeling to predict the in vivo outcome of an oral drug product is gaining a lot of interest. Fully relying on these models as a surrogate tool requires continuous optimization and validation. To do so, intraluminal and systemic data are desirable to judge the predicted outcomes. The aim of this study was to predict the systemic concentrations of ibuprofen after oral administration of an 800 mg immediate-release (IR) tablet to healthy subjects in fasted-state conditions. A mechanistic oral absorption model coupled with a two-compartmental pharmacokinetic (PK) model was built in Phoenix WinNonlinWinNonlin® software and in the GastroPlus™ simulator. It should be noted that all simulations were performed in an ideal framework as we were in possession of a plethora of in vivo data (e.g., motility, pH, luminal and systemic concentrations) in order to evaluate and optimize these models. All this work refers to the fact that important, yet crucial, gastrointestinal (GI) variables should be integrated into biopredictive dissolution testing (low buffer capacity media, considering phosphate versus bicarbonate buffer, hydrodynamics) to account for a valuable input for physiologically-based pharmacokinetic (PBPK) platform programs. While simulations can be performed and mechanistic insights can be gained from such simulations from current software, we need to move from correlations to predictions (IVIVC → IVIVP) and, moreover, we need to further determine the dynamics of the GI variables controlling the dosage form transit, disintegration, dissolution, absorption and metabolism along the human GI tract. Establishing the link between biopredictive in vitro dissolution testing and mechanistic oral absorption modeling (i.e., physiologically-based biopharmaceutics modeling (PBBM)) creates an opportunity to potentially request biowaivers in the near future for orally administered drug products, regardless of its classification according to the Biopharmaceutics Classification System (BCS).

Keywords: oral absorption; in silico modeling; GastroPlus; Phoenix WinNonlin; pharmacokinetics; clinical studies; ibuprofen; manometry; gastrointestinal; mechanistic modeling; PBPK; PBBM

1. Introduction

Although advances have been made and insights have improved throughout the years, there is still a lot of gastrointestinal (GI) variables that are poorly understood that should be investigated for their influence on drug release and systemic exposure after oral intake of a drug product [1,2]. The knowledge has improved about the intestinal behavior of an active pharmaceutical ingredient (API) in terms of solubility, dissolution, permeation, supersaturation, and precipitation, as demonstrated in different clinical aspiration studies performed over the last ten years [3–7]. In these studies, drug concentrations were measured in healthy volunteers after aspiration of GI fluids after oral administration. Subsequently, drug concentrations were determined in these aspirates in parallel with collecting blood samples to assess systemic exposure. As these studies contributed to formulation behavior in the GI tract, it was not always straightforward to correlate the measured drug concentrations in the upper part of the small intestine with concentrations appearing in blood. The knowledge about the impact of the surrounding dynamic GI environment on drug- and formulation behavior remains rather scarce and requires further investigation. The constantly changing climate of GI pH and motility patterns can alter drug behavior along the GI tract in such a way that it is necessary to investigate these mechanisms and, in a next step, to take these variables into account in in vitro and in silico predictive models to facilitate oral drug development [8–11]. GI motility is defined by the different contractile phases of the migrating motor complex (MMC): phase I is an inert period with little activity; phase II features sporadic contractions gradually ascending in magnitude; and phase III is characterized by powerful, high-frequency contractile bursts that promote emptying of contents where peak flow rates are observed [12]. In recent work, a clinical aspiration study was performed that aimed to measure the impact of physiological variables on the systemic exposure of orally-administered ibuprofen (immediate-release tablets, 800 mg) [13,14]. The outcome of this study demonstrated how phase III contractions and fluctuating pH (caused by the low buffer capacity) in the human intestinal tract had a major impact on ibuprofen's dissolution and, consequently, absorption in fasted ($n = 20$) and fed state ($n = 17$).

Based on these new insights, it has become clear that working in a biorelevant setting (i.e., simulated GI media, multi-compartmental in vitro models, solubility/permeability interplay) will result in more accurate predictions. From that perspective, the OrBiTo community took the initiative to design a decision tree which makes it handy for formulation scientists to select the most appropriate biopredictive dissolution test depending on the biopharmaceutical properties of the drug compound and the type of formulation [15]. This decision tree clearly focuses on some biorelevant aspects of the GI tract that play a pivotal role in and have a significant impact on the luminal behavior of a drug product; these variables should not be neglected in a biopredictive dissolution test. For instance, in the case of weakly basic compounds, the implementation of a GI transfer should be included in order to capture the supersaturated state of the drug after transfer from the stomach compartment to the intestinal compartment. Besides the optimization of in vitro tools, mechanism-based in silico models should be optimized and validated at the same time. The outcome of the in vitro dissolution tests can serve, in a second step, as input for physiologically-based pharmacokinetic (PBPK) platforms to simulate the systemic exposure of the drug. While a lot of progress has been made by mechanism-based in silico models to identify key issues in the development of new oral drug products [11,16–19], there are still many aspects that are poorly understood that need to be optimized/integrated to maximize the utility of these models towards predicting the systemic outcome of novel and generic drug candidates. Commercially available software packages such as the Simcyp® simulator, GastroPlus™, and PK-Sim® are just a few programs that are frequently used in the non-clinical stage of drug product development to get an idea about the in vivo performance of the drug product when administered to patients. The underlying syntax/algorithm of these packages describes the mass transport of the drug throughout the different built-in compartments and should be adequately reflecting the physiological processes of the human body. From an academic perspective, it is our mission to see (i) if the underlying mathematical equations are making any sense and (ii) if they are representing the physiological variables in a proper and biorelevant manner (physiological range). For instance, all these programs describe the stomach compartment as a single, well-stirred compartment, assuming that a drug will be homogeneously distributed along the entire stomach after oral administration. Based on measured gastric concentrations of the non-absorbable markers, phenol red and paromomycin, it was clearly shown that these markers were not homogeneously distributed among the different regions of the stomach (i.e., fundus, body and antrum). Therefore, we developed a mechanistic oral absorption model in the Berkeley-Madonna® software package (Version 8.3.18) that could only explain the observed luminal data when the stomach was handled as a two-compartmental model that was connected with a bypass flow to reflect the immediate fast transfer of liquid from stomach to small intestine after drinking a solution of these markers [20].

For this study, we aimed to reflect the luminal and systemic concentrations of ibuprofen under fasting state conditions starting with the simplest model, assuming a first-order kinetic process for dissolution, gastric emptying and absorption. In a second step, the model was revised, and dissolution was handled as pH dependent and gastric emptying was treated as a first-order process until the time of appearance of phase 3 contractions post-dose—after which, the remaining dose was directly transferred to the duodenal compartment. The mechanistic model focused on the integration of phase III contractions to simulate a house-keeper wave that is responsible for the direct release of ibuprofen particles from the stomach into the small intestine. In the different compartments of the small intestine, the dissolution of ibuprofen is driven by the regional pH, determining the fraction dissolved and undissolved. Afterward, a statistical analysis was performed to see how both scenarios matched with the observed luminal and systemic concentrations. In addition to this model, an advanced compartmental absorption and transit (ACAT™) model was developed in GastroPlus™ to assess the impact of dynamic pH, fluid volumes and gastric emptying on the systemic performance of ibuprofen. A comparison of these simulations was made with simulations performed by default settings.

2. Materials and Methods

2.1. Reference Intraluminal and Systemic Data of Ibuprofen

2.1.1. Intraluminal and Systemic Profiling of Ibuprofen in Healthy Volunteers

The study was held at the University of Michigan Hospital after receiving approval by the internal review board (IRB) at both University of Michigan and FDA (HUM00085066) under the project (HHSF223201310144C (Sun D. and Amidon G.L., Principle Investigators)—09/30/15–12/31/18 "Modernization of in vivo-in vitro Oral Bioperformance Prediction and Assessment: A research study to evaluate the performance of an ibuprofen oral dosage form in the gastrointestinal tract of healthy adult volunteers") [13,14]. Briefly, 13 healthy volunteers (men and women) were recruited; 7 out of 13 subjects participated in the study twice to generate intra-subject variability data. All volunteers provided written informed consent to participate in this study. After a fasting period, a multi-lumen GI tube from MUI Scientific (Mississauga, ON, Canada) was introduced via the mouth to the small intestine. Abdominal fluoroscopy was performed to ensure the GI tube was properly positioned in the different regions of the GI tract (i.e., stomach, duodenum, proximal and distal jejunum). The subject was asked to remain in bed while the GI tube was equilibrated by performing a baseline GI motility test for approximately 3–5 h (Medical Measurement Systems (MMS), Williston, VT, USA). Prior to the administration of the ibuprofen tablet, an intravenous catheter was introduced in the antecubital area of the subject for blood collection. The catheter was kept open with a heparin and saline solution. The subjects were asked to empty his/her bladder prior to the start of the study. At approximately 4:00 AM, the subject was given a single oral dose of ibuprofen (800 mg tablet). The study drug was administered with 250 mL of water containing USP grade phenol red (0.1 mg/mL). The actual amount of water consumed was measured and recorded. Volunteers were not obliged to drink the total amount of administered water to avoid any feeling of nausea at the start of the study. GI samples (stomach, duodenum and jejunum) were collected at 0, 0.25, 0.5, 0.75, 1, 1.5, 2, 2.5, 3, 4, 5, 6, and 7 h. Blood samples (4 mL/time point) were collected at 0, 0.167, 0.33, 0.5, 0.75, 1, 1.5, 2, 2.5, 3, 4, 5, 6, 7, 8, 12 and 28 h. Plasma was separated from blood samples by centrifugation and stored at −80 °C until analysis. The pH of GI fluid samples was immediately measured and recorded. The GI fluid samples were centrifuged at a speed of 17,000× g for 10 min and the supernatant was placed in the new tube for drug concentration analysis.

2.1.2. Recording of Post-Dose Phase III Contractions

MMC phase III motility periods were identified from the water-perfused manometric measurements using spectral density estimation and penalized logistic regression as described in detail by Hens and co-workers and will be briefly discussed here [13]. After positioning, the catheter was connected to a computer console that generated real-time manometry recordings in the different segments of the GI tract (Medical Measurement Systems, Dover, NH, USA). The manometric channels attached to the catheter were perfused with water at a rate of 2 mL/min and served as intestinal pressure recording ports to assess intestinal motility. Each segment contained four motility channels to monitor pressure events. Baseline intestinal motility was evaluated for 3–5 h prior to study drug administration of the tablet. Subsequently, GI motility was measured continuously for 7 h. Powerful antral phase III contractions were defined as the occurrence of regular 2–3 contractions per minute for at least 2 min with an average amplitude of 75 mmHg. Duodenal phase III contractions were characterized by 11–12 contractions per minute with an average amplitude of 33 mmHg which can last for at least 3 min. As the contractile activity propagates, it becomes less spatiotemporally organized resulting in slower propulsion rates in the distal small bowel. The corresponding spectral density estimate of a phase III period will have high energy levels in the 10–12 cycles/min components, leading to a concentrated spectrum. During non-phase III motility, the spectral density will have a more diffuse spectrum. Using penalized logistic regression, it was clearly observed that the proportion of energy in the 9–12 cycle/min frequencies is an important predictor of phase III motility.

2.1.3. Thermodynamic Equilibrium Solubility of Ibuprofen in Fasted-State Human Gastric and Intestinal Fluids (Fahgf/Fahif)

The thermodynamic solubility of ibuprofen was determined by the shake-flask method (25 RPM), incubating gastrointestinal fluids for 24 h with an excess amount of ibuprofen (Acros Organics, Morris Plains, NJ, USA) at 37 °C. The fluids that were used for measuring the thermodynamic solubility of ibuprofen were aspirated gastric, duodenal and jejunal fluids of three different time points of subject B005-F2. Following the 24 h incubation, samples were centrifuged for 15 min at 17,000 g (AccuSpin Micro 17, Fisher Scientific, Pittsburgh, PA, USA). The supernatant was diluted 10-fold with methanol (Fisher Scientific, Pittsburgh, PA, USA) and again centrifuged for 5 min in order to discard any proteins that could interfere with the HPLC analysis (see below). Solubility measurements were performed in triplicate.

2.1.4. Bioanalysis of Ibuprofen by HPLC

Solubility samples were analyzed by HPLC–UV (Hewlett Packard series 1100 HPLC Pump, Santa Clara, CA, USA), combined with Agilent Technologies 1200 Series Autosampler (Santa Clara, CA, USA). A volume of 5 µL was injected into the HPLC system connected to a UV lamp that was able to detect ibuprofen at a wavelength of 220 nm (Agilent 1100 Series UV lamp, Santa Clara, CA, USA). An isocratic run containing 70% acetonitrile (VWR International, West Chester, PA, USA) and 30% purified water (both containing 0.1% TFA) was used to detect ibuprofen at a retention time of 2.9 min using a reversed-phase C-18 column (Eclipse Plus C18, 4.6 × 150 mm, 5.5 µm, Agilent Technologies) and a 1 mL/min flow rate. The calibration curve was made in methanol based on a stock solution of ibuprofen in methanol (1 mM). Linearity was observed between 10.32 µg/mL and 0.32 µg/mL. The observed peaks were integrated using ChemStation software (Agilent Technologies, B.04.03 version). The developed analytical method met the FDA requirements for bioanalytical method validation [21].

2.2. Mechanistic Oral Absorption Modeling in Phoenix WinNonlin®

WinNonlin User-Customized Mechanistic Model to Stress the Pivotal Underlying GI Variables: InVivo_GIS versus InVivo_GISPlus

A compartmental model including stomach, duodenum and jejunum with first-order transit and absorption rates was designed to describe the time evolution of ibuprofen mass and concentrations in duodenum, jejunum and plasma. The following assumptions were made with respect to the 'in vivo Gastrointestinal System model (InVivo_GIS)':

1. Ibuprofen dissolution was considered negligible in the stomach chamber due to the acidic pH (pH < pKa). The administered oral tablet disintegrates in the stomach and particles will not be dissolved but emptied in the next segment, i.e., the duodenum. In addition, no significant absorption can occur from the stomach.
2. Gastric emptying follows a first-order kinetic process.
3. Dissolution follows a first-order process in the duodenal and jejunal segment. The dissolution rates are proportional to the remaining amount of solid ibuprofen.
4. Duodenal and jejunal compartments are well-mixed, resulting in homogenous drug concentrations.
5. The permeability of the intestinal membrane is high for ibuprofen, indicating that dissolved ibuprofen will be immediately absorbed. Only solid particles transit from the duodenum to the jejunum.
6. Transit from the duodenum to the jejunum is faster than the transit from the jejunum to the more distal parts.
7. Drug degradation does not occur in the GI lumen.

This basic model was further extended to explore the influence of intestinal pH and motility. Therefore, we developed a model which we will refer to as the 'InVivo_GISPlus':

1. Gastric emptying follows a first-order kinetic up to the next post-dose phase III contractions when all the remaining stomach content is suddenly emptied in the duodenum.
2. Dissolution follows a first-order process in the duodenal and jejunal segment. The dissolution rates are proportional to the remaining amount of solid ibuprofen. The dissolution rate is modeled as a function of luminal pH values. Ibuprofen solubility is re-calculated at each time point with the duodenum or jejunal pH at that specific moment.

Model schemes are represented in Figure 1. The system of differential equations was written as the American Standard Code for Information Interchange (ASCII) code and run in Phoenix WinNonlin® V8 (Certara, Princeton, NJ, USA).

Six differential equations were used, describing the amount of solid ibuprofen as a function of time in the stomach ($M_{stomach}^{solid}$), in the duodenum ($M_{duodenum}^{solid}$), and in the jejunum ($M_{jejunum}^{solid}$), as well as the amount of dissolved ibuprofen as a function of time in the duodenum ($M_{duodenum}^{dissolved}$), in the jejunum ($M_{jejunum}^{dissolved}$) and in plasma (M_{plasma}). Integrated model parameters were:

- Duodenal and jejunum average fluid volume values during the sampling time, V1 and V2, respectively;
- Transit rate coefficients from the duodenal to the jejunal segment, K_TD; and from the jejunum to the more distal segment, K_TJ;
- First-order rate coefficient of gastric emptying, K_{empt};
- Dissolution rate coefficient, K_Diss;
- First-order absorption rate constants, K_a.

In each subject, the elimination rate coefficient (K_{el}) and the distribution volume in plasma (V3) were fixed to the value obtained after performing a non-compartmental PK analysis. Time to the next phase III wave post-dose (TMMC) was fixed to the experimentally determined value [22]. The individual pH values in duodenum and jejunum at each time point were used in InVivo_GISPlus model to recalculate ibuprofen's solubility at each time point. The absorption rate coefficient was fixed to a high value of 12 h^{-1} based knowing that ibuprofen does not have any permeability-related issues (fraction absorbed ~1) [22]. This value was based on ibuprofen permeability in rat small intestine [23] that was scaled up to human P_{eff} value with the human-rat correlation described by Zakeri-Milani et al. [24]. The 13 mathematical equations to describe the mass transport of ibuprofen in the InVivo_GISPlus model are summarized in the Supplemental Information. Both models InVivo_GIS and InVivo_GISplus were fitted simultaneously to duodenal, jejunal and plasma concentrations.

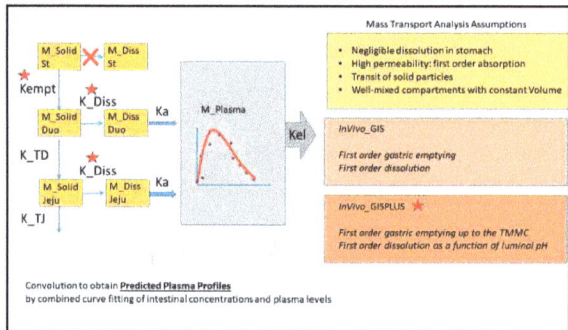

Figure 1. Mass transport analysis scheme and assumptions of InVivo_GIS and InVivo_GISPLUS models. K_{empt}: first-order emptying rate coefficient; K_a: first-order absorption rate coefficient; K_TD and K_TJ: first order transit coefficients from duodenum to jejunum and from jejunum to distal segments, respectively; TMMC: time to the next Phase III wave post-dose; K_Diss: first-order dissolution rate constants.

2.3. Mechanistic Oral Absorption Modeling in GastroPlus™

2.3.1. GastroPlus™ Advanced Compartmental Absorption Transit (ACAT™) Mechanistic Absorption Model

Simulations were performed by the commercially available PBPK modeling platform GastroPlus™ 9.6 (Simulations Plus, Inc., Lancaster, CA, USA) and all simulations were judged based on and compared with the observed luminal and systemic concentrations of ibuprofen after oral administration of 800 mg ibuprofen (Shreveport, LA, USA; IBU™—Ibuprofen Tablets, USP, 800 mg) to twenty healthy subjects in fasted state.

The advanced compartmental and absorption transit (ACAT™) was applied with slight adjustments related to pH, gastric emptying and fluid dynamics. This model is described in detail by Hens and Bolger [25]. To implement a dynamic pH and fluid volume as a function of time, a mixed-multiple dosage form was selected. The mixed-multiple dosage form consisted of 13 different .cat files, personalized by a different pH and volume value to simulate a dynamic fluid and pH model over time. The implemented pH values were the same average values according to the values as measured during the clinical aspiration study. The implemented values for the fluid volume were extracted from Mudie and co-workers [26]. The gastric transit time was set at 2.04 h, which conforms with the average time to phase III contractions post-dose, as observed in the clinical aspiration study of ibuprofen.

MedChem Designer 5.0 (Simulations Plus, Inc., Lancaster, CA, USA) was applied to draw the molecular structure of ibuprofen. Data describing the drug's physicochemical and biopharmaceutical properties were obtained from literature or from estimates calculated by ADMET predictor 9.0 (Simulations Plus, Inc., Lancaster, CA, USA). All physicochemical and biopharmaceutics parameters that were used to perform the simulations are described in Table 1.

Table 1. Physicochemical, biopharmaceutical and pharmacokinetic disposition properties to perform simulations in GastroPlus™ for ibuprofen.

Input Parameter	Value/Selection Dynamic Settings	Value/Selection Default Settings	Reference
Physicochemical Properties			
Molecular weight (g/mol)	206.29	206.29	ADMET Predictor 9.0
pKa (acidic)	4.54	4.54	ADMET Predictor 9.0
Octanol/water partition coefficient (log$P$)	3.65	3.65	ADMET Predictor 9.0
Biopharmaceutics Properties			
Human effective permeability (P_{eff}) ($\times 10^{-4}$ cm/s)	4.1	4.1	[27]
Particle size radius (um)	62	62	In-house data
Dose volume (mL)	250	250	[13]
pH at reference solubility	6.2	6.2	[28]
Solubility at reference pH (mg/mL)	1.99	1.99	[28]
Solubility in Fasted state human gastric fluid (FaHGF) (mg/mL)—pH 1.46	0.0048	0.0048	[29]
Solubility in Fasted state human intestinal fluid (FaHIF) (duodenum) (mg/mL)—pH 3.74	0.0102	0.0102	[29]
Solubility in FaHIF (jejunum) (mg/mL)—pH 4.6	1.2	1.2	[30]
Distribution and Clearance			
Pharmacokinetic model	Two-compartmental	Two-compartmental	[31]
Clearance (L/h)	4.05	4.05	[31]
K_{10} (1/h)	1.16	1.16	[31]
K_{12} (1/h)	4.55	4.55	[31]
K_{21} (1/h)	3.46	3.46	[31]
Advanced Compartmental and Absorption Transit model (ACAT™) Model Parameters			
Gastric transit time (h)	2.04	0.25	[13]
Dynamic fluid volume model	Based on 100% of the volumes measured in human MRI study after drinking a glass of water (240 mL)	Default static values under the physiology tab 'Human—Physiological—Fasted'	[26]
Dynamic pH model	Based on average pH values derived from gastric, duodenal and jejunal aspirated fluids after oral administration of 800 mg of ibuprofen	Default static values under the physiology tab 'Human—Physiological—Fasted'	[13]

A two-compartmental PK model was used to describe the distribution and clearance of ibuprofen. Values for rate constants (K_{10}, K_{12}, K_{21}) were optimized based on literature data that reported systemic data of ibuprofen after intravenous (IV) administration of 800 mg ibuprofen with an infusion rate of approximately 6 min (between 5 and 7 min) [31]. Estimations of these rate constants were performed by the PKPlus™ module.

2.3.2. Data Presentation

The observed intraluminal and systemic concentration–time profiles are presented as the mean ± standard deviation (SD) for all participating subjects and are extracted from previous work [13,14]. Pharmacokinetic and intraluminal parameters are reported and compared with the simulated outcomes.

3. Results and Discussion

3.1. Mechanistic Oral Absorption Modeling in WinNonlin

Figure 2 shows the simulated outcomes (model-fitted values) when applying the InVivo_GIS (purple lines) versus the InVivo_GISPlus (red lines).

When comparing both simulated profiles derived from the two models, it is clear that including luminal pH values and the 'house-keeper' phase III wave contractions provide better predicted (i.e., model-fitted) values. This is not only the case for the simulated plasma concentrations—capturing plasma C_{max}—but also for the improved predictions with respect to luminal levels reflecting the oscillations associated with pH changes. Applying dynamic pH values and, therefore, showing an improved reflection of the intraluminal behavior was also observed when using the InVivo_GISPlus model to simulate the average concentration–time profiles in the duodenum, jejunum and plasma concentrations (Figure 3).

To quantitatively assess the improved predictions with the InVivo_GISPlus model, a comparison between the outcomes derived from the InVivo_GIS and InVivo_GISPlus was made and the simulated results were compared with the observed data and the prediction error was expressed as an absolute percentage deviation. Table 2 summarizes the mean absolute percentage deviation between predicted and experimental values in the main pharmacokinetic parameters (C_{max}, T_{max}, and AUC) in the three compartments, namely the duodenum, jejunum, and plasma.

Table 2. Average absolute deviation percentage between predicted and experimental values of C_{max}, T_{max} and AUC in the duodenum, jejunum and plasma.

Plasma	InVivo_GIS	InVivo_GISPlus
C_{max}	48.3	19.8
T_{max}	50.8	15.7
AUC	11.0	13.1
Duodenum	**InVivo_GIS**	**InVivo_GISPlus**
C_{max}	50.8	15.7
T_{max}	62.0	27.4
AUC	82.8	88.3
Jejunum	**InVivo_GIS**	**InVivo_GISPlus**
C_{max}	46.91	25.47
T_{max}	50.83	15.75
AUC	78.68	28.19

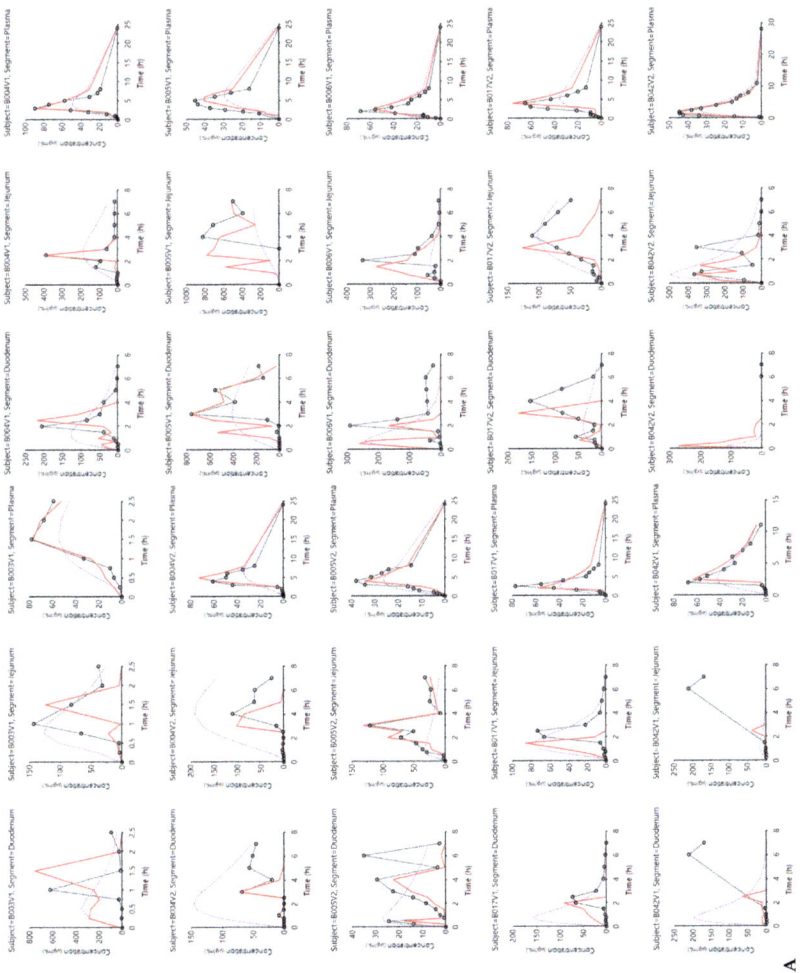

Figure 2. *Cont.*

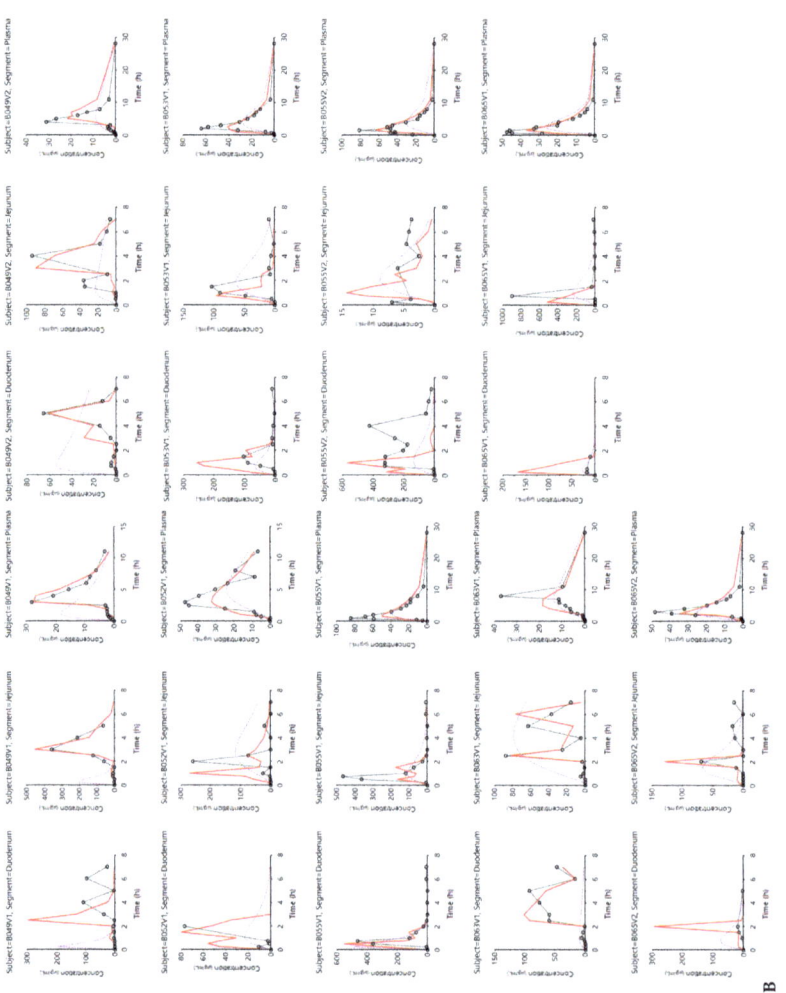

Figure 2. (**A**) and (**B**) describe the experimental and model-fitted concentration values of ibuprofen for all subjects. Experimental (black dots) and model-fitted concentration values of ibuprofen in the duodenal, jejunal and systemic compartments for each and every subject in fasting state conditions. Each row includes the observed and simulated concentration–time profiles in the duodenal, jejunal and plasma segments in three separate columns. The purple line reflects the InVivo_GIS model-predicted values, whereas the red line corresponds with the simulated (model-fitted) values derived from the InVivo_GISPlus model. The experimental values are reflected by the dark grey lines and dots.

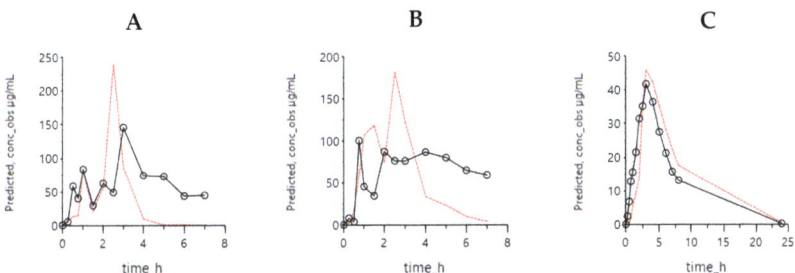

Figure 3. Simulated outcomes of the average concentrations using the InVivo_GISPlus model. Average experimental ibuprofen concentrations are shown by the black dots in the duodenum (**A**), jejunum (**B**) and plasma (**C**) across all the subjects. Simulated values of the InVivo_GISPlus model are represented with red lines. The experimental values are reflected by the dark black lines and dots.

Table 3 shows the applied settings of each model parameter to adequately simulate the corresponding intraluminal and systemic concentration–time profiles for each individual.

Table 3. InVivo_GISPlus individual and average parameter values. Median values and the fitted values for the average subjects are also shown for comparison. SD: standard deviation; CV: coefficient of variation. K_{empt} is the gastric emptying rate constant; K_TD and K_TJ represent the transit rate constants in the duodenal and jejunal compartment, respectively; K_Diss represent the intestinal dissolution rate constant; V1 and V2 represent the duodenal and jejunal residual volumes, respectively.

Parameter	K_{EMPT} (1/h)	K_TD (1/h)	K_TJ (1/h)	K_Diss mL/(ug*h)	V1 (mL)—Duodenal	V2 (mL)—Jejunal
Average	0.84	1.99	0.13	0.10	155.11	70.64
SD	1.27	3.01	0.25	0.36	128.44	80.48
CV%	151.84	150.83	196.68	361.28	82.81	113.93
B003V1	0.39	0.20	0.130	0.101	80.4	20.0
B004V1	0.08	0.59	0.059	1.48×10^{-3}	73.9	18.5
B004V2	0.02	1.86	0.209	5.05×10^{-3}	195.4	209.2
B005V1	0.51	0.22	0.010	1.61×10^{-4}	15.3	2.5
B005V2	0.18	0.45	0.224	3.62×10^{-4}	350.5	84.5
B006V1	0.95	1.84	0.042	3.51×10^{-4}	123.2	64.6
B017V1	0.16	0.41	0.081	5.75×10^{-3}	62.8	10.2
B017V2	0.07	0.08	0.036	1.11×10^{-3}	77.6	19.5
B042V1	0.13	10.26	0.000	7.31×10^{-2}	29.0	5.2
B042V2	0.05	0.19	0.086	1.52×10^{-3}	150.0	80.6
B049V1	0.05	0.19	0.086	1.52×10^{-3}	262.3	10.6
B049V2	0.05	0.19	0.086	1.52×10^{-3}	150.0	80.6
B052V1	2.79	2.99	0.019	6.96×10^{-4}	19.0	27.6
B053V1	1.24	1.79	0.039	3.48×10^{-4}	137.8	215.8
B055V1	4.05	0.47	0.100	9.00×10^{-5}	126.6	50.0
B055V2	3.65	0.07	0.001	4.33×10^{-4}	119.6	93.4
B063V1	1.00×10^{-3}	4.12	1.140	1.96×10^{-3}	115.9	56.3
B065V1	0.20	2.51	0.092	0.121	500.0	283.1
B065V2	1.28	9.48	0.002	1.59	357.7	10.1
Median	0.18	0.47	8.1×10^{-2}	1.52×10^{-3}	123.24	49.99
Average Subject	0.45	0.47	7.9×10^{-2}	9.34×10^{-4}	136.53	56.89

The estimated volumes are higher than the reported values in duodenum and jejunum measured by magnetic resonance imaging (MRI) [26]. Nevertheless, it should be noted that the applied average value could be interpreted as the volume of fluid directly in contact with the solid particles during that specific period. Considering that continuous secretion and absorption of water in the small intestine occurs, the volume of fluid flowing through the segment can be high. A potential interpretation to translate the obtained parameters to the in vitro GIS device could be that the average fluid volume in contact with solid ibuprofen in duodenum and jejunum is in total 220 mL over an 8 h period to complete absorption. That would correspond to a 0.5 mL/min volumetric flow to be implemented in the in vitro GIS system.

As ibuprofen will be heavily dependent on the pH along the GI tract to dissolve, the dissolution rate was plotted against the residual pH values. Figure 4 depicts the intestinal dissolution rate (estimated from the InVivo_GISPlus model) versus the measured average pH (duodenum and jejunum) for each individual as a function of time.

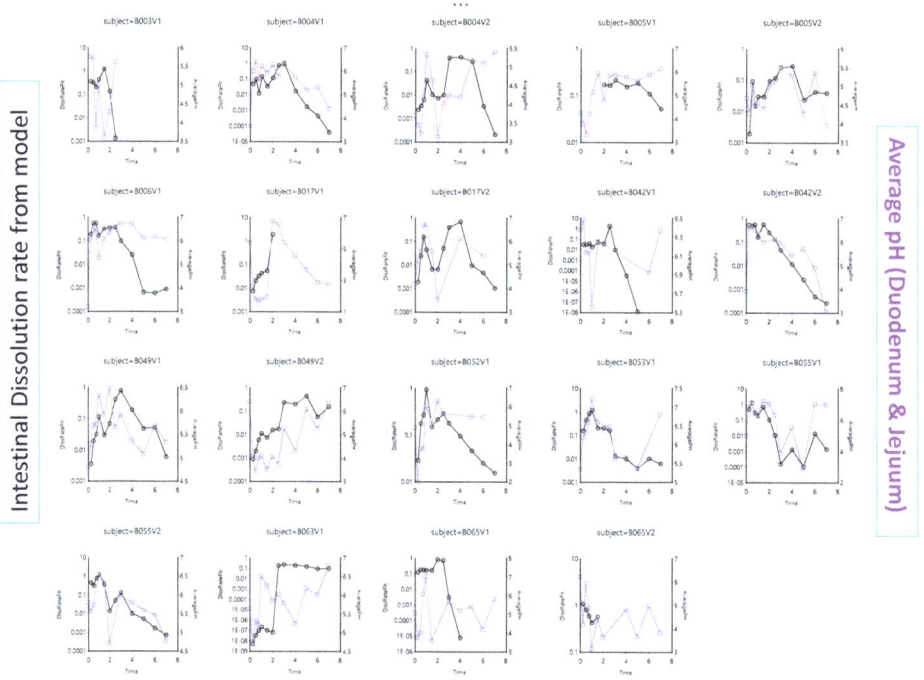

Figure 4. Average intestinal pH values in each subject (purple line and squares) and the intestinal dissolution rate (black line and dots) estimated from InVivo_GISPLUS model.

The in vivo dissolution rates in each subject can be estimated from the differential equations derived from the InVivo_GISPlus model. As Figure 4 shows, the pH fluctuations sometimes dictate directly the dissolution rate. The overlap is not perfect as other variables (such as the fluid volume) also affect the dissolution rate. However, in this model, a static volume was considered. If the dissolution rate increases, the amount of ibuprofen entering the systemic circulation will increase as well. Therefore, the intestinal dissolution rate was plotted against the absorption rate, deconvoluted from the plasma concentration–time profiles. This was done for each individual (Figure 5).

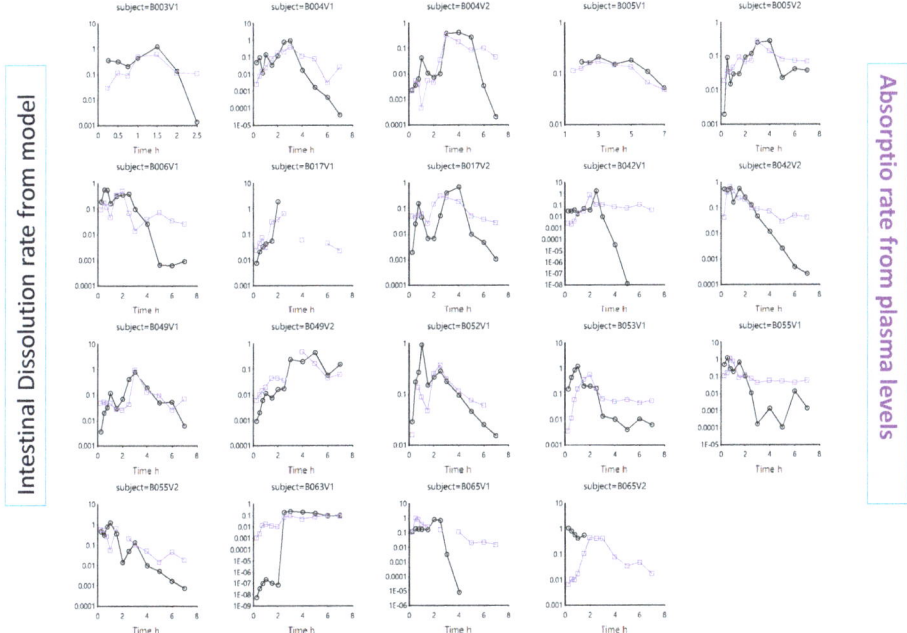

Figure 5. The intestinal in vivo ibuprofen dissolution rate estimated from InVivo_GISPLUS model and the absorption rate obtained from Wagner–Nelson deconvolution profiles in each individual. Absorption rates were derived from previous work by Bermejo and co-workers [22].

This work also aimed to demonstrate the impact of gastric emptying on the systemic exposure of the drug. In this case, and as shown by Hens et al., the time of phase III contractions post-dose will determine the arrival of ibuprofen in the intestinal tract. The faster these contractions will be initiated, the higher the plasma C_{max} will be. It is hypothesized that a fast onset of this house-keeper wave will remove more drug content directly from the stomach into the small intestine, resulting in high amount of drug that will be available for absorption (assuming pH > pKa). Whenever these phase III contractions are rather postponed (e.g., due to the intake of food), drug release from the stomach to the small intestine will be rather pulsatile than instantaneous, resulting in a lower driving force for intestinal absorption which ultimately leads to a lower plasma C_{max}. The variability in gastric emptying of solid particles was also observed by Locatelli and colleagues when visualizing the gastric emptying process of pellets by scintigraphy studies [32]. The variability in emptying as a function of time was compared with the variability in emptying that was simulated by the InVivo_GISPlus model for each subject and demonstrated a similar trend (Figure 6).

3.2. Mechanistic Oral Absorption Modeling in GastroPlus™

The first commercial software program to attempt a comprehensive description of the GI tract in the context of a PBPK model was GastroPlus™ (Simulations Plus, Inc., Lancaster, CA, USA). The first version of GastroPlus™ was established in August 1998 and was based on the work of Lawrence X. Yu and Gordon L. Amidon [33]. The model consisted of "continuous stirring tank reactor" compartments to describe the transit of a drug from one segment in the GI tract to the other, with simple estimations of (i) dissolution based on aqueous solubility and (ii) absorption rate coefficients based on existing pharmacokinetic data. In 2001, an advanced compartmental absorption and transit (ACAT™) model was developed and defined each compartment's volume and transit by mass balance approximations. Later on, in 2018, Hens and Bolger aimed to convert the static settings of the ACAT™ model to more dynamic settings [25]. They developed a dynamic fluid and pH model in the GastroPlus™ simulator to reflect the dynamic alternations of fluid volumes and pH values in the different compartments of the GI tract. Especially in the case of BCS class 2 compounds, suffering from poor aqueous solubility and high permeability, these dynamic settings will result in improved predictions towards the in vivo outcome of the drug product when comparing these simulations with the simulations obtained when static, default settings were applied. The benefit of these dynamic settings has already been shown for posaconazole, a weakly basic drug [25].

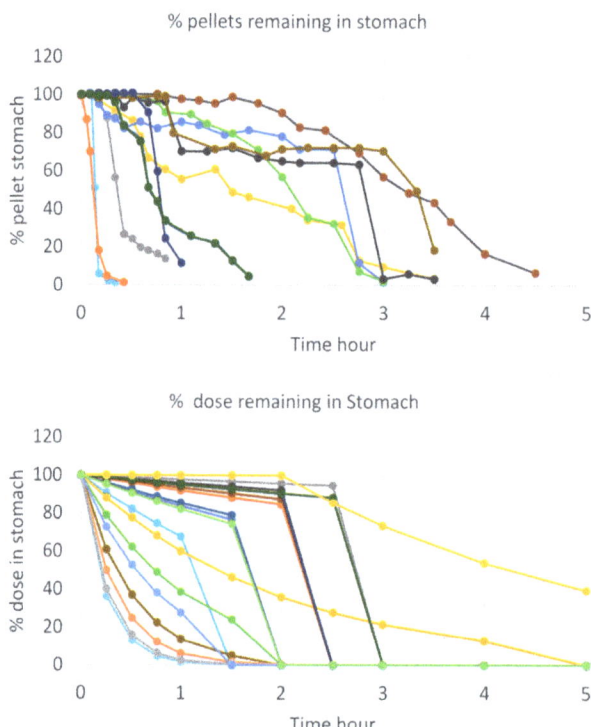

Figure 6. (Upper plot) Data from 19 individual scintigraphy studies of gastric emptying of pellets collected by Locatelli et al. [32]. (Bottom plot) Individual solid ibuprofen particle gastric emptying kinetics predicted by InVivo_GISPLUS model.

3.2.1. Solubility versus pH: pH-Driven Dissolution

Thermodynamic solubility of ibuprofen was determined in three different aspirated fluids (i.e., gastric, duodenal and jejunal) of subject B005-F2. The ADMET Predictor 9.0 was used to predict the acidic pKa and how solubility would be defined in the physiological range. The observed versus simulated solubility values closely matched as depicted in Figure 7.

The solubility factor is equal to the ratio of the maximum solubility to the intrinsic solubility for this specific acidic pKa. This demonstrates the ability of ibuprofen to easily dissolve at pH levels above its pKa, converting to its ionized form which is more soluble than its non-ionized form.

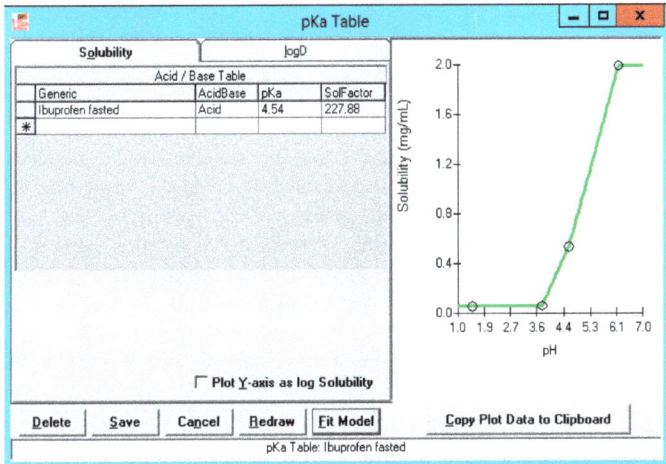

Figure 7. Solubility versus pH profile for ibuprofen. The green line represents the predicted solubility versus pH curve, whereas the blue dots represent the measured solubility values in fasted-state human GI fluids. The upper blue dot is a solubility value of ibuprofen measured in fasted-state duodenal fluid by Heikkilä and co-workers [28].

It should be noted that in this clinical study, authors monitored the residual bulk pH in the GI tract (stomach, duodenum, and jejunum) and measured the solution concentrations of ibuprofen in these different regions. The pH values of the aspirates were extremely fluctuating as a consequence of the low buffer capacity [13]. As research scientists in pharmaceutical industry don't have any access to these values and mostly make use of high buffer capacity media to explore drug dissolution, overestimations in predicting the plasma C_{max} will be made (see below: Advanced compartmental absorption and transit simulations: static simulations with default settings). However, there is more evidence that biopredictive dissolution setting should focus on integrating relevant aspects that have a major impact on the fraction dissolved of a drug. For instance, lowering the buffer capacity of the media and highlighting the interplay between surface and bulk pH is a critical aspect that should not be neglected. This has been observed for modified-release, but also for immediate-release formulations [34–37]. Pepin and co-workers modeled the dissolution profiles of acalabrutinib (weak base, pKas 3.54 (B), 5.77 (B), 12.1 (A)) using an in-house Excel® tool and concluded that making use of the bulk apparent drug solubility will lead to an over-estimation of the drug dissolution rate at all pH values below the highest drug pKa [38]. By taking into account product particle size distribution (P-PSD) and the surface pH of drug particles, accurate simulated dissolution rates were simulated. In addition, in the case of ionizable compounds such as ibuprofen, the pH at the surface of dissolving particles (pH_0) is a complex function between buffer- and drug-related properties. In the case of ibuprofen, in vitro results demonstrated that the surface pH is lower than the bulk pH (ranging from pH 4.8–5.8) in 5 mM bicarbonate depending upon hydrodynamics which can hamper the dissolution process as such. This was observed by Al-Gousous and co-workers, who observed differences in bulk and surface pH (and thus bulk and surface solubility) resulting in slower dissolution kinetics of ibuprofen when using low bicarbonate-buffered, dissolution media [39]. Therefore, the use of the human buffer bicarbonate will be more favorable to adequately reflect the luminal dissolution kinetics and to represent the relevant interactions between buffer species and drug molecules [39–41]. Biopredictive dissolution tests performed by Cristofoletti et al. demonstrated that ibuprofen dissolution in a lower buffer capacity medium (i.e., 5 mM phosphate buffer) affected bulk pH and its own dissolution kinetics [42,43]. Considering P-PSD and the self-buffering capacity of ibuprofen resulted in the best simulation with respect to plasma C_{max} and AUC for two Nurofen® tablets of 200 mg orally administered to healthy adults. In another clinical study by Hofmann and colleagues [44], ibuprofen suspensions (varying in particle size radius) were intraduodenally administered in healthy subjects. After administration, duodenal pH was monitored in parallel with systemic exposure of ibuprofen. The administration of small particles led to a more pronounced pH drop than for large particles under the same infusion conditions. Still, absorption rates were higher for these smaller particles compared to the larger particles, but no significant differences in plasma C_{max} were observed, suggesting that variability in the systemic outcome of the drug is more related to the rate of gastric emptying (motility-driven) and/or intestinal transit times. Besides the bulk/surface pH, the hydrodynamics of the GI tract also have an enormous impact on the dissolution rate. Performing dissolution experiments for 200 mg of ibuprofen in 5 mM phosphate buffer at 75, 50 and 30 rotations per minute (RPM) in the USP II apparatus, demonstrated maximum cumulative fractions dissolved of 0.83, 0.84 and 0.26, respectively. Based on computational fluid dynamics (CFD), the presented shear rates in the GI tract are more in line with the shear rates that are reproduced when lower rotation speeds are applied [6].

In conclusion, some important, yet crucial, GI variables should be integrated into biopredictive dissolution testing (low buffer capacity media, phosphate versus bicarbonate buffer, hydrodynamics) to account for a valuable input for PBPK platform programs.

3.2.2. Simulation of Distribution and Clearance of Ibuprofen: A Two-Compartmental Pharmacokinetic (PK) Approach

Simulation of distribution and clearance of ibuprofen was performed in the PKPlus™ module based on literature data that showed the clearance of ibuprofen after an intravenous administration of an 800 mg dose of ibuprofen with a perfusion rate of approximately 6 min. For this study, 12 healthy subjects (aged between 18 and 65 years old) were recruited [31]. One-, two- and three-compartmental models were compared, and the best fit was observed for a two-compartmental PK model based on the Akaike Information Criterion (AIC) and R^2. As no extensive first-pass metabolism is observed for ibuprofen [45], a two-compartmental approach is definitely sufficient in describing the distribution and clearance of ibuprofen. Observed versus simulated data are depicted in Figure 8.

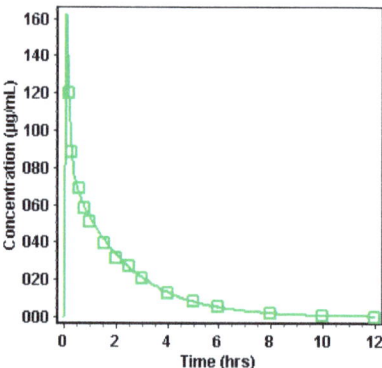

Figure 8. Observed (green squares) versus predicted (green line) concentrations of ibuprofen after intravenous administration of an 800 mg dose to 12 healthy subjects [31]. Simulations were performed by using a two-compartmental PK model.

3.2.3. Advanced Compartmental Absorption and Transit Simulations: Static Simulations with Default Settings

In the first set of modeling experiments, the default settings of GastroPlus™ were applied in order to assess predictions when a static volume and pH is applied in each compartment of the ACAT™ model (Table 4).

Table 4. Default setting values for volume (mL) and pH in the GastroPlus™ simulator.

GI Compartment	Volume (mL)	pH	Transit Time (h)
1. Stomach	48.92	1.3	0.25
2. Duodenum	44.57	6	0.26
3. Jejunum 1	166.6	6.2	0.94
4. Jejunum 2	131	6.4	0.75
5. Ileum 1	102	6.6	0.58
6. Ileum 2	75.35	6.9	0.42
7. Ileum 3	53.57	7.4	0.29
8. Caecum	50.49	6.4	4.48
9. Ascending Colon	53.55	6.8	13.44

Regarding the fact that (i) there is no dissolution-limiting step at pH > 6 and that (ii) large volumes are always present during the simulation time, fast onset of dissolution was observed in the intestinal compartments (Figure 9).

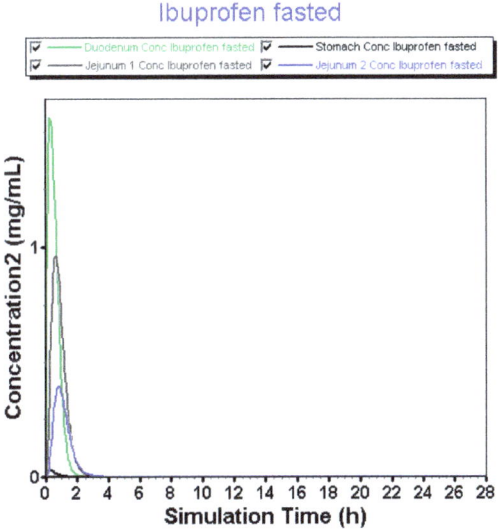

Figure 9. Simulated concentration–time profiles of ibuprofen in the different GI compartments of the GastroPlus™ simulator.

Solution concentrations in the stomach are negligible due to the integrated acidic pH (pH 1.3) that will prevent almost any dissolution of ibuprofen in the gastric compartment. After transfer, ibuprofen will rapidly dissolve in the more neutral pH environment of the intestinal tract. There is a trend that the dissolution is the highest in the duodenum followed by the first part of the jejunum and the second part of the jejunum (diluting effect). When the 800 mg dose appears in the first compartment of the GI tract, dissolution will be enhanced due to the large volume (44.57 mL) and high pH (pH 6). As the solubility of ibuprofen is approximately 2 mg/mL at pH 6.2 (Figure 7), an enormous amount of ibuprofen will immediately dissolve and be available for absorption without any limitations. As the concentration at the surface of the ibuprofen particles (C_s) drives the dissolution rate under sink conditions (pH < 6.2), whereas the bulk concentration (C_b) comes into play in the case when there are no sink conditions [39].

This is an ongoing process until it hits the transit time to move forward for the remaining undissolved particles towards the next compartment. Obviously, this luminal behavior will be reflected in the systemic compartment, as depicted in Figure 10.

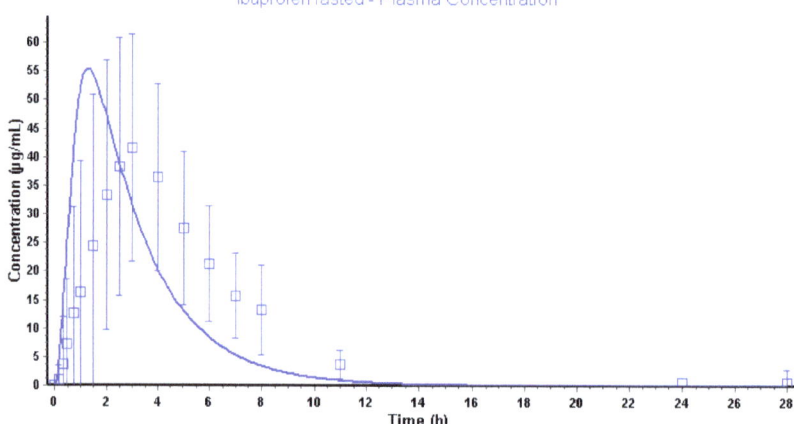

Figure 10. Observed (blue squares) and simulated (blue line) plasma concentrations of ibuprofen after oral administration of an 800 mg dose.

Pharmacokinetic parameters are shown in Table 5.

Table 5. Pharmacokinetic disposition parameters between observed and simulated data applying the default settings.

Pharmacokinetic (PK) Parameters	Observed Pharmacokinetic Data	Simulated Pharmacokinetic Data
Plasma C_{max} (µg/mL)	41.7	55.5
Plasma T_{max} (h)	3.00	1.31
Plasma $AUC_{0-\infty}$ (µg·h/mL)	259	189
Plasma AUC_{0-28h} (µg·h/mL)	255	189

Using the default settings, simulations performed by GastroPlus™ are overestimating the observed pharmacokinetic parameters with respect to plasma C_{max} and plasma T_{max}. Although predictions are in the same concentration range, there is still a 33% higher predicted plasma C_{max} compared to the observed plasma C_{max}. Moreover, the simulated plasma T_{max} is appearing tremendously earlier related to the fast dissolution in the intestinal compartments. The clinical aspiration study clearly demonstrated the presence of ibuprofen in the GI tract up to 7 h. This simulation, however, informs us that the amount absorbed of ibuprofen is 100% in approximately 2 h (Figure 11).

In conclusion, there is a mismatch between the simulations and the observed data, highly related to physiological variables (i.e., pH, fluid volumes and gastric emptying) that were considered as pivotal covariates explaining intersubject variability in oral and systemic drug behavior of ibuprofen. Therefore, in the next set of simulations, these variables will be optimized.

3.2.4. Advanced Compartmental Absorption and Transit Simulations: Dynamic Simulations with Adjusted Settings

In the second set of simulations experiments, the goal was to better (in terms of accuracy) reflect the intraluminal behavior taking into account some important physiological aspects that were not considered during the simulations when default settings were applied. All data derived from the clinical aspiration study were analyzed in previous work and revealed how GI motility and pH have a major impact on plasma C_{max} and T_{max}, respectively. As intraluminal pH is not static at all in the human GI tract, the ACAT™ model was adjusted using a constantly changing pH as a function of time, in line with the values observed in the clinical aspiration study. This was applied to all segments of the

GI tract (i.e., stomach, duodenum and jejunum). Moreover, the gastric transit time was delayed from 0.25 h to 2.04 h. As the observed house-keeper wave was on average 2.04 h [22], the gastric transit time was postponed to this specific value. The strong burst of phase III contractions is a surrogate for the rapid emptying of gastric content into the upper small intestine and was demonstrated to have an important impact on the plasma C_{max} of ibuprofen for this specific study.

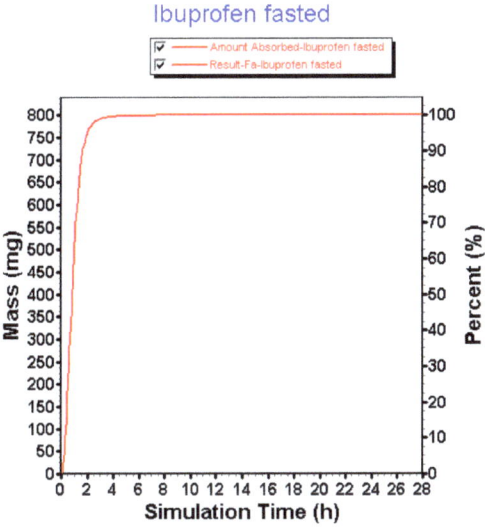

Figure 11. Amount absorbed of ibuprofen under the default settings in the GastroPlus™ simulator.

Application of mixed-multiple doses as dosage form in GastroPlus™ makes it possible to implement different .cat files for each time point (every 15 min) all containing a different fluid volume and pH as observed by MRI data and pH values of aspirated fluids, respectively. All these separate .cat files were uploaded in the GastroPlus™ simulator and were used in chronological order. Figure 12 demonstrates the simulated and observed plasma data.

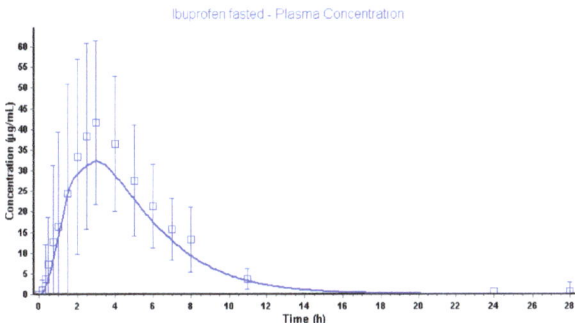

Figure 12. Simulated and observed plasma concentrations of ibuprofen applying the dynamic ACAT™ model.

Pharmacokinetic disposition parameters are shown in Table 6.

The application of the dynamic settings resulted in a predicted plasma C_{max} differing 22% compared to the observed plasma C_{max}. The predicted plasma T_{max} was similar to the observed plasma T_{max}. The exposure (expressed as the area under the curve (AUC)) is the same as observed for the simulations performed with the default settings, highly likely because the amount of dose that is absorbed is 100%. However, the dissolution and absorption of ibuprofen were more sustained using dynamic settings (Figure 13).

Table 6. Pharmacokinetic disposition parameters between observed and simulated data applying the default settings.

Pharmacokinetic (PK) Parameters	Observed Pharmacokinetic Data	Simulated Pharmacokinetic Data
Plasma C_{max} (µg/mL)	41.7	32.5
Plasma T_{max} (h)	3.0	3.0
Plasma $AUC_{0-\infty}$ (µg·h/mL)	259	189
Plasma AUC_{0-28h} (µg·h/mL)	255	189

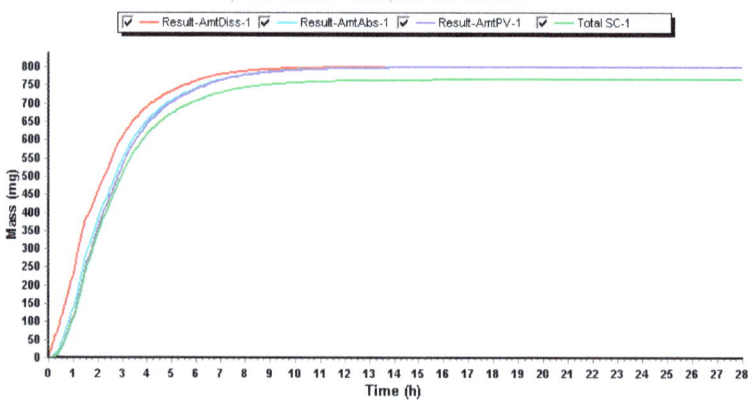

Figure 13. The amount dissolved, absorbed, reaching the portal vein and reaching the systemic circulation after mechanistically modeling of ibuprofen concentrations in GastroPlus™.

When comparing the fraction absorbed from the observed date (by deconvolution) versus the fraction observed that was simulated in GastroPlus™ using the dynamic settings, a positive overlap was observed (Figure 14).

Figure 15 represents the simulated and observed intraluminal profiles in the different regions of the GI tract.

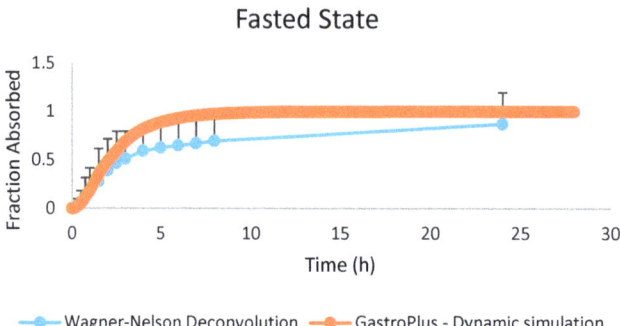

Figure 14. The observed fraction absorbed (based on Wagner–Nelson deconvolution) versus the simulated fraction absorbed from the GastroPlus™ simulator.

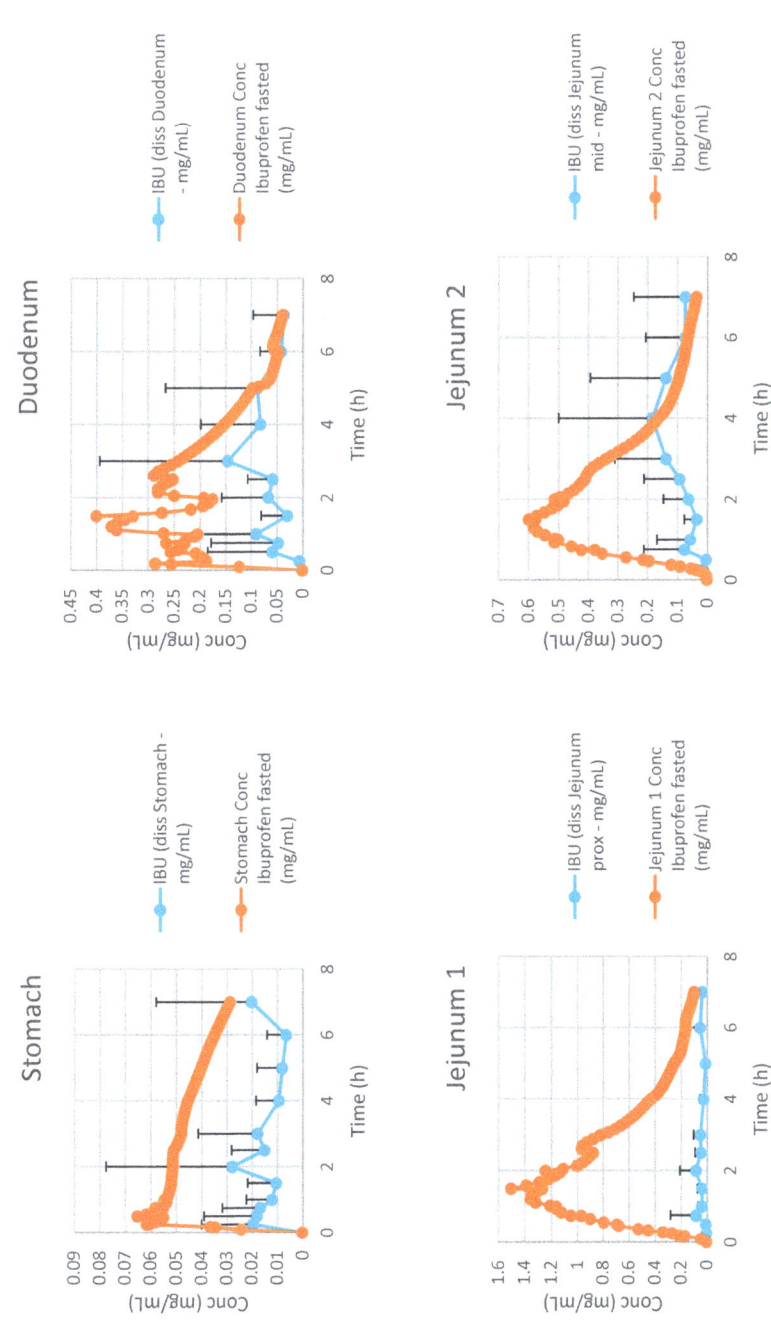

Figure 15. Simulated and observed intraluminal concentrations of ibuprofen in the different segments of the GI tract. Observed data are presented as the mean ± SD.

Simulated results are in line with the observed data, although slightly overestimated with respect to the jejunal concentrations. The reason for this phenomenon can be attributed to the fact that GastroPlus™ handles the small intestine as different compartments, all characterized by specific transit times. As the human jejunum and ileum are quite large (2.5 m and 3.5 m, respectively), the presence of fluid pockets may play a significant role in the amount of drug that will dissolve. It is estimated that the jejunum consists of 13 mL of fluids based on the MRI data of Mudie and co-workers [26], which is more than enough for ibuprofen to dissolve. However, in vivo, these volumes are presented as small, separate water pockets that may hamper the drug to reach its equilibrium solubility. The impact of pockets is less concerned for the duodenal compartment as this segment is only 25 cm long and, based on these simulations, the absence of water pockets seems to have less impact on drug dissolution as the predictions are in line with the in vivo duodenal concentrations. Therefore, these simulations may open public debate to discuss the relevance of simulating these pockets in computational modeling as recently done by Yu and co-workers [46], who developed a dynamic fluid compartmental and absorption transit (DFCAT) model. Related to the compound characteristics (e.g., solubility and permeability), stochastic modeling of these fluid pockets could influence the predicted outcome of the drug product. Figure 16 represents the amounts of ibuprofen dissolved versus undissolved when applying a dynamic versus static fluid model (pH values of the different compartments were the same for both simulations).

We hypothesize that the present fluids will impact the amount of drug dissolved, even though the drug has no limited capacity with respect to dissolution (BCS class 1/2a/3) and regardless of favorable pH to initiate dissolution of the drug in the intestine (BCS class 2a) [47]. Future studies should shed light on the relevance and importance of this topic.

The rate of gastric emptying will alter systemic exposure in such a way that it is favorable to have a fast release of ibuprofen into the small intestine which will generate a high driving force for intestinal absorption. In contrast, when gastric emptying is delayed and ibuprofen will be sustained released from the stomach, the driving force will not be as big as for a direct onset of gastric emptying. Figure 17 demonstrates the parameter sensitivity analysis (PSA) with respect to the 'gastric transit time'. These data are in line with the observed data from the clinical study where a fast onset of post-dose phase III contractions resulted in a higher plasma C_{max}.

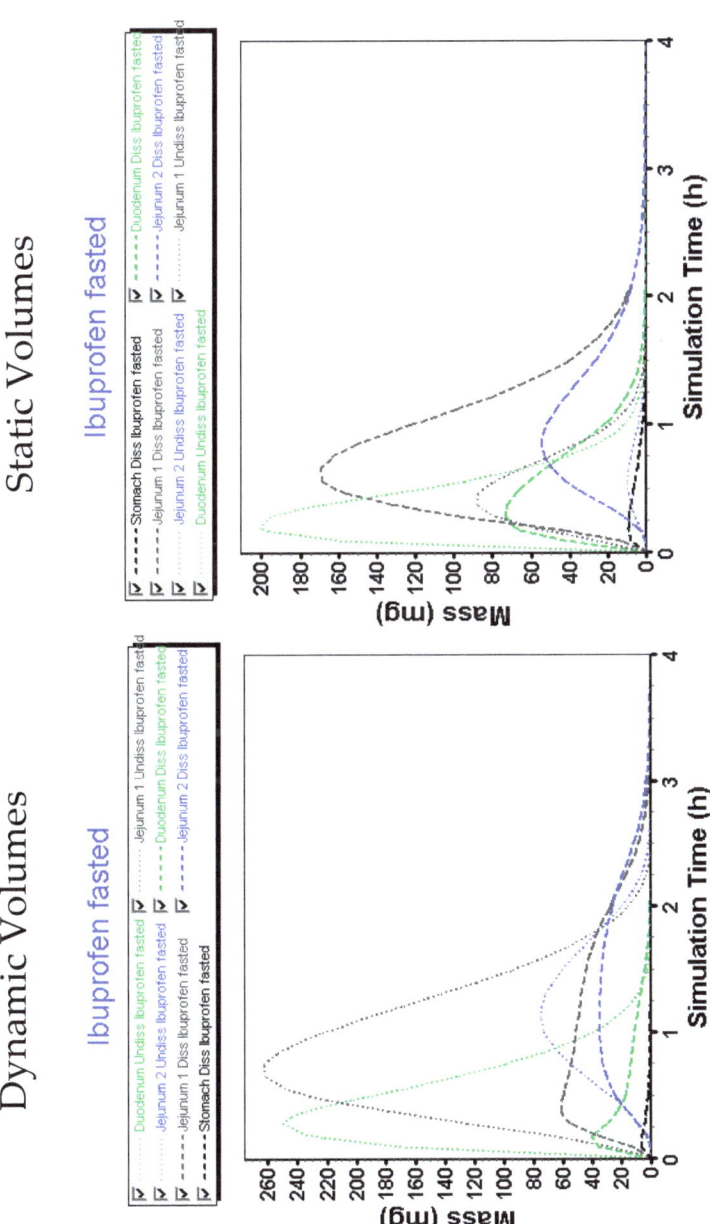

Figure 16. Simulated GI profiles when applying a static (i.e., constant) versus a dynamic fluid model.

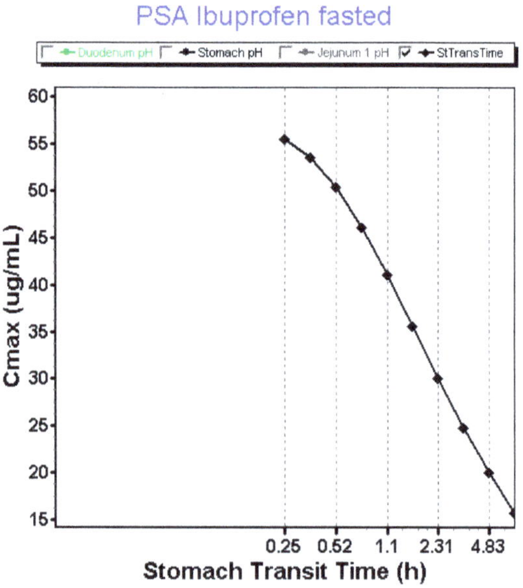

Figure 17. Impact of stomach transit time on the plasma C_{max} for ibuprofen after oral administration of an 800 mg dose in fasted state. PSA: parameter sensitivity analysis.

4. Conclusions and Future Directions: Requesting Biowaivers?

In conclusion, this work demonstrated a mechanistic modeling approach to explain the intraluminal and systemic performance of an orally administered ibuprofen drug product (RLD) in fasted-state conditions. The simulations that were performed highlighted the importance of considering gastric emptying, fluid volumes, motility, and pH as indispensable covariates that should be included in the models to ensure realistic predictions of systemic plasma concentrations of ibuprofen. Both these simulations were done in a user-customized model (Phoenix WinNonlin®) and in a commercially available software package (GastroPlus™). In both cases, we demonstrated the importance of integrating physiological variables to mechanistically understand and observe the impact of these parameters on ibuprofen intestinal absorption. With respect to fluid volumes, simulations in GastroPlus™ demonstrated the impact of dynamic fluids, as measured by an MRI study, on the dissolved amounts of ibuprofen throughout the different GI compartments. There should be further developed with respect to the 'complexity' of in silico models to predict the in vivo outcome plasma levels of a drug. Clear guidelines should assist formulation scientists in whether specific physiological variables should be considered and should be integrated into computational models, highly depending on the purpose of the simulation. Parameter and sensitivity analyses can serve as useful tools to assess the sensitivity of physiological variables predicting the in vivo performance of an oral drug product. Even today, the dynamics of these GI processes are relatively poorly described quantitatively and do not adequately reflect the in vivo GI conditions and thus the plasma performance of the orally administered ibuprofen. While simulations can be performed and mechanistic insight gained from such simulations from current software, we need to further determine the dynamics of the GI variables controlling the dosage form transit, disintegration, dissolution absorption and metabolism along the GI tract in order to move from correlation to prediction (IVIVC → IVIVP). The obtained underlying cumulative dissolution profile derived from the GastroPlus™ simulator (Figure 13) and the simulated concentration–time profiles from the Phoenix WinNonlin® platform (Figure 2) will serve as a reference to optimize our in-house biopredictive dissolution device, the Gastrointestinal Simulator (GIS). Establishing the link between biopredictive in vitro dissolution testing and mechanistic oral absorption modeling (i.e., physiologically-based biopharmaceutics modeling (PBBM)) opens an opportunity to potentially request biowaivers in the near future for orally administered drug products, regardless of its classification according to the BCS [47–50].

Supplementary Materials: Both mathematical equations for simulations performed in Phoenix WinNonlin® as well as the dynamic .cat files for simulations in GastroPlus™ are provided for the reader. These .cat files are compatible with all versions of GastroPlus™. All these files can be found at the following link for free: https://zenodo.org/record/3562430#.XfSmtOhKg-U.

Author Contributions: Conceptualization, M.B., B.H. and G.L.A.; Data curation, M.B., J.D., D.M., P.P., Y.T., K.S. and G.L.A.; Formal analysis, B.H., J.D., D.M., Y.T., K.S. and G.L.A.; Funding acquisition, G.L.A.; Investigation, P.P.; Software, M.B.; Writing-original draft, B.H. All authors have read and agreed to the published version of the manuscript.

Funding: This work was partially supported by grant # HHSF223201510157C and grant # HHSF223201310144C by the U.S. Food and Drug Administration (FDA). B.H. acknowledges the financial support from the Flemish Research Council (FWO—applicant number postdoctoral researcher: 12R2119N).

Acknowledgments: These data were presented at the 2019 annual American Association of Pharmaceutical Scientists (AAPS) meeting on 3 November 2019 in San Antonio, TX.

Conflicts of Interest: The authors declare no conflict of interest. Yasuhiro Tsume is from Merck & Co., Inc., the company had no role in the design of the study; in the collection, analyses, or interpretation of data; in the writing of the manuscript, and in the decision to publish the results.

References

1. Hens, B.; Corsetti, M.; Spiller, R.; Marciani, L.; Vanuytsel, T.; Tack, J.; Talattof, A.; Amidon, G.L.; Koziolek, M.; Weitschies, W.; et al. Exploring Gastrointestinal Variables Affecting Drug and Formulation Behavior: Methodologies, Challenges and Opportunities. *Int. J. Pharm.* **2016**, *59*, 79–97. [CrossRef] [PubMed]
2. DeSesso, J.M.; son, C.F. Anatomical and physiological parameters affecting gastrointestinal absorption in humans and rats. *Food Chem. Toxicol.* **2001**, *39*, 209–228. [CrossRef]
3. Hens, B.; Brouwers, J.; JacobCorsetti, M.; Augustijns, P. Supersaturation and Precipitation of Posaconazole Upon Entry in the Upper Small Intestine in Humans. *J. Pharm. Sci.* **2016**, *105*, 2677–2684. [CrossRef] [PubMed]
4. Hens, B.; Corsetti, M.; Brouwers, J.; Augustijns, P. Gastrointestinal and Systemic Monitoring of Posaconazole in Humans After Fasted and Fed State Administration of a Solid Dispersion. *J. Pharm. Sci.* **2016**, *105*, 2904–2912. [CrossRef] [PubMed]
5. Hens, B.; Brouwers, J.; Corsetti, M.; Augustijns, P. Gastrointestinal behavior of nano- and microsized fenofibrate: In vivo evaluation in man and in vitro simulation by assessment of the permeation potential. *Eur. J. Pharm. Sci.* **2015**, *77*, 40–47. [CrossRef]
6. Hens, B.; Sinko, P.D.; Job, N.; Dean, M.; Al-Gousous, J.; Salehi, N.; Ziff, R.M.; Tsume, Y.; Bermejo, M.; Paixão, P.; et al. Formulation predictive dissolution (fPD) testing to advance oral drug product development: An introduction to the US FDA funded "21st Century BA/BE" project. *Int. J. Pharm.* **2018**, *548*, 120–127. [CrossRef]
7. Psachoulias, D.; Vertzoni, M.; Goumas, K.; Kalioras, V.; Beato, S.; Butler, J.; Reppas, C. Precipitation in and supersaturation of contents of the upper small intestine after administration of two weak bases to fasted adults. *Pharm. Res.* **2011**, *28*, 3145–3158. [CrossRef]
8. Kostewicz, E.S.; Abrahamsson, B.; Brewster, M.; Brouwers, J.; Butler, J.; Carlert, S.; Dickinson, P.A.; Dressman, J.; Holm, R.; Klein, S.; et al. In vitro models for the prediction of in vivo performance of oral dosage forms. *Eur. J. Pharm. Sci.* **2014**, *57*, 342–366. [CrossRef]
9. Ehrhardt, C.; Kim, K. (Eds.) *Drug Absorption Studies: In Situ, In Vitro and In Silico Models*; Biotechnology: Pharmaceutical Aspects; Springer: New York, NY, USA, 2008; ISBN 978-0-387-74900-6.
10. Hens, B.; Bermejo, M.; Tsume, Y.; Gonzalez-Alvarez, I.; Ruan, H.; Matsui, K.; Amidon, G.E.; Cavanagh, K.; Kuminek, G.; Benninghoff, G.; et al. Evaluation and optimized selection of supersaturating drug delivery systems of posaconazole (BCS class 2b) in the gastrointestinal simulator (GIS): An in vitro-in silico-in vivo approach. *Eur. J. Pharm. Sci.* **2018**, *115*, 258–269. [CrossRef]

11. Kostewicz, E.S.; Aarons, L.; Bergstrand, M.; Bolger, M.B.; Galetin, A.; Hatley, O.; Jamei, M.; Lloyd, R.; Pepin, X.; Rostami-Hodjegan, A.; et al. PBPK models for the prediction of in vivo performance of oral dosage forms. *Eur. J. Pharm. Sci.* **2014**, *57*, 300–321. [CrossRef]
12. Deloose, E.; Janssen, P.; Depoortere, I.; Tack, J. The migrating motor complex: Control mechanisms and its role in health and disease. *Nat. Rev. Gastroenterol. Hepatol.* **2012**, *9*, 271–285. [CrossRef] [PubMed]
13. Hens, B.; Tsume, Y.; Bermejo, M.; Paixao, P.; Koenigsknecht, M.J.; Baker, J.R.; Hasler, W.L.; Lionberger, R.; Fan, J.; Dickens, J.; et al. Low Buffer Capacity and Alternating Motility along the Human Gastrointestinal Tract: Implications for in vivo Dissolution and Absorption of Ionizable Drugs. *Mol. Pharm.* **2017**, *14*, 4281–4294. [CrossRef]
14. Koenigsknecht, M.J.; Baker, J.R.; Wen, B.; Frances, A.; Zhang, H.; Yu, A.; Zhao, T.; Tsume, Y.; Pai, M.P.; Bleske, B.E.; et al. In vivo Dissolution and Systemic Absorption of Immediate Release Ibuprofen in Human Gastrointestinal Tract under Fed and Fasted Conditions. *Mol. Pharm.* **2017**, *14*, 4295–4304. [CrossRef] [PubMed]
15. Andreas, C.J.; Rosenberger, J.; Butler, J.; Augustijns, P.; McAllister, M.; Abrahamsson, B.; Dressman, J. Introduction to the OrBiTo decision tree to select the most appropriate in vitro methodology for release testing of solid oral dosage forms during development. *Eur. J. Pharm. Biopharm.* **2018**, *130*, 207–213. [CrossRef] [PubMed]
16. Berlin, M.; Ruff, A.; Kesisoglou, F.; Xu, W.; Wang, M.H.; Dressman, J.B. Advances and challenges in PBPK modeling—Analysis of factors contributing to the oral absorption of atazanavir, a poorly soluble weak base. *Eur. J. Pharm. Biopharm.* **2015**, *93*, 267–280. [CrossRef] [PubMed]
17. Chow, E.C.Y.; Talattof, A.; Tsakalozou, E.; Fan, J.; Zhao, L.; Zhang, X. Using Physiologically Based Pharmacokinetic (PBPK) Modeling to Evaluate the Impact of Pharmaceutical Excipients on Oral Drug Absorption: Sensitivity Analyses. *AAPS J.* **2016**, *18*, 1500–1511. [CrossRef] [PubMed]
18. Hens, B.; Talattof, A.; Paixão, P.; Bermejo, M.; Tsume, Y.; Löbenberg, R.; Amidon, G.L. Measuring the Impact of Gastrointestinal Variables on the Systemic Outcome of Two Suspensions of Posaconazole by a PBPK Model. *AAPS J.* **2018**, *20*, 57. [CrossRef] [PubMed]
19. Margolskee, A.; Darwich, A.S.; Pepin, X.; Aarons, L.; Galetin, A.; Rostami-Hodjegan, A.; Carlert, S.; Hammarberg, M.; Hilgendorf, C.; Johansson, P.; et al. IMI—Oral biopharmaceutics tools project—Evaluation of bottom-up PBPK prediction success part 2: An introduction to the simulation exercise and overview of results. *Eur. J. Pharm. Sci.* **2017**, *96*, 610–625. [CrossRef]
20. Paixão, P.; Bermejo, M.; Hens, B.; Tsume, Y.; Dickens, J.; Shedden, K.; Salehi, N.; Koenigsknecht, M.J.; Baker, J.R.; Hasler, W.L.; et al. Gastric emptying and intestinal appearance of nonabsorbable drugs phenol red and paromomycin in human subjects: A multi-compartment stomach approach. *Eur. J. Pharm. Biopharm.* **2018**, *129*, 162–174. [CrossRef]
21. *Food & Drug Administration Guidance for Industry: Bioanalytical Method Validation*; U.S. Food and Drug Administration (U.S. FDA): Silver Spring, MD, USA, 2001.
22. Bermejo, M.; Paixão, P.; Hens, B.; Tsume, Y.; Koenigsknecht, M.; Baker, J.; Hasler, W.; Lionberger, R.; Jianghong, F.; Dickens, J.; et al. The Impact of Gastrointestinal Motility and Luminal pH On the Oral Absorption of Ibuprofen in Humans—Part 1: Fasted State Conditions. *Mol. Pharm.* **2018**, *5*, 5454–5467. [CrossRef]
23. Lozoya-Agullo, I.; Zur, M.; Beig, A.; Fine, N.; Cohen, Y.; González-Álvarez, M.; Merino-Sanjuán, M.; González-Álvarez, I.; Bermejo, M.; Dahan, A. Segmental-dependent permeability throughout the small intestine following oral drug administration: Single-pass vs. Doluisio approach to in-situ rat perfusion. *Int. J. Pharm.* **2016**, *515*, 201–208. [CrossRef] [PubMed]
24. Zakeri-Milani, P.; Valizadeh, H.; Tajerzadeh, H.; Azarmi, Y.; Islambolchilar, Z.; Barzegar, S.; Barzegar-Jalali, M. Predicting human intestinal permeability using single-pass intestinal perfusion in rat. *J. Pharm. Pharm. Sci.* **2007**, *10*, 368–379. [PubMed]
25. Hens, B.; Bolger, M.B. Application of a Dynamic Fluid and pH Model to Simulate Intraluminal and Systemic Concentrations of a Weak Base in GastroPlus™. *J. Pharm. Sci.* **2019**, *108*, 305–315. [CrossRef] [PubMed]
26. Mudie, D.M.; Murray, K.; Hoad, C.L.; Pritchard, S.E.; Garnett, M.C.; Amidon, G.L.; Gowland, P.A.; Spiller, R.C.; Amidon, G.E.; Marciani, L. Quantification of gastrointestinal liquid volumes and distribution following a 240 mL dose of water in the fasted state. *Mol. Pharm.* **2014**, *11*, 3039–3047. [CrossRef] [PubMed]

27. Tsume, Y.; Langguth, P.; Garcia-Arieta, A.; Amidon, G.L. In silico prediction of drug dissolution and absorption with variation in intestinal pH for BCS class II weak acid drugs: Ibuprofen and ketoprofen. *Biopharm. Drug Dispos.* **2012**, *33*, 366–377. [CrossRef]
28. Heikkilä, T.; Karjalainen, M.; Ojala, K.; Partola, K.; Lammert, F.; Augustijns, P.; Urtti, A.; Yliperttula, M.; Peltonen, L.; Hirvonen, J. Equilibrium drug solubility measurements in 96-well plates reveal similar drug solubilities in phosphate buffer pH 6.8 and human intestinal fluid. *Int. J. Pharm.* **2011**, *405*, 132–136. [CrossRef]
29. Augustijns, P.; Wuyts, B.; Hens, B.; Annaert, P.; Butler, J.; Brouwers, J. A review of drug solubility in human intestinal fluids: Implications for the prediction of oral absorption. *Eur. J. Pharm. Sci.* **2014**, *57*, 322–332. [CrossRef]
30. Walravens, J.; Brouwers, J.; Spriet, I.; Tack, J.; Annaert, P.; Augustijns, P. Effect of pH and comedication on gastrointestinal absorption of posaconazole: Monitoring of intraluminal and plasma drug concentrations. *Clin. Pharm.* **2011**, *50*, 725–734. [CrossRef]
31. Pavliv, L.; Voss, B.; Rock, A. Pharmacokinetics, safety, and tolerability of a rapid infusion of i.v. ibuprofen in healthy adults. *Am. J. Health Syst. Pharm.* **2011**, *68*, 47–51. [CrossRef]
32. Locatelli, I.; Mrhar, A.; Bogataj, M. Gastric emptying of pellets under fasting conditions: A mathematical model. *Pharm. Res.* **2009**, *26*, 1607–1617. [CrossRef]
33. Yu, L.X.; Amidon, G.L. A compartmental absorption and transit model for estimating oral drug absorption. *Int. J. Pharm.* **1999**, *186*, 119–125. [CrossRef]
34. Fadda, H.M.; Merchant, H.A.; Arafat, B.T.; Basit, A.W. Physiological bicarbonate buffers: Stabilisation and use as dissolution media for modified release systems. *Int. J. Pharm.* **2009**, *382*, 56–60. [CrossRef] [PubMed]
35. Al-Gousous, J.; Tsume, Y.; Fu, M.; Salem, I.I.; Langguth, P. Unpredictable Performance of pH-Dependent Coatings Accentuates the Need for Improved Predictive in vitro Test Systems. *Mol. Pharm.* **2017**, *14*, 4209–4219. [CrossRef]
36. Al-Gousous, J.; Amidon, G.L.; Langguth, P. Toward Biopredictive Dissolution for Enteric Coated Dosage Forms. *Mol. Pharm.* **2016**, *13*, 1927–1936. [CrossRef] [PubMed]
37. Karkossa, F.; Klein, S. Individualized in vitro and in silico methods for predicting in vivo performance of enteric-coated tablets containing a narrow therapeutic index drug. *Eur. J. Pharm. Biopharm.* **2019**, *135*, 13–24. [CrossRef] [PubMed]
38. Pepin, X.J.H.; Sanderson, N.J.; Blanazs, A.; Grover, S.; Ingallinera, T.G.; Mann, J.C. Bridging in vitro dissolution and in vivo exposure for acalabrutinib. Part I. Mechanistic modelling of drug product dissolution to derive a P-PSD for PBPK model input. *Eur. J. Pharm. Biopharm.* **2019**, *142*, 421–434. [CrossRef] [PubMed]
39. Al-Gousous, J.; Salehi, N.; Amidon, G.E.; Ziff, R.M.; Langguth, P.; Amidon, G.L. Mass Transport Analysis of Bicarbonate Buffer: Effect of the CO2-H2CO3 Hydration-Dehydration Kinetics in the Fluid Boundary Layer and the Apparent Effective p Ka Controlling Dissolution of Acids and Bases. *Mol. Pharm.* **2019**, *16*, 2626–2635. [CrossRef]
40. Al-Gousous, J.; Sun, K.X.; McNamara, D.P.; Hens, B.; Salehi, N.; Langguth, P.; Bermejo, M.; Amidon, G.E.; Amidon, G.L. Mass Transport Analysis of the Enhanced Buffer Capacity of the Bicarbonate-CO2 Buffer in a Phase-Heterogenous System: Physiological and Pharmaceutical Significance. *Mol. Pharm.* **2018**, *15*, 5291–5301. [CrossRef]
41. Krieg, B.J.; Taghavi, S.M.; Amidon, G.L.; Amidon, G.E. In vivo predictive dissolution: Transport analysis of the CO_2, bicarbonate in vivo buffer system. *J. Pharm. Sci.* **2014**, *103*, 3473–3490. [CrossRef]
42. Cristofoletti, R.; Dressman, J.B. FaSSIF-V3, but not compendial media, appropriately detects differences in the peak and extent of exposure between reference and test formulations of ibuprofen. *Eur. J. Pharm. Biopharm.* **2016**, *105*, 134–140. [CrossRef]
43. Cristofoletti, R.; Hens, B.; Patel, N.; Esteban, V.V.; Schmidt, S.; Dressman, J. Integrating Drug- and Formulation-Related Properties with Gastrointestinal Tract Variability Using a Product-Specific Particle Size Approach: Case Example Ibuprofen. *J. Pharm. Sci.* **2019**, *108*, 3842–3847. [CrossRef] [PubMed]
44. Hofmann, M.; Thieringer, F.; Nguyen, M.A.; Månsson, W.; Galle, P.R.; Langguth, P. A novel technique for intraduodenal administration of drug suspensions/solutions with concurrent pH monitoring applied to ibuprofen formulations. *Eur. J. Pharm. Biopharm.* **2019**, *136*, 192–202. [CrossRef] [PubMed]

45. Atkinson, H.C.; Stanescu, I.; Frampton, C.; Salem, I.I.; Beasley, C.P.H.; Robson, R. Pharmacokinetics and Bioavailability of a Fixed-Dose Combination of Ibuprofen and Paracetamol after Intravenous and Oral Administration. *Clin. Drug Investig.* **2015**, *35*, 625–632. [CrossRef] [PubMed]
46. Yu, A.; Jackson, T.; Tsume, Y.; Koenigsknecht, M.; Wysocki, J.; Marciani, L.; Amidon, G.L.; Frances, A.; Baker, J.R.; Hasler, W.; et al. Mechanistic Fluid Transport Model to Estimate Gastrointestinal Fluid Volume and Its Dynamic Change Over Time. *AAPS J.* **2017**, *19*, 1682–1690. [CrossRef]
47. Amidon, G.L.; Lennernäs, H.; Shah, V.P.; Crison, J.R. A Theoretical Basis for a Biopharmaceutic Drug Classification: The Correlation of in vitro Drug Product Dissolution and in vivo Bioavailability. *Pharm. Res.* **1995**, *12*, 413–420. [CrossRef]
48. Heimbach, T.; Suarez-Sharp, S.; Kakhi, M.; Holmstock, N.; Olivares-Morales, A.; Pepin, X.; Sjögren, E.; Tsakalozou, E.; Seo, P.; Li, M.; et al. Dissolution and Translational Modeling Strategies Toward Establishing an in vitro-In vivo Link—A Workshop Summary Report. *AAPS J.* **2019**, *21*, 29. [CrossRef]
49. Suarez-Sharp, S.; Li, M.; Duan, J.; Shah, H.; Seo, P. Regulatory Experience with in vivo in vitro Correlations (IVIVC) in New Drug Applications. *AAPS J.* **2016**, *18*, 1379–1390. [CrossRef]
50. Suarez-Sharp, S.; Cohen, M.; Kesisoglou, F.; Abend, A.; Marroum, P.; Delvadia, P.; Kotzagiorgis, E.; Li, M.; Nordmark, A.; Bandi, N.; et al. Applications of Clinically Relevant Dissolution Testing: Workshop Summary Report. *AAPS J.* **2018**, *20*, 93. [CrossRef]

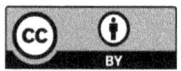

© 2020 by the authors. Licensee MDPI, Basel, Switzerland. This article is an open access article distributed under the terms and conditions of the Creative Commons Attribution (CC BY) license (http://creativecommons.org/licenses/by/4.0/).

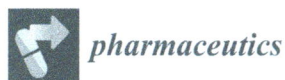

Article

BCS Class IV Oral Drugs and Absorption Windows: Regional-Dependent Intestinal Permeability of Furosemide

Milica Markovic [1], Moran Zur [1], Inna Ragatsky [1], Sandra Cvijić [2] and Arik Dahan [1,*]

1. Department of Clinical Pharmacology, School of Pharmacy, Faculty of Health Sciences, Ben-Gurion University of the Negev, Beer-Sheva 8410501, Israel; milica@post.bgu.ac.il (M.M.); moranfa@post.bgu.ac.il (M.Z.); inna.ragatsky@gmail.com (I.R.)
2. Department of Pharmaceutical Technology and Cosmetology, Faculty of Pharmacy, University of Belgrade, Vojvode Stepe 450, 11221 Belgrade, Serbia; sandra.cvijic@pharmacy.bg.ac.rs
* Correspondence: arikd@bgu.ac.il; Tel.: +972-8-647-9483; Fax: +972-8-647-9303

Received: 16 November 2020; Accepted: 30 November 2020; Published: 2 December 2020

Abstract: Biopharmaceutical classification system (BCS) class IV drugs (low-solubility low-permeability) are generally poor drug candidates, yet, ~5% of oral drugs on the market belong to this class. While solubility is often predictable, intestinal permeability is rather complicated and highly dependent on many biochemical/physiological parameters. In this work, we investigated the solubility/permeability of BCS class IV drug, furosemide, considering the complexity of the entire small intestine (SI). Furosemide solubility, physicochemical properties, and intestinal permeability were thoroughly investigated in-vitro and in-vivo throughout the SI. In addition, advanced in-silico simulations (GastroPlus®) were used to elucidate furosemide regional-dependent absorption pattern. Metoprolol was used as the low/high permeability class boundary. Furosemide was found to be a low-solubility compound. Log D of furosemide at the three pH values 6.5, 7.0, and 7.5 (representing the conditions throughout the SI) showed a downward trend. Similarly, segmental-dependent in-vivo intestinal permeability was revealed; as the intestinal region becomes progressively distal, and the pH gradually increases, the permeability of furosemide significantly decreased. The opposite trend was evident for metoprolol. Theoretical physicochemical analysis based on ionization, pK_a, and partitioning predicted the same trend and confirmed the experimental results. Computational simulations clearly showed the effect of furosemide's regional-dependent permeability on its absorption, as well as the critical role of the drug's absorption window on the overall bioavailability. The data reveals the absorption window of furosemide in the proximal SI, allowing adequate absorption and consequent effect, despite its class IV characteristics. Nevertheless, this absorption window so early on in the SI rules out the suitability of controlled-release furosemide formulations, as confirmed by the in-silico results. The potential link between segmental-dependent intestinal permeability and adequate oral absorption of BCS Class IV drugs may aid to develop challenging drugs as successful oral products.

Keywords: BCS class IV drugs; segmental-dependent intestinal permeability; intestinal absorption; oral drug delivery; biopharmaceutics; physiologically-based pharmacokinetic (PBPK) modeling; furosemide

1. Introduction

The biopharmaceutical classification system (BCS) developed by Amidon et al. revealed that the solubility/dissolution of the drug and its intestinal permeability are the two key factors that dictate drug absorption following oral administration [1,2]. Drug solubility in the gastrointestinal milieu may change in different intestinal segments, e.g., due to pH changes, in a fairly predictable manner; depending on the pKa, the solubility of acidic drugs may increase as the luminal pH rises in more distal regions of the small intestine, and vice versa for basic drugs [3–5]. On the other hand, time- and segmental-dependent intestinal permeability is more complicated and harder to predict [1]. Mechanisms contributing to segmental-dependent permeability throughout the gastrointestinal tract (GIT) include different morphology along the GIT, variable intestinal mucosal cell differentiation, changes in the drug concentration (in case of carrier-mediated transport), modulation of tight junction permeability, and luminal contents and properties, e.g., pH, transporter expression, variability in the structure/composition of the intestinal membrane itself, and more [6–11].

The four BCS classes highlight the limiting factors of the absorption process: (1) Class I, high-solubility high-permeability drugs, indicate the easier and straightforward development process, and complete absorption is expected; (2) Class II, low-solubility high-permeability drugs, indicate that a solubility/dissolution limitation is expected; (3) Class III, high-solubility low-permeability drugs, indicate that the intestinal absorption of this class of drugs will be limited by the permeability rate; and (4) Class IV, low-solubility low-permeability drugs [12]. Since Class IV drugs suffer from inadequate solubility and permeability, they have very poor oral bioavailability and are inclined to exhibit very large inter- and intrasubject variability. Therefore, unless the drug dose is very low, they are generally poor oral drug candidates. Yet, according to some estimates, ~5% of the world's top oral drugs belong to this class [13–15]. In some cases, this is due to the absorption window, which is often critical for the success or failure of a certain drug. In order to gather information about the drug absorption window, extensive work and thorough analysis of luminal conditions and drug absorption is needed, within different locations throughout the GIT. Here, we present such analysis for BCS class IV drug, furosemide [16].

Furosemide is a powerful loop diuretic and is indicated for treating edematous conditions associated with heart, renal, and hepatic failure, as well as for the treatment of hypertension [17,18]. Drug therapy with furosemide is often complex, due to apparent erratic oral systemic availability and unpredictable responses to an administered dose [19]. Even though furosemide is a class IV drug, it is a very common and widely prescribed drug on the market.

In this work, we aimed to investigate the reason for apparent success of furosemide as a marketed product, despite its poor biopharmaceutical properties, and classification as BCS class IV drug, in order to allow development of future class IV compounds. We posit that segmental-dependent permeability of furosemide may contribute to its absorption complexity and provide a certain absorption window in which the drug has suitable permeability and, hence, gets absorbed. For this reason, we investigated the in-vivo intestinal permeability of furosemide throughout different segments of the small intestine. Solubility studies, as well as theoretical physicochemical analysis of furosemide and advanced modern in-silico GastroPlus® simulations, were performed, in order to elucidate the mechanistic reasons behind the experimental results. Furosemide data were compared to the β-blocker metoprolol, the Food and Drug Administration (FDA) reference drug for the low/high permeability class boundary. Overall, this experimental setup allowed us to reveal important insights on the performance of furosemide, despite its unfavorable drug-like properties, and discuss extrapolation of these insights to other BCS class IV drug candidates.

2. Methods

2.1. Materials

Furosemide, metoprolol, phenol red, potassium chloride, potassium phosphate monobasic, potassium phosphate dibasic, sodium chloride, acetic acid, maleic acid, *n*-octanol, and trifluoroacetic acid (TFA) were all purchased from Sigma Chemical Co. (St. Louis, MO, USA). Acetonitrile and water, ultra-performance liquid chromatography (UPLC) grade were purchased from Merck KGaA, Darmstadt, Germany. Remaining chemicals were of analytical reagent grade.

2.2. Solubility Studies

The pH-dependent solubility studies were performed using the shake flask method, as previously reported [20–23]. The equilibrium solubility of furosemide was determined at both 37 °C and at room temperature (25 °C), in phosphate buffer pH 7.5, acetate buffer pH 4.0, and maleate buffer pH 1.0. Surplus quantity of furosemide was introduced to glass vials holding buffer solutions with different pH; the pH of those solutions was measured following drug addition to the buffers and, consequently, placed in the shaking incubator (100 rpm) at 37 °C. The vials were centrifuged (10,000 rpm, 10 min), and the supernatant was instantly analyzed by UPLC. The dose number for furosemide was calculated using the established equation: $D_0 = M/V_0/C_s$; M being the highest single-unit dose strength of furosemide (taken as 80 mg [24]), V_0 is the initial volume of water (250 mL), and C_s is the solubility at each pH; the drug is considered highly soluble if the $D_0 < 1$.

2.3. Evaluation of Octanol-Buffer Partition Coefficients (Log D)

Furosemide and metoprolol experimental octanol-buffer partition coefficients (Log D) were studied at pH 6.5, 7.0, and 7.5 using the shake-flask method [8,11]. Drug solutions in octanol-saturated phosphate buffer (pH 6.5, 7.0, 7.5) were equilibrated at 37 °C for 48 h. The octanol and water phase were divided via centrifugation, and the drug content in the water phase was quantified using UPLC; the furosemide/metoprolol concentration in the octanol phase was determined by mass balance.

2.4. Physicochemical Analysis

The theoretical fraction extracted into octanol (f_e) was calculated using the following equation [25,26].

$$f_e = \frac{f_u P}{1 + f_u P},$$

in which P represents the octanol-water partition coefficient of the unionized drug form, and f_u is the fraction unionized of the drug at a certain pH. Experimental Log P values were taken from the literature for both furosemide (2.29) [27] and metoprolol (2.19) [28]. The f_u versus pH was plotted according to the Henderson-Hasselbalch equation, using the pK_a literature values: 9.68 for metoprolol [29] and 3.8 for furosemide [24].

2.5. Rat Single-Pass Intestinal Perfusion

Effective permeability coefficient (P_{eff}) of furosemide versus metoprolol in various intestinal segments was assessed using the single-pass rat intestinal perfusion (SPIP) in-vivo model. The murine studies were completed according to the approved protocol by Ben-Gurion University of the Negev Animal Use and Care Committee (Protocol IL-08-01-2015). The animals (male Wistar rats weighing 230–260 g, Harlan, Israel) were housed and handled according to Ben-Gurion University of the Negev Unit for Laboratory Animal Medicine Guidelines. All animals were fasted overnight (12–18 h) with free access to water; rats were randomly allocated to different experimental groups. The intestinal perfusion study was performed according to the previous reports [7,9,30–32]. Animals were anesthetized via intramuscular injection of 1 mL/kg ketamine-xylazine solution (9%:1%) and placed on a heated (37 °C) surface (Harvard Apparatus Inc., Holliston, MA, USA); the rat abdomen was uncovered via a midline incision (~3 cm). Permeability (P_{eff}) was measured in proximal jejunum (starting 2 cm lower from the ligament of Treitz), mid-small intestine (SI) segment (isolated between the end of the upper and the beginning of the lower segments), and distal segment of the ileum (ending 2 cm above the cecum) accounting for the complexity of the entire SI [7]. Intestinal segments were cannulated on both ends and perfused with drug-free buffer. Working solutions containing furosemide (320 µg/mL), metoprolol (400 µg/mL), and phenol red (a non-absorbable marker for water flux measurements) were prepared with potassium phosphate monobasic and sodium phosphate dibasic, to achieve pH of 6.5, 7.0 and 7.5; osmolarity (290 mOsm/L) and ionic strength in all buffers was maintained throughout the study.

Drug solutions were incubated in a 37 °C water bath. Steady-state environment was ensured by perfusing the drug-containing buffer for 1 h, followed by additional 1 h of perfusion, during which sampling was done every 10 min. The pH of the collected samples was measured in the outlet sample to verify that there was no pH change throughout the perfusion. All samples were assayed by UPLC. The length of each perfused intestinal segment was measured in the end of the experiment. The effective permeability (P_{eff}; cm/s) through the rat SI wall was calculated according to the following equation:

$$P_{eff} = \frac{-Q\ln(C'_{out}/C'_{in})}{2\pi RL},$$

in which Q is the perfusion buffer flow rate (0.2 mL/min); C'_{out}/C'_{in} is the ratio of the outlet/inlet drug concentration adjusted for water transport; R is the radius of the intestinal segment (conventionally used as 0.2 cm); and L is the exact length of the perfused SI segment as was measured at the experiment endpoint [7,33,34].

2.6. Analytical Methods

Concentration of furosemide and metoprolol was evaluated using an UPLC instrument Waters Acquity UPLC H-Class (Milford, MA, USA), with a photodiode array detector and Empower software. Furosemide and metoprolol were separated on Acquity UPLC XTerra C18 3.5 µm 4.6 mm × 250 mm column (Waters Co., Milford, MA, USA). Gradient mobile phase, going from 70:30% to 90:10% *v/v* 0.1% trifluoroacetic acid in water/acetonitrile, respectively, on a flow rate of 1 mL/min (25 °C). The inter- and intraday coefficients of variation were < 1.0% and 0.5%, respectively.

2.7. Statistics

Solubility studies were performed in four replicates; Log D studies were performed in six replicates, whereas animal perfusion studies were *n* = 4. Values are expressed as means ± standard deviation (SD). To determine statistically significant differences among the experimental groups, a 2-tailed nonparametric Mann–Whitney U test for 2-group comparison was used; $p < 0.05$ was termed significant.

2.8. In-Silico Simulations

Computer simulations of furosemide absorption and concomitant plasma concentrations following oral administration in humans were conducted using GastroPlus™ software package (v. 9.7.0009, 2019, Simulations Plus Inc., Lancaster, CA, USA). The required input data regarding drug physicochemical and pharmacokinetic properties were experimentally determined, taken from literature or in-silico predicted. Human permeability values throughout the SI were calculated from the experimental rat single-pass intestinal perfusion data, using the software integrated "permeability converter". Drug disposition was best described by three-compartmental pharmacokinetic model, whereas the relevant parameters (clearance (*CL*), volume of distribution (*Vd*) and distribution constants between central and peripheral compartments) were estimated using PKPlus software module, based on the in-vivo plasma concentration data for an intravenous (i.v.) bolus dose [35]. The application of three-compartmental model to describe furosemide pharmacokinetics has already been reported in literature [36,37]. Graphical data from literature were digitized using DigIt™ program (version 1.0.4, 2001–2008, Simulations Plus, Inc., Lancaster, CA, USA). Physiological parameters were the software default values representing fasted state physiology of a healthy human representative.

The software simulates drug absorption from the GIT using the integrated Advanced Compartment Absorption and Transit (ACAT) GIT model that consists of nine compartments (stomach, duodenum, two segments of jejunum, three segments of ileum, caecum, and ascendant colon). These compartments are linked in series, and the amount of drug dissolved and absorbed from each compartment is calculated by the system of differential equations. More details on the ACAT model can be found in the literature [38,39]. Regarding the fact that furosemide is a poorly-soluble drug, the model accounted for the effect of bile salt on drug solubility and diffusion coefficient. Drug dissolution rate under physiological conditions was predicted using the software default Johnson dissolution equation (based on modified Nernst-Bruner equation) [40].

The validity of the model (i.e., the selection of input values) was validated by comparison of the prediction results (bioavailability (F), maximum plasma concentration (C_{max}), time to reach C_{max} (t_{max}), and area under the plasma concentration-time curve ($AUC_{0-\infty}$)) with published data from the in-vivo studies for peroral (p.o.) drug administration. Percent prediction error (%PE) between the predicted and mean in-vivo observed data from a clinical study was calculated using the following equation:

$$\%PE = \frac{(\text{Observed value} - \text{Predicted value}) \times 100}{\text{Observed value}}.$$

In the next step, the generated model was used to mechanistically interpret furosemide regional absorption pattern, and to estimate the outcomes for various hypothetical drug dissolution scenarios (illustrating drug dissolution from immediate-release (IR) and controlled-release (CR) oral formulations). In the last case, hypothetical dissolution profiles were used as additional inputs to describe drug release rate in-vivo, and the selected dosage form was "CR dispersed" to allow input of the tabulated dissolution data.

3. Results

The solubility values obtained for furosemide at 37 °C and at room temperature (25 °C) are summarized in Table 1, as well as the corresponding dose number (D_0). Furosemide showed pH-dependent solubility, in accordance with its acidic nature. It can be seen that, while at pH 7.5, furosemide has suitable solubility (as evident by D_0 lower than 1), at the lower pH values, 1.0 and 4.0, it is poorly soluble. When taking 80 mg as the highest dose strength, although $D_0 < 1$ was obtained at pH 7.5, at pH 1.0 and 4.0, the D_0 is higher than 1; hence, furosemide was found to be a low-solubility compound according to the BCS.

Table 1. Furosemide solubility values (µg/mL) at the tree pH values 1.0, 4.0, and 7.5, at 37 °C (upper panel), and at room temperature (25 °C; lower panel), as well as the corresponding dose number (D_0) calculated for an 80-mg dose. Data presented as mean ± SD; $n = 6$.

	At 37 °C	
pH	Solubility (µg/mL)	Corresponding D_0
1	19.4 ± 3.7	16.5
4	65.5 ± 9.0	4.8
7.5	8340.1 ± 81.6	0.04
	At 25 °C	
pH	Solubility (µg/mL)	Corresponding D_0
1	40.3 ± 16.2	7.9
4	56.7 ± 12.2	5.6
7.5	8550.6 ± 149.4	0.04

Octanol-buffer partition coefficient values of furosemide and metoprolol at the three pH values 6.5, 7.0, and 7.5 (representing the conditions throughout the small intestine) are presented in Figure 1. Both drugs presented a clear pH-dependent Log D values across the studied pH range, with opposite trends; while furosemide's partitioning decreases as the pH rises, metoprolol shows higher partitioning into octanol at higher pH (metoprolol is the acceptable reference drug for the low/high permeability class boundary). In addition, furosemide's Log D at pH 6.5 was higher than that of metoprolol at the same pH; this is a surprising finding since Log D may sometimes be used as a surrogate for passive permeability. Indeed, at higher pH values (7.0 and 7.5), metoprolol Log D increases, while furosemide decreases, and metoprolol Log D becomes higher than furosemide.

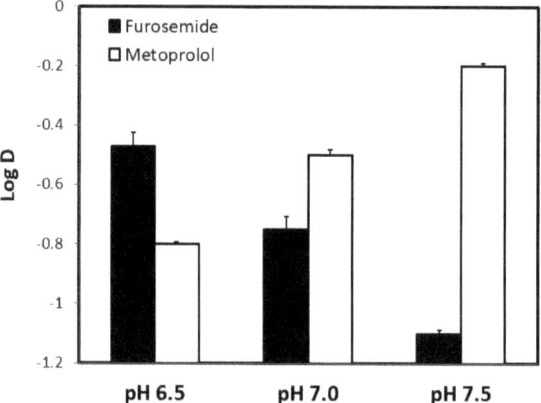

Figure 1. The octanol-buffer partition coefficients, Log D, for furosemide and metoprolol at the three pH values 6.5, 7.0, and 7.5. Data are presented as the mean ± S.D.; n = 6 in each experimental group.

Furosemide and metoprolol physicochemical properties are presented in Table 2. Figure 2 presents furosemide versus metoprolol theoretical fraction unionized (f_u) and fraction extracted into octanol (f_e) as a function of pH. The plots have a standard sigmoidal shape, with opposite trends for furosemide vs. metoprolol. The f_e vs. pH plot follows the same pattern to the f_u plot, only with a shift to the right (higher pH values) for acidic drug (furosemide), and to the left (lower pH values) for basic (metoprolol) drugs. The shift magnitude in both cases equals Log(P − 1) at the midpoint of the f_e and f_u curves [25,26]. The experimental drug octanol-buffer partitioning at the three pH values (6.5, 7.0, and 7.5) are illustrated in Figure 2, as well, and it can be seen that they were in excellent agreement with the theoretical plots.

Table 2. Physicochemical parameters and chemical structure of furosemide and metoprolol.

Drug	Chemical Structure	pK$_a$	Log P	PSA
Furosemide		3.8	2.3	127.7
Metoprolol		9.7	2.2	53.2

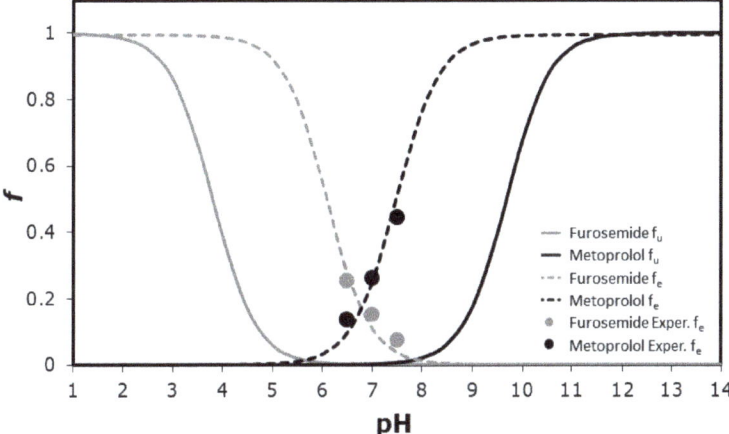

Figure 2. The theoretical fraction unionized (f_u) and fraction extracted into octanol (f_e) plots as a function of pH for furosemide and metoprolol, as well as experimental buffer-octanol partitioning of the drugs in the three pH values 6.5, 7.0, and 7.5 ($n = 5$).

The effective permeability coefficient (P_{eff}, cm/sec) values of furosemide and metoprolol determined using the single-pass intestinal perfusion (SPIP) rat model, in three intestinal segments, namely proximal jejunum (pH 6.5), mid small intestine (pH 7.0), and distal ileum (pH 7.5), are presented in Figure 3. It can be seen that significant regional-dependent permeability of furosemide throughout the small intestine was evident: the permeability of furosemide gradually decreases, while the permeability of metoprolol gradually increases, as the SI segments become more distal.

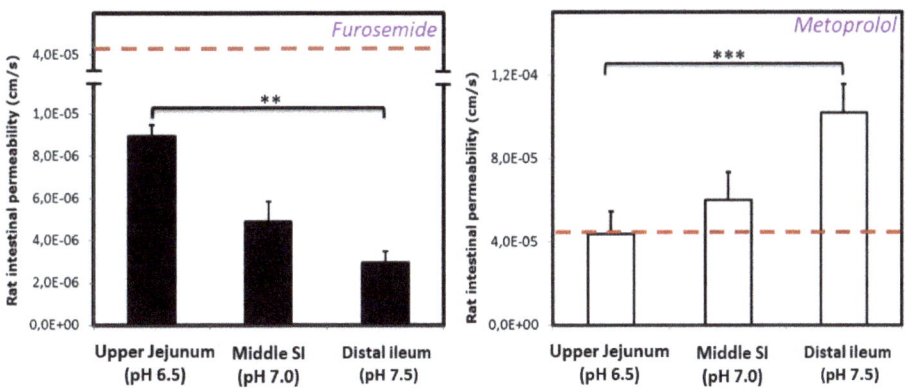

Figure 3. Effective permeability values (P_{eff}; cm/s) obtained for furosemide and metoprolol after in-situ single pass perfusion to the rat proximal jejunum at pH 6.5, mid-small intestine at pH 7.0, and to the distal ileum at pH 7.5. Mean ± S.D.; $n = 4$ in each experimental group; ** $p < 0.01$, *** $p < 0.001$.

The input data regarding drug physicochemical and pharmacokinetic properties, used for in-silico simulations, are presented in Table 3. The simulated furosemide plasma concentration profile following p.o. administration is depicted in Figure 4, along with the mean profiles observed in the in-vivo studies. In addition, the observed and model predicted pharmacokinetic parameters are compared in Table 4. The presented data demonstrate that the generated model adequately describes furosemide absorption and disposition. The course of the predicted plasma profile fairly resembles the observed data. However, certain variations are observed between the mean in-vivo data from different studies referring to the same drug dose (Figure 4, Table 4). Indeed, it has been reported that furosemide oral absorption is highly variable between individuals, e.g., C_{max} varied three-fold, and t_{max} varied five-fold [36,37,41]; moreover, individual AUC values for 40 mg furosemide oral dose varied between 1.57 and 3.76 µg·h/mL (more than two-fold) [36,37,41], and even larger AUC values were observed in another study with the same drug dose (2.23–6.10 µg·h/mL) [42], indicating that, regardless of the high PE(%) values in Table 4, the model predicted value of 3.66 µg·h/mL is not an overestimate of the extent of drug absorption. In addition, extensive intrasubject variability was observed for orally dosed furosemide, and these variations were attributed to the absorption process (i.e., day to day variations in physiological factors) since the repeated i.v. doses showed only marginal intrasubject variability [36,37,41]. Considering pronounced inter- and intraindividual variability in furosemide oral absorption, the simulated profile can be seen as a reasonable estimate (Figure 4). Moreover, the predicted fraction of oral drug absorption (cc. 52%) is in accordance with the values reported in the literature [36,37].

Table 3. The selected input parameters for furosemide absorption GastroPlus® simulation.

Parameter	Value	Source
Molecular weight (g/mol)	330.75	/
Log D (pH 7.5)	−1.0818	experimental values
Solubility at 37 °C (µg/mL)	19.4 (pH 1.0)	
	65.5 (pH 4.0)	
	8340.1 (pH 7.5)	
pK_a (acid)	3.8	[24]
Human effective permeability, P_{eff} (cm/s)	0.4043×10^{-4} (duodenum, jejunum)	values converted using GastroPlus™ integrated "permeability converter" based on experimental rat perfusion data
	0.2246×10^{-4} (ileum 1 and 2)	
	0.1392×10^{-4} (ileum 3, caecum, colon)	
Diffusion coefficient (cm²/s)	0.7289×10^{-5}	GastroPlus™ calculated value (based on molecular weight)
Mean precipitation time (s)	900	GastroPlus™ default values
Particle density (g/mL)	1.2	
Particle radius (µm)	25	
Blood/plasma concentration ratio	1	
Plasma fraction unbound (%)	1	[24]
Clearance, CL (L/h/kg)	0.121	calculated using GastroPlus™ PKPlus module, based on the i.v. data [35]
Volume of distribution, Vd (L/kg)	0.043	
Distribution constant k_{12} (1/h)	0.964	
Distribution constant k_{21} (1/h)	1.614	
Distribution constant k_{13} (1/h)	0.925	
Distribution constant k_{32} (1/h)	0.708	
Regional pH in the GIT	1.3; 6.0; 6.2; 6.4; 6.6; 6.9; 7.4; 6.4; 6.8	GastroPlus™ default values for stomach, duodenum, jejunum 1, jejunum 2, ileum 1, ileum 2, ileum 3, caecum, and ascendant colon
Regional volume of fluid in the GIT (mL)	46.56; 40.54; 150.00; 119.30; 91.71; 68.88; 48.57; 46.44; 49.21	
Regional transit time in the GIT (h)	0.25; 0.26; 0.93; 0.74; 0.58; 0.42; 0.29; 4.13; 12.38	

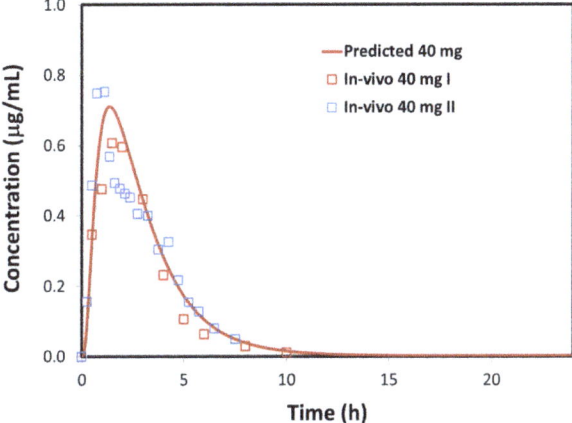

Figure 4. GastroPlus® simulated (line) versus mean observed (markers) plasma concentration profiles following p.o. administration of furosemide. Mean observed values represent 40 mg immediate-release (IR) tablet profile I [43] and 40 mg IR tablet profile II [37].

Table 4. Comparison between GastroPlus® simulated and in-vivo observed furosemide pharmacokinetic parameters following p.o. drug administration.

Parameter	40 mg p.o. Dose				
	In-Vivo I [a]	In-Vivo II [b]	Predicted	PE(%) I	PE(%) II
C_{max} (µg/mL)	0.61	0.75	0.71	−17.14	5.54
t_{max} (h)	1.5	1.12	1.36	9.33	−22.22
$AUC_{0 \rightarrow \infty}$ (µg·h/mL)	2.13	2.44	3.66	−71.25	−50.06
$AUC_{0 \rightarrow 24 h}$ (µg·h/mL)	2.11	2.33	2.52	−19.25	−8.15
F (%)	NA	NA	52.2	NA	NA

[a] Refers to the mean plasma profile from [43] (40 mg IR tablet); [b] refers to the mean plasma profile from [37] (40 mg IR tablet); NA, not available/not applicable.

The predicted furosemide dissolution and absorption profiles following an IR oral formulation (IR tablet) are illustrated in Figure 5. The generated profiles clearly indicate that drug permeability is the limiting factor for absorption under fasted state GIT conditions. Namely, although furosemide is a low-solubility drug, due to ionization at the elevated pH conditions in the proximal SI, drug dissolution from an IR formulation is expected to be fast (>85% in 30 min). Therefore, furosemide absorption from an IR formulation is mainly governed by poor permeability. The predicted regional-dependent absorption distribution (Figure 6) further highlights the role of furosemide segmental absorption on the overall drug bioavailability. As implied by the regional-dependent permeability data, but also considering the surface area available for absorption, furosemide absorption predominantly happens in the proximal parts of the SI (76.6% of the total amount absorbed into the enterocytes), and only a minor fraction of drug (23.2% of the total amount absorbed into the enterocytes) passes into systemic circulation through mid and distal GIT regions.

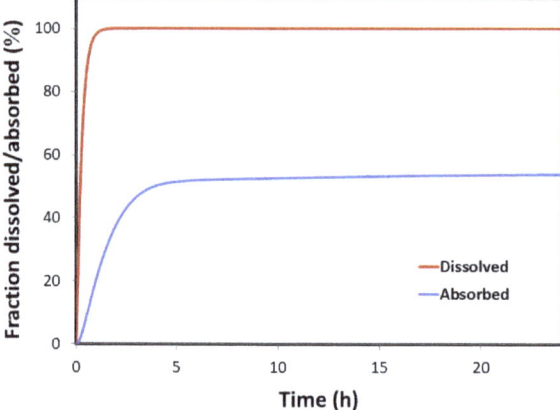

Figure 5. GastroPlus® simulated dissolution and absorption profiles following p.o. administration of 40 mg furosemide dose (dissolution profile was simulated using the software default Johnson equation).

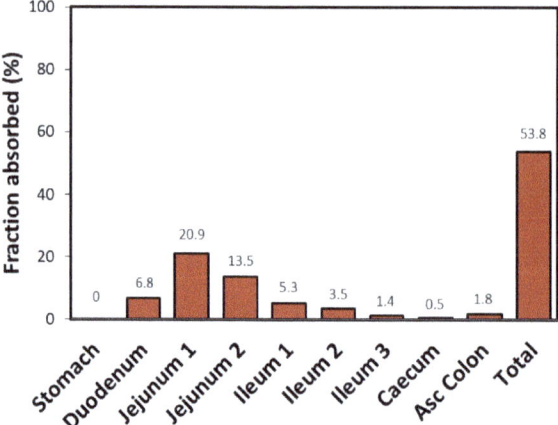

Figure 6. GastroPlus® simulated regional absorption of furosemide following p.o. administration of 40 mg drug dose (the simulated values refer to the fraction of drug dose that entered into the enterocytes).

The prediction results corresponding to various dissolution scenarios are presented in Figure 7b–d and Table 5. According to the simulated data, furosemide release rate from an oral formulation highly impacts the concomitant absorption process, whereas prolonged drug release rate leads to marked delay in the rate and extent of drug absorption. The estimated pharmacokinetic parameters (Table 5) indicate that furosemide bioavailability would show more than a 10-fold decrease in case the complete drug dissolution is achieved within 24 h in comparison to 15 min. A similar trend is observed for C_{max} and AUC values (17.75- and 17.38-fold decrease, respectively), while t_{max} would be prolonged (about two-fold). It is interesting to note that t_{max} increases with decrease in drug dissolution up to some point, but further decrease in drug dissolution (e.g., 85% in more than 6 h) would not cause additional delay in peak plasma concentration. This is because, after cc. 2 h, the drug leaves proximal parts of the intestine, where majority of furosemide absorption takes place, and, later on, in mid and especially distal intestine, only a small fraction of drug can be absorbed, as illustrated in Figure 7d.

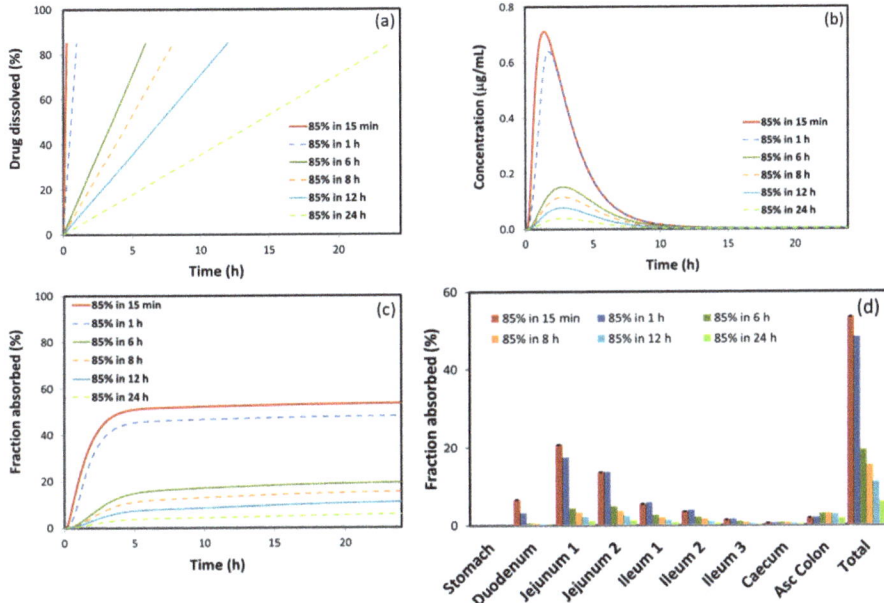

Figure 7. GastroPlus® simulated furosemide dissolution profiles (**a**); and (**b**) the corresponding simulated plasma profiles; (**c**) absorption profiles; and (**d**) regional absorption distribution.

Table 5. GastroPlus® predicted pharmacokinetic parameters for different furosemide virtual dissolution profiles from 40 mg p.o. dosage forms.

Dissolution	C_{max} (µg/mL)	t_{max} (h)	$AUC_{0\to\infty}$ (µg·h/mL)	F (%)
85% in 15 min	0.71	1.36	3.65	51.91
85% in 1 h	0.64	1.76	3.71	46.35
85% in 6 h	0.15	2.80	0.80	16.64
85% in 8 h	0.11	2.80	0.61	12.73
85% in 12 h	0.08	2.80	0.41	8.65
85% in 24 h	0.04	2.80	0.21	4.36

4. Discussion

BCS class IV drugs (e.g., sulfamethoxazole, ritonavir, paclitaxel, and furosemide) exhibit numerous unfavorable characteristics (low solubility and permeability, high presystemic metabolism, efflux transport), which make their oral drug delivery challenging. In addition to this, class IV drugs often demonstrate inter/intra-subject variability. Indeed, following oral administration, the absorption and bioavailability of furosemide are highly variable (37–51%) [35,41]. It has been suggested that this variability is highly depend on the absorption process [41], which in turn is dependent on drug aqueous solubility and intestinal permeability following oral administration [1,44]. It has also been hypothesized that variable gastric/intestinal first-pass metabolism can be a factor in causing incomplete and irregular furosemide absorption in humans [45]. Despite the unfavorable class IV drug characteristics, furosemide was shown to be exceptionally useful and successful marketed drug product for the treatment of edema [17]. For this reason, we decided to investigate furosemide's solubility and in-vivo regional-dependent permeability throughout the GIT, as main parameters that guide absorption of oral drugs.

It was shown that a correlation between human P_{eff} in the jejunum and physicochemical parameters advocates that there is a high pH-dependent influence on the passive intestinal permeability in-vivo [46]. Indeed, furosemide in-vivo permeability data demonstrate a downward trend towards the distal intestinal segments as the pH gradually increases, a trend that can be expected for acidic drugs, since the pH in the intestinal lumen gradually increases towards distal SI regions (Figure 3). Many BCS class IV drugs are substrates for efflux transporters [47]. There is some evidence that furosemide might be a substrate for efflux transporters [48,49]; thus, such permeability trend could also be influenced by the P-glycoprotein (P-gp) transporter in which expression levels are increased from proximal to distal SI segments [6,50–52]. Since metoprolol's intestinal permeability is passive and does not involve carrier-mediated absorption, it exhibited pH-dependent intestinal permeability, with reverse tendency compared to furosemide; as a basic drug, metoprolol showed upward increase in permeability towards distal SI segments with rising pH values (Figure 3). At any point throughout the SI, furosemide exhibited significantly lower permeability than the benchmark (metoprolol's jejunum permeability), which confirms its BCS low-permeability classification and incomplete absorption. Despite the fact that furosemide is a low-permeability drug, the higher permeability in the proximal intestinal regions provides a window for furosemide absorption, and we posit that this is one of the main reasons for furosemide's sufficient bioavailability and success as a marketed drug. Theoretical f_u and f_e as a function of pH were found to be in excellent correlation to these in-vivo data. In addition, in-silico modeling indicated that furosemide dissolution from an IR formulation would be fairly complete before the drug leaves proximal SI (Figure 5), although the drug is generally classified as low-soluble, enabling timely delivery of the dissolved drug to the distinct absorption site. Complete furosemide dissolution under physiological conditions is also confirmed by the experimental solubility results (Table 1).

Furosemide Log D studies showed higher partition coefficient in comparison to metoprolol at pH 6.5, whereas, in the in-vivo intestinal perfusion experiment, furosemide showed significantly lower jejunum permeability than metoprolol (Figure 1). A possible reason for this difference in the partitioning and in-vivo permeability can be the polar surface area (PSA) of both drugs [53]. A sigmoidal relationship between the fraction absorbed following oral administration and the dynamic polar surface area was reported in the past [54–56]. It was shown that orally administered drugs with large PSA (>120) are hardly absorbed by the passive transcellular route, while drugs with a small PSA (<60) are almost completely absorbed [55,56]. This is in agreement with our results, as furosemide has much higher PSA (127.7) than metoprolol (53.2) [54,55]. Another reason for the difference in the partitioning and in-vivo permeability may be the presence of active efflux transport involved in the intestinal permeability. The influence of efflux transport at pH 6.5 (proximal intestinal segments) could decrease furosemide's permeability in-vivo, which was not accounted for in the octanol partitioning studies.

The Log P value of furosemide (2.3) is in the close proximity to that of metoprolol (2.2), pointing to high permeability (Table 2). However, the Log P calculation is based on the unionized drug fraction, and, since furosemide has acidic nature it is likely that, once it passes the acidic stomach environment, it will mostly be in ionized form (the pH throughout the GIT varies from 5.9–6.3 in the proximal SI to 7.4–7.8 in distal SI segments; pH in the colon is fluctuating between pH 5–8 [57]); therefore the high furosemide Log P is not in correspondence with permeability in-vivo. Thus, we posit that no single parameter can be used for measuring the drug absorption process, but rather, a combination of physicochemical parameters and in-vitro and in-vivo findings, as well as careful consideration of inclusion criteria prior to making decisions. Despite the high Log P value for furosemide, it was indeed confirmed that furosemide is a BCS class IV drug, based on both the solubility data (Table 1) and the intestinal permeability (Figure 3).

Suitable formulation is the main approach to create an efficacious drug product for the administration of BCS class IV drugs [47]. Absorption windows in the proximal intestinal segments can restrict the oral drug bioavailability and can be a significant limitation for the development of CR drug formulation. The underlying reasons are mechanistically explained by our in-silico results (Figure 7). As mentioned, furosemide permeability results revealed acceptable permeability in the proximal segments of the SI, which is presumably the reason why furosemide has appropriate drug bioavailability, despite being a BCS class IV drug. However, since CR products release the drug over 12–24 h, mostly in the colon, (transit time throughout the small intestine is 3–4 h [58]), the fact that furosemide is mainly absorbed from proximal SI segments, (with decreased permeability at distant GIT segments) prevents the formulation of furosemide as a CR product, as shown previously [21,59,60]. However, we believe that formulations based on gastro-retentive dosage forms (GRDF) can be shown as prosperous for furosemide [61]. There are several similar examples in the literature where absorption window occurs in the upper GI, and this has been used to create GDRF formulations to improve the drug absorption, such as riboflavin [62] and levodopa [59,63].

Several types of bariatric surgeries (specifically Roux-en-Y gastric bypass and mini bypass) result in bypassing the upper SI. In cases where the absorption window is indeed in this upper SI region, the absorption following the bariatric surgery can be hampered vastly, since the actual segment responsible for the majority of absorption is bypassed [64–66].

5. Conclusions

Regional-dependent permeability throughout the small intestine was evident for furosemide. The permeability of furosemide gradually decreases throughout the small intestine as a function of the pH change in the intestinal lumen. However, at any point throughout the small intestine, furosemide exhibited significantly lower permeability than the benchmark of metoprolol's permeability in the jejunum, which may explain the incomplete absorption of the drug. We propose that, for a drug to be classified as BCS low-permeability, its intestinal permeability should not match/exceed the low/high class benchmark anywhere throughout the intestinal tract, as well as is not restricted necessarily to the jejunum. Nevertheless, low-permeable drugs should not be treated as 'unfavorable' by default; instead, therapeutic potential and suitable formulation strategies should be considered on a case-by-case basis, taking into account the overall results of in-vitro, in-vivo, and in-silico testing, throughout the entire gastrointestinal tract.

Author Contributions: M.M., M.Z., I.R., S.C. and A.D. worked on conceptualization, methodology, investigation, analyzed the data, and outlined the manuscript. S.C. worked on software investigation. Writing: S.C., A.D. and M.M. prepared the original draft of the article, and M.Z. and I.R. contributed to the writing-review and editing of the full version. All authors have read and agreed to the published version of the manuscript.

Funding: This work received no external funding.

Conflicts of Interest: The authors declare no conflict of interest.

References

1. Amidon, G.L.; Lennernäs, H.; Shah, V.P.; Crison, J.R. A theoretical basis for a biopharmaceutic drug classification: The correlation of in vitro drug product dissolution and in vivo bioavailability. *Pharm. Res.* **1995**, *12*, 413–420. [CrossRef]
2. Dahan, A.; Miller, J.M.; Amidon, G.L. Prediction of solubility and permeability class membership: Provisional BCS classification of the world's top oral drugs. *AAPS J.* **2009**, *11*, 740–746. [CrossRef]
3. Dahan, A.; Beig, A.; Lindley, D.; Miller, J.M. The solubility-permeability interplay and oral drug formulation design: Two heads are better than one. *Adv. Drug Deliv. Rev.* **2016**, *101*, 99–107. [CrossRef]
4. Dahan, A.; Miller, J.M. The solubility-permeability interplay and its implications in formulation design and development for poorly soluble drugs. *AAPS J.* **2012**, *14*, 244–251. [CrossRef]
5. Miller, J.M.; Beig, A.; Carr, R.A.; Webster, G.K.; Dahan, A. The solubility-permeability interplay when using cosolvents for solubilization: Revising the way we use solubility-enabling formulations. *Mol. Pharm.* **2012**, *9*, 581–590. [CrossRef]
6. Dahan, A.; Amidon, G.L. Segmental dependent transport of low permeability compounds along the small intestine due to P-Glycoprotein: The role of efflux transport in the oral absorption of BCS class III drugs. *Mol. Pharm.* **2009**, *6*, 19–28. [CrossRef]

7. Dahan, A.; West, B.T.; Amidon, G.L. Segmental-dependent membrane permeability along the intestine following oral drug administration: Evaluation of a triple single-pass intestinal perfusion (TSPIP) approach in the rat. *Eur. J. Pharm. Sci.* **2009**, *36*, 320–329. [CrossRef]
8. Fairstein, M.; Swissa, R.; Dahan, A. Regional-dependent intestinal permeability and BCS classification: Elucidation of pH-related complexity in rats using pseudoephedrine. *AAPS J.* **2013**, *15*, 589–597. [CrossRef]
9. Lozoya-Agullo, I.; Zur, M.; Beig, A.; Fine, N.; Cohen, Y.; Gonzalez-Alvarez, M.; Merino-Sanjuan, M.; Gonzalez-Alvarez, I.; Bermejo, M.; Dahan, A. Segmental-dependent permeability throughout the small intestine following oral drug administration: Single-pass vs. Doluisio approach to in-situ rat perfusion. *Int. J. Pharm.* **2016**, *515*, 201–208. [CrossRef]
10. Markovic, M.; Zur, M.; Dahan, A.; Cvijić, S. Biopharmaceutical characterization of rebamipide: The role of mucus binding in regional-dependent intestinal permeability. *Eur. J. Pharm. Sci.* **2020**, *152*, 105440. [CrossRef]
11. Zur, M.; Hanson, A.S.; Dahan, A. The complexity of intestinal permeability: Assigning the correct BCS classification through careful data interpretation. *Eur. J. Pharm. Sci.* **2014**, *61*, 11–17. [CrossRef]
12. U.S. Department of Health and Human Services, Food and Drug Administration; Center for Drug Evaluation and Research (CDER). *Waiver of In-Vivo Bioavailability and Bioequivalence Studies for Immediate-Release Solid Oral Dosage Forms Based on a Biopharmaceutics Classification System; Guidance for Industry*; Center for Drug Evaluation and Research (CDER): Silver Spring, MD, USA, 2017.
13. Dahan, A.; Wolk, O.; Kim, Y.H.; Ramachandran, C.; Crippen, G.M.; Takagi, T.; Bermejo, M.; Amidon, G.L. Purely in silico BCS classification: Science based quality standards for the world's drugs. *Mol. Pharm.* **2013**, *10*, 4378–4390. [CrossRef]
14. Takagi, T.; Ramachandran, C.; Bermejo, M.; Yamashita, S.; Yu, L.X.; Amidon, G.L. A provisional biopharmaceutical classification of the top 200 oral drug products in the United States, Great Britain, Spain, and Japan. *Mol. Pharm.* **2006**, *3*, 631–643. [CrossRef]
15. Wolk, O.; Agbaria, R.; Dahan, A. Provisional in-silico biopharmaceutics classification (BCS) to guide oral drug product development. *Drug Des. Dev. Ther.* **2014**, *8*, 1563–1575. [CrossRef]
16. Lindenberg, M.; Kopp, S.; Dressman, J.B. Classification of orally administered drugs on the World Health Organization model list of essential medicines according to the biopharmaceutics classification system. *Eur. J. Pharm. Biopharm.* **2004**, *58*, 265–278. [CrossRef]
17. Furosemide Tablets, United States Pharmacopeia Label. Available online: https://www.accessdata.fda.gov/drugsatfda_docs/label/2016/018487s043lbl.pdf (accessed on 11 July 2020).
18. Ellison, D.H.; Felker, G.M. Diuretic Treatment in Heart Failure. *N. Engl. J. Med.* **2017**, *377*, 1964–1975. [CrossRef]
19. Hammarlund-Udenaes, M.; Benet, L.Z. Furosemide pharmacokinetics and pharmacodynamics in health and disease—An update. *J. Pharmacokinet. Biopharm.* **1989**, *17*, 1–46. [CrossRef]
20. Dahan, A.; Wolk, O.; Zur, M.; Amidon, G.L.; Abrahamsson, B.; Cristofoletti, R.; Groot, D.W.; Kopp, S.; Langguth, P.; Polli, J.E.; et al. Biowaiver monographs for immediate-release solid oral dosage forms: Codeine phosphate. *J. Pharm. Sci.* **2014**, *103*, 1592–1600. [CrossRef]
21. Markovic, M.; Zur, M.; Fine-Shamir, N.; Haimov, E.; González-Álvarez, I.; Dahan, A. Segmental-dependent solubility and permeability as key factors guiding controlled release drug product development. *Pharmaceutics* **2020**, *12*, 295. [CrossRef]
22. Zur, M.; Cohen, N.; Agbaria, R.; Dahan, A. The biopharmaceutics of successful controlled release drug product: Segmental-dependent permeability of glipizide vs. metoprolol throughout the intestinal tract. *Int. J. Pharm.* **2015**, *489*, 304–310. [CrossRef]
23. Zur, M.; Gasparini, M.; Wolk, O.; Amidon, G.L.; Dahan, A. The low/high BCS permeability class boundary: Physicochemical comparison of metoprolol and labetalol. *Mol. Pharm.* **2014**, *11*, 1707–1714. [CrossRef]
24. Granero, G.E.; Longhi, M.R.; Mora, M.J.; Junginger, H.E.; Midha, K.K.; Shah, V.P.; Stavchansky, S.; Dressman, J.B.; Barends, D.M. Biowaiver monographs for immediate release solid oral dosage forms: Furosemide. *J. Pharm. Sci.* **2010**, *99*, 2544–2556. [CrossRef] [PubMed]
25. Wagner, J.G.; Sedman, A.J. Quantitaton of rate of gastrointestinal and buccal absorption of acidic and basic drugs based on extraction theory. *J. Pharmacokinet. Biopharm.* **1973**, *1*, 23–50. [CrossRef]
26. Winne, D. Shift of pH-absorption curves. *J. Pharmacokinet. Biopharm.* **1977**, *5*, 53–94. [CrossRef]
27. Berthod, A.; Carda-Broch, S.; Garcia-Alvarez-Coque, M.C. Hydrophobicity of ionizable compounds. A theoretical study and measurements of diuretic octanol−water partition coefficients by countercurrent chromatography. *Anal. Chem.* **1999**, *71*, 879–888. [CrossRef]

28. Henchoz, Y.; Guillarme, D.; Martel, S.; Rudaz, S.; Veuthey, J.L.; Carrupt, P.A. Fast log P determination by ultra-high-pressure liquid chromatography coupled with UV and mass spectrometry detections. *Anal. Bioanal. Chem.* **2009**, *394*, 1919–1930. [CrossRef]
29. Teksin, Z.S.; Hom, K.; Balakrishnan, A.; Polli, J.E. Ion pair-mediated transport of metoprolol across a three lipid-component PAMPA system. *J. Control. Release Off. J. Control. Release Soc.* **2006**, *116*, 50–57. [CrossRef]
30. Lozoya-Agullo, I.; Gonzalez-Alvarez, I.; Zur, M.; Fine-Shamir, N.; Cohen, Y.; Markovic, M.; Garrigues, T.M.; Dahan, A.; Gonzalez-Alvarez, M.; Merino-Sanjuán, M.; et al. Closed-loop doluisio (colon, small intestine) and single-pass intestinal perfusion (colon, jejunum) in rat—Biophysical model and predictions based on Caco-2. *Pharm. Res.* **2017**, *35*, 2. [CrossRef]
31. Lozoya-Agullo, I.; Zur, M.; Fine-Shamir, N.; Markovic, M.; Cohen, Y.; Porat, D.; Gonzalez-Alvarez, I.; Gonzalez-Alvarez, M.; Merino-Sanjuan, M.; Bermejo, M.; et al. Investigating drug absorption from the colon: Single-pass vs. Doluisio approaches to in-situ rat large-intestinal perfusion. *Int. J. Pharm.* **2017**, *527*, 135–141. [CrossRef]
32. Lozoya-Agullo, I.; Zur, M.; Wolk, O.; Beig, A.; Gonzalez-Alvarez, I.; Gonzalez-Alvarez, M.; Merino-Sanjuan, M.; Bermejo, M.; Dahan, A. In-situ intestinal rat perfusions for human Fabs prediction and BCS permeability class determination: Investigation of the single-pass vs. the Doluisio experimental approaches. *Int. J. Pharm.* **2015**, *480*, 1–7. [CrossRef]
33. Dahan, A.; Miller, J.M.; Hilfinger, J.M.; Yamashita, S.; Yu, L.X.; Lennernas, H.; Amidon, G.L. High-permeability criterion for BCS classification: Segmental/pH dependent permeability considerations. *Mol. Pharm.* **2010**, *7*, 1827–1834. [CrossRef]
34. Wolk, O.; Markovic, M.; Porat, D.; Fine-Shamir, N.; Zur, M.; Beig, A.; Dahan, A. Segmental-dependent intestinal drug permeability: Development and model validation of in silico predictions guided by in vivo permeability values. *J. Pharm. Sci.* **2019**, *108*, 316–325. [CrossRef]
35. Kelly, M.R.; Cutler, R.E.; Forrey, A.W.; Kimpel, B.M. Pharmacokinetics of orally administered furosemide. *Clin. Pharmacol. Ther.* **1974**, *15*, 178–186. [CrossRef]
36. Benet, L.Z. Pharmacokinetics/pharmacodynamics of furosemide in man: A review. *J. Pharmacokinet. Biopharm.* **1979**, *7*, 1–27. [CrossRef]
37. Hammarlund, M.M.; Paalzow, L.K.; Odlind, B. Pharmacokinetics of furosemide in man after intravenous and oral administration. Application of moment analysis. *Eur. J. Clin. Pharmacol.* **1984**, *26*, 197–207. [CrossRef]
38. Agoram, B.; Woltosz, W.S.; Bolger, M.B. Predicting the impact of physiological and biochemical processes on oral drug bioavailability. *Adv. Drug Deliv. Rev.* **2001**, *50*, S41–S67. [CrossRef]
39. Lin, L.; Wong, H. Predicting oral drug absorption: Mini review on physiologically-based pharmacokinetic models. *Pharmaceutics* **2017**, *9*, 41. [CrossRef]
40. Lu, A.T.K.; Frisella, M.E.; Johnson, K.C. Dissolution modeling: Factors affecting the dissolution rates of polydisperse powders. *Pharm. Res.* **1993**, *10*, 1308–1314. [CrossRef]
41. Grahnén, A.; Hammarlund, M.; Lundqvist, T. Implications of intraindividual variability in bioavailability studies of furosemide. *Eur. J. Clin. Pharmacol.* **1984**, *27*, 595–602. [CrossRef]
42. Waller, E.S.; Hamilton, S.F.; Massarella, J.W.; Sharanevych, M.A.; Smith, R.V.; Yakatan, G.J.; Doluisio, J.T. Disposition and absolute bioavailability of furosemide in healthy males. *J. Pharm. Sci.* **1982**, *71*, 1105–1108. [CrossRef]
43. Beermann, B.; Midskov, C. Reduced bioavailability and effect of furosemide given with food. *Eur. J. Clin. Pharmacol.* **1986**, *29*, 725–727. [CrossRef]
44. Dahan, A.; Lennernäs, H.; Amidon, G.L. The fraction dose absorbed, in humans, and high jejunal human permeability relationship. *Mol. Pharm.* **2012**, *9*, 1847–1851. [CrossRef]
45. Lee, M.G.; Chiou, W.L. Evaluation of potential causes for the incomplete bioavailability of furosemide: Gastric first-pass metabolism. *J. Pharm. Biopharm.* **1983**, *11*, 623–640. [CrossRef]
46. Dahlgren, D.; Lennernas, H. Intestinal permeability and drug absorption: Predictive experimental, computational and in vivo approaches. *Pharmaceutics* **2019**, *11*, 411. [CrossRef]
47. Ghadi, R.; Dand, N. BCS class IV drugs: Highly notorious candidates for formulation development. *J. Control. Release Off. J. Control. Release Soc.* **2017**, *248*, 71–95. [CrossRef]
48. Flanagan, S.D.; Cummins, C.L.; Susanto, M.; Liu, X.; Takahashi, L.H.; Benet, L.Z. Comparison of furosemide and vinblastine secretion from cell lines overexpressing multidrug resistance protein (P-glycoprotein) and multidrug resistance-associated proteins (MRP1 and MRP2). *Pharmacology* **2002**, *64*, 126–134. [CrossRef]

49. Takahashi, M.; Washio, T.; Suzuki, N.; Igeta, K.; Fujii, Y.; Hayashi, M.; Shirasaka, Y.; Yamashita, S. Characterization of gastrointestinal drug absorption in cynomolgus monkeys. *Mol. Pharm.* **2008**, *5*, 340–348. [CrossRef]
50. Cao, X.; Yu, L.X.; Barbaciru, C.; Landowski, C.P.; Shin, H.C.; Gibbs, S.; Miller, H.A.; Amidon, G.L.; Sun, D. Permeability dominates in vivo intestinal absorption of P-gp substrate with high solubility and high permeability. *Mol. Pharm.* **2005**, *2*, 329–340. [CrossRef]
51. Englund, G.; Rorsman, F.; Rönnblom, A.; Karlbom, U.; Lazorova, L.; Gråsjö, J.; Kindmark, A.; Artursson, P. Regional levels of drug transporters along the human intestinal tract: Co-expression of ABC and SLC transporters and comparison with Caco-2 cells. *Eur. J. Pharm. Sci.* **2006**, *29*, 269–277. [CrossRef]
52. Zimmermann, C.; Gutmann, H.; Hruz, P.; Gutzwiller, J.-P.; Beglinger, C.; Drewe, J. Mapping of multidrug resistance gene 1 and multidrug resistance-associated protein isoform 1 to 5 mRNA expression along the human intestinal tract. *Drug Metab. Dispos.* **2005**, *33*, 219. [CrossRef]
53. Winiwarter, S.; Bonham, N.M.; Ax, F.; Hallberg, A.; Lennernäs, H.; Karlén, A. Correlation of human jejunal permeability (in vivo) of drugs with experimentally and theoretically derived parameters. A multivariate data analysis approach. *J. Med. Chem.* **1998**, *41*, 4939–4949. [CrossRef]
54. Clark, D.E. Rapid calculation of polar molecular surface area and its application to the prediction of transport phenomena. 1. Prediction of intestinal absorption. *J. Pharm. Sci.* **1999**, *88*, 807–814. [CrossRef]
55. Palm, K.; Luthman, K.; Ungell, A.-L.; Strandlund, G.; Beigi, F.; Lundahl, P.; Artursson, P. Evaluation of dynamic polar molecular surface area as predictor of drug absorption: Comparison with other computational and experimental predictors. *J. Med. Chem.* **1998**, *41*, 5382–5392. [CrossRef]
56. Ertl, P.; Rohde, B.; Selzer, P. Fast calculation of molecular polar surface area as a sum of fragment-based contributions and its application to the prediction of drug transport properties. *J. Med. Chem.* **2000**, *43*, 3714–3717. [CrossRef]
57. Koziolek, M.; Grimm, M.; Becker, D.; Iordanov, V.; Zou, H.; Shimizu, J.; Wanke, C.; Garbacz, G.; Weitschies, W. Investigation of pH and temperature profiles in the GI tract of fasted human subjects using the intellicap(®) system. *J. Pharm. Sci.* **2015**, *104*, 2855–2863. [CrossRef]
58. Davis, S.S.; Hardy, J.G.; Fara, J.W. Transit of pharmaceutical dosage forms through the small intestine. *Gut* **1986**, *27*, 886–892. [CrossRef]
59. Streubel, A.; Siepmann, J.; Bodmeier, R. Drug delivery to the upper small intestine window using gastroretentive technologies. *Curr. Opin. Pharmacol.* **2006**, *6*, 501–508. [CrossRef]
60. Clear, N.J.; Milton, A.; Humphrey, M.; Henry, B.T.; Wulff, M.; Nichols, D.J.; Anziano, R.J.; Wilding, I. Evaluation of the Intelisite capsule to deliver theophylline and frusemide tablets to the small intestine and colon. *Eur. J. Pharm. Sci. Off. J. Eur. Fed. Pharm. Sci.* **2001**, *13*, 375–384. [CrossRef]
61. Darandale, S.S.; Vavia, P.R. Design of a gastroretentive mucoadhesive dosage form of furosemide for controlled release. *Acta Pharm. Sin. B* **2012**, *2*, 509–517. [CrossRef]
62. Kagan, L.; Lapidot, N.; Afargan, M.; Kirmayer, D.; Moor, E.; Mardor, Y.; Friedman, M.; Hoffman, A. Gastroretentive accordion pill: Enhancement of riboflavin bioavailability in humans. *J. Control. Release Off. J. Control. Release Soc.* **2006**, *113*, 208–215. [CrossRef]
63. Klausner, E.A.; Eyal, S.; Lavy, E.; Friedman, M.; Hoffman, A. Novel levodopa gastroretentive dosage form: In-vivo evaluation in dogs. *J. Control. Release* **2003**, *88*, 117–126. [CrossRef]
64. Israel, S.; Elinav, H.; Elazary, R.; Porat, D.; Gibori, R.; Dahan, A.; Azran, C.; Horwitz, E. Case report of increased exposure to antiretrovirals following sleeve gastrectomy. *Antimicrob. Agents Chemother.* **2020**, *64*. [CrossRef]
65. Porat, D.; Dahan, A. Medication management after bariatric surgery: Providing optimal patient care. *J. Clin. Med.* **2020**, *9*, 1511. [CrossRef]
66. Porat, D.; Markovic, M.; Zur, M.; Fine-Shamir, N.; Azran, C.; Shaked, G.; Czeiger, D.; Vaynshtein, J.; Replyanski, I.; Sebbag, G.; et al. Increased paracetamol bioavailability after sleeve gastrectomy: A crossover pre- vs. post-operative clinical trial. *J. Clin. Med.* **2019**, *8*, 1949. [CrossRef]

Publisher's Note: MDPI stays neutral with regard to jurisdictional claims in published maps and institutional affiliations.

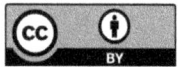

© 2020 by the authors. Licensee MDPI, Basel, Switzerland. This article is an open access article distributed under the terms and conditions of the Creative Commons Attribution (CC BY) license (http://creativecommons.org/licenses/by/4.0/).

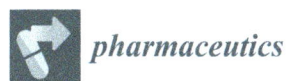

Article

Pharmacokinetic Models to Characterize the Absorption Phase and the Influence of a Proton Pump Inhibitor on the Overall Exposure of Dacomitinib

Ana Ruiz-Garcia [1], Weiwei Tan [2], Jerry Li [2], May Haughey [2], Joanna Masters [2], Jennifer Hibma [2] and Swan Lin [2,*]

[1] Metrum Research Group, San Diego, CA 92121, USA; anar@metrumrg.com
[2] Department of Pharmacometrics, Pfizer Inc, San Diego, CA 92121, USA; weiwei.tan@pfizer.com (W.T.); jerry.li@pfizer.com (J.L.); may.haughey@pfizer.com (M.H.); joanna.c.masters@pfizer.com (J.M.); jennifer.e.hibma@pfizer.com (J.H.)
* Correspondence: swan.lin@pfizer.com; Tel.: +1-(858)-622-7377

Received: 17 March 2020; Accepted: 3 April 2020; Published: 7 April 2020

Abstract: Introduction: Dacomitinib is an epidermal growth factor receptor (EGFR) inhibitor approved for the treatment of metastatic non-small cell lung cancer (NSCLC) in the first line in patients with EGFR activating mutations. Dacomitinib is taken orally once daily at 45 mg with or without food, until disease progression or unacceptable toxicity occurs. Oncology patients often can develop gastroesophageal reflux disease (GERD), which may require management with an acid-reducing agent. Proton pump inhibitors (PPIs), such as rabeprazole, inhibit sodium-potassium adenosine triphosphatase (H^+/K^+-ATPase) pumps that stimulate acid secretion in the stomach and have a prolonged pharmacodynamic effect that extends beyond 24 h post-administration. The aim of this work was to characterize the absorption of dacomitinib via modeling with a particular interest in quantifying the impact of rabeprazole on the pharmacokinetics (PK) of dacomitinib. Materials and Methods: The pooled dataset consisted of five clinical pharmacology healthy volunteer studies, which collected serial pharmacokinetic concentration-time profiles of dacomitinib. Non-linear mixed effects modeling was carried out to characterize dacomitinib pharmacokinetics in the presence and absence of the concomitant use of a PPI, rabeprazole. Several absorption models, some more empirical, and some more physiologically based, were tested: transit compartment, first-order absorption with and without lag time, and variations of combined zero- and first-order absorption kinetics models. Results: The presence of a PPI was a significant covariate affecting the extent (F) and rate (ka) of dacomitinib absorption, as previously reported in the dedicated clinical study. A transit compartment model was able to best describe the absorption phase of dacomitinib.

Keywords: zero-order absorption; first-order absorption; combined zero- and first-order absorption; transit compartment absorption model

1. Introduction

Dacomitinib is currently approved for the first-line treatment of patients with metastatic non-small cell lung cancer (NSCLC) with epidermal growth factor receptor (EGFR) exon 19 deletion or exon 21 L858R substitution mutations [1]. Dacomitinib is a selective, adenosine triphosphate (ATP)-competitive, irreversible, small-molecule inhibitor of the HER (ErbB) family of receptor tyrosine kinases (RTKs), including the epidermal growth factor receptor (EGFR, HER1), the HER2 receptor (ErbB2), the HER4 receptor (ErbB4), and their oncogenic variants (e.g., EGFR with del exon 19 or L858R mutations) [2–4]. Dacomitinib has demonstrated the inhibition of HER1, HER2, and HER4 in biochemical kinase assays, the dose-dependent inhibition of HER1 and phosphorylation of HER2 RTK in tumor xenografts, and the inhibition of tumor growth or tumor regression in experimental models of cancer [5].

In clinical studies in healthy volunteers, following a single oral administration of dacomitinib at 45 mg under fasted conditions, the median time to reach the maximum observed plasma concentration (T_{max}) of dacomitinib ranged from 8 to 10 h after dosing. Dacomitinib undergoes extensive extravascular distribution, with a geometric mean (percent coefficient of variation, CV%) apparent volume of distribution (V_z/F) ranging from 2415 to 4005 L (19–33%). The in vitro binding of dacomitinib to human plasma proteins is approximately 98%. Following a single 45 mg oral dose of dacomitinib, the mean plasma half-life of dacomitinib ranged from 55 to 90 h, and the geometric mean apparent plasma clearance of dacomitinib was approximately 27 to 38 L/h [6–10].

In a Phase 1 crossover study, dacomitinib was administered as a single 45-mg oral dose under fasting conditions to subjects who had received seven daily doses of rabeprazole until steady-state was reached [6]. The median T_{max} of dacomitinib was approximately 12 h, longer than the T_{max} of 8 h seen with dacomitinib alone. Furthermore, exposure to dacomitinib, represented by area under the curve from 0 to 96 h (AUC_{0-96}) and maximum concentration (C_{max}), was reduced with coadministration with rabeprazole at steady state than when dacomitinib was given alone, with adjusted geometric mean ratios (GMR) for AUC_{0-96} and C_{max} of 60.8% and 49.5%, respectively.

The aim of this work was to characterize the PK of dacomitinib via modeling using healthy volunteer data, with a particular interest in quantifying the impact of rabeprazole, administered at a dose of 40 mg daily for 7 days prior to the administration of dacomitinib, on the absorption of dacomitinib.

2. Materials and Methods

The present population PK analysis was based on pooled data from 5 clinical studies in healthy volunteers. All healthy volunteers in the pooled dataset were male. A brief description of each study is provided in this section and in Table 1. For all PK assessments, the date and time of the clinic visit, and the dose, date, and time of the PK sample collection were captured on the case report form (CRF). The dates and times were used to derive the time that elapsed between the PK sample draw and last dose administered (hours post-dose).

Plasma samples were analyzed for the concentrations of dacomitinib at Intertek Pharmaceutical Services (San Diego, CA; formerly known as Alta Analytical Laboratory) using a validated, sensitive, and specific liquid chromatography atmospheric pressure ionization with tandem mass spectrometry (LC-API/MS/MS) method. The assay complied with Pfizer standard operating procedures (SOPs). The performance of the method during validation is documented at the clinical research organization (CRO)/Pfizer method validation report. Plasma specimens were stored at approximately −20 or −70 °C until analysis and assayed within the period of established stability data generated during validation. Calibration standard responses were linear over the range of 1.00 ng/mL to 200 ng/mL for dacomitinib using a weighted (l/concentration2) linear least squares regression. The lower limit of quantification (LLOQ) for dacomitinib was 1.00 ng/mL. Clinical specimens with plasma concentrations below the LLOQ were reported as below limit of quantification (BLQ).

Table 1. Dacomitinib population PK pooled dataset—summary of studies.

Protocol No.	Study Design and Objective	Treatment Groups	No. of Subjects	Duration of Treatment	Study Start/Status
1015	Randomized, single-dose, 2-sequence, and 3-period crossover Phase 1 study. To estimate the BA of a single 45-mg dose of dacomitinib under fed and fasted conditions. To estimate the BA of a single 45-mg dose of dacomitinib administered under antacid drug treatment relative to fasted conditions. To evaluate the safety and tolerability of the proposed formulation in healthy subjects.	Healthy volunteers (Route: oral; Dose Regimen: single 45-mg dose of dacomitinib) 3 conditions (A: antacid treatment, B: fasted, and C: fed)	Planned: 24 Randomized: 24	Single dose each treatment period; 12 Study Days each treatment period with at least a 16-day washout period between each dose.	25 Oct 2012/21 Jan 2013
1021	Open-label, single-fixed sequence, 2-period Phase 1 assessment in extensive CYP2D6 metabolizer subjects. To estimate the effect of paroxetine, on the PK of a single 45-mg dose of dacomitinib. To assess the safety and tolerability of dacomitinib when given alone and when co-administered with paroxetine.	Healthy volunteers (Route: oral; Dose Regimen: Dacomitinib: 45-mg QD. Paroxetine: 30 mg QD) Schedule shown in "Duration of Treatment."	Planned: 14 Randomized: 14	Period 1 (11 days): single 45-mg dose of dacomitinib on Day 1. Period 2 (14 days): single 30-mg doses of paroxetine QD for 3 days, then single 45-mg dose of dacomitinib plus a single 30-mg dose of paroxetine on Day 4. On Days 5 to 10, single 30-mg doses of paroxetine were administered QD. There was washout period of at least 21 days between periods.	28 Mar 2011/08 Jun 2011
1022	Randomized, single-dose, 2-sequence, 2-period crossover Phase 1 study. To determine the relative BA of the proposed 45-mg dacomitinib tablet to 3 × the clinical 15-mg tablet. To assess the inter-subject variability in dacomitinib plasma PK of the proposed 45-mg dacomitinib tablet compared to 3 × the clinical 15-mg tablet in the fasted state. To evaluate the safety and tolerability of the proposed 45-mg dacomitinib tablet and the clinical formulation.	Two treatment periods: Treatment A: 3 × 15-mg single oral dose of, clinical tablets. Treatment B: 45 mg single oral dose of the proposed 45 mg dacomitinib tablet.	Planned: 32 Randomized: 32	Single dose each treatment period; 12 Study Days each treatment period with at least a 16-day washout period between each dose.	04 Apr 2011/20 May 2011
1039	Open-label, randomized, 2-period, 2-treatment, 2-sequence, cross-over, single-dose Phase 1 study. To estimate the effect of a single 45-mg dose of dacomitinib on the PK of a single 30-mg dose of dextromethorphan. To assess the PK of a single dose of dacomitinib and to assess safety and tolerability of dacomitinib and dextromethorphan.	Healthy volunteers (Route: oral; Dose Regimen: Treatment A: A single 30-mg dose of dextro-methorphan. Treatment B: A 45-mg dacomitinib, followed 4 h later by 30 mg of dextro-methorphan)	Planned: 14 Randomized: 14	Two treatment periods followed by a washout period of at least 14 days.	30 Oct 2009/17 Dec 2009
1051	Open-label, non-randomized, 1 period Phase 1 study to characterize the PK of dacomitinib. To characterize the PK of a single 45 mg oral dose of dacomitinib administered under fasted conditions to healthy Chinese volunteers. To evaluate the safety and tolerability of a single 45 mg oral dose of dacomitinib administered under fasted conditions to healthy Chinese volunteers.	Healthy Chinese volunteers (Route: oral; Dose Regimen: single 45-mg dose of dacomitinib)	Planned: 14 Randomized: 14	Single oral dose; total of 12 Study Days.	31 Jul 2014/04 Sep 2014

Abbreviations: BA = bioavailability; CYP = cytochrome P450; PK = pharmacokinetics; QD = once daily.

2.1. Pooled Analysis Dataset

The following studies were included in the pooled dataset and are summarized in Table 1. All studies were approved by an Independent Ethics Committee. All subjects provided written, informed consent prior to study entry. The studies were conducted in accordance with the Declaration of Helsinki and International Conference on Harmonization Good Clinical Practice Guidelines, in addition to meeting all local regulatory requirements. Adverse events (AEs) were monitored throughout the studies and recorded by the investigator, including severity (mild, moderate, or severe), and likely relationship to study treatment for all observed or volunteered AEs. Safety was also assessed by clinical laboratory tests, physical examination, measurement of vital signs (pulse rate and blood pressure), and electrocardiograms (ECGs).

2.1.1. Study 1015

Study 1015 was an open-label, randomized, single-dose, 2-sequence, and 3-period crossover Phase 1 study to investigate the effect of food and the effect of increased gastric pH achieved by treatment with a proton pump inhibitor (PPI) on the PK behavior of dacomitinib in healthy adult subjects [6]. Subjects received a single 45-mg dose of dacomitinib under 3 different conditions or treatments (antacid treatment using rabeprazole, fasted, and fed), with treatments in Period 2 and Period 3 (fed/fasted) assigned in random order with a washout period of at least 16 days between treatments. PK samples were collected at specified times over 264 h post-dose in each period to determine plasma concentrations of dacomitinib.

The pooled data for this population PK analysis include all dacomitinib PK data from subjects who received a single 45-mg dose of dacomitinib with or without PPI under fasted condition and did not include the PK collections under fed conditions.

2.1.2. Study 1021

Study 1021 was an open-label, single fixed sequence, 2 period Phase 1 study in healthy subjects who were CYP2D6 extensive metabolizers [7]. During Period 1, subjects received a single 45-mg dose of dacomitinib. During Period 2, subjects received a single 30-mg dose of paroxetine (a CYP2D6 inhibitor) once daily (QD) for 3 days (Days 1 to 3). On Day 4, subjects were co-administered a 45-mg single dose of dacomitinib plus a single 30-mg dose of paroxetine. Single 30-mg doses of paroxetine were administered QD for the next 6 days (Days 5 to 10). There was a washout period of at least 21 days between dose administration in Periods 1 and 2. Subjects were genotyped for CYP2D6 polymorphism. PK samples were collected at specified time points over 240 h post-dose in each period to determine the plasma concentrations of dacomitinib.

The pooled data for this population PK analysis included all dacomitinib PK data from subjects received a single 45-mg dose of dacomitinib without paroxetine under fasted conditions and did not include the PK collections when dacomitinib was given in combination with paroxetine.

2.1.3. Study 1022

Study 1022 was a single-center, randomized, single-dose crossover study to determine the relative bioavailability of the proposed commercializable 45-mg dacomitinib tablet compared to three 15-mg clinical tablets in the fasted state in healthy subjects [8]. A total of 32 healthy men were enrolled and received treatment. PK samples were collected at specified time points over 264 h post-dose in each period to determine plasma concentrations of dacomitinib.

The pooled data for this population PK analysis included all dacomitinib PK data from all subjects who received a single 45-mg dose of dacomitinib in this study.

2.1.4. Study 1039

Study 1039 was a single-center, randomized, single-dose, 2-treatment crossover study to investigate the effect of dacomitinib co-administration on dextromethorphan exposure, a CYP2D6 probe drug, in healthy adult subjects [9]. Subjects received 2 treatments (Treatment A was single 30-mg oral dose of dextromethorphan; and Treatment B was 45 mg single oral dose of dacomitinib followed 4 h later by a single 30-mg oral dose of dextromethorphan) in random order following an 8-h fast with a washout period of at least 14 days between treatments. Subjects were genotyped for CYP2D6 polymorphism. Serial PK samples were collected at specified times over 144 h (dacomitinib) and 48 h (dextromethorphan) post-dose in each period to determine the plasma concentrations of dextromethorphan, dextrorphan, and dacomitinib. When dacomitinib was co-administered with dextromethorphan, the exposure (AUC and C_{max}) of dextromethorphan was markedly increased (855.4% and 873.5%, respectively). These results suggest that dacomitinib may increase the exposure of other drugs primarily metabolized by CYP2D6.

The pooled data for this population PK analysis include all dacomitinib PK data from all subjects that received a single 45-mg dose of dacomitinib in this study. It should be noted that dextromethorphan did not impact dacomitinib PK; therefore, all dacomitinib PK data from this study was included.

2.1.5. Study 1051

Study 1051 was a single-center, open-label, 1-period, single-dose study to determine the PK of dacomitinib, in healthy male adult Chinese subjects following a single oral dose of 45 mg dacomitinib administered under fasted conditions [10]. Serial PK samples were collected at specified time points over 11 days to determine the plasma concentrations of dacomitinib. A total of 14 healthy Asian subjects were enrolled, received treatment, and were evaluated for PK.

The pooled data for this population PK analysis include all dacomitinib PK data from all subjects that received a single 45-mg dose of dacomitinib in this study.

2.2. Modeling Software and Analysis

All modeling was performed using the NONMEM version 7.4.3 software (ICON Development Solutions, Ellicott City, MD, USA). The stepwise covariate model building procedure (SCM) was executed using Perl-speaks-NONMEM (PsN), version 4.9.0 [11]. For data manipulation, visual predictive checks (VPCs), post-processing, and plotting, R version 3.5.1 (R Foundation for Statistical Computing, Vienna, Austria) was used [12]. The NONMEM population PK dataset included patient identification, dosing information, the time of sample collection, serum concentrations, and other relevant information (e.g., demographics, laboratory test values).

During model building, the goodness of fit (GOF) of different models to the data was evaluated using the following criteria: (1) change in the objective function value (OFV), (2) visual inspection of scatter plots, (3) precision of the parameter estimates, and (4) decreases in both inter-individual variability (IIV) and residual variability. These criteria were used only when the minimization step was successful and standard errors of parameter estimates were obtained using the covariance step. The difference in the OFV between 2 hierarchical models has an approximate χ^2 (chi-square) probability distribution with the number of degrees of freedom (df) equal to the difference in the number of parameters between the models. Based on the χ^2 distribution with df = 1, a change in OFV of 10.83 corresponds to a significance level (α) of 0.001.

The stochastic approximation expectation-maximization (SAEM) estimation method with interaction available in NONMEM was used in the analysis. This method leads to population parameters converging towards the maximum of the exact likelihood. The OFV that is displayed during SAEM analysis is not valid for assessing minimization or for hypothesis testing. It is highly stochastic, and does not represent a marginal likelihood that is integrated over all possible empirical Bayes prediction of the interindividual random effect (ETA, η), but rather, is the likelihood for a given set of ηs. After the stochastic portion was completed, a suitable objective function for hypothesis testing and standard errors was obtained by importance sampling method (IMP) at the final population parameter values [13]. During model building, the GOF of different models to the data was evaluated.

The stability of the models throughout the model development process was closely evaluated. Inspection of the covariance matrix of the estimates at every stage of model development was performed to verify that extreme pairwise correlations of the parameters were not encountered and avoid ill conditioning. Additionally, it was ensured that the condition number of the covariance matrix of the parameter estimates (i.e., the ratio of the largest to smallest eigenvalues, obtained from the PRINT = E option on the covariance block) was less than 1000 [14].

The IIV in the PK parameters was modeled using multiplicative exponential random effects of the form:

$$\theta_i = \theta \cdot e^{\eta_i} \quad (1)$$

where θ (THETA) is the typical individual (population mean) value of the parameter and η_i denotes the interindividual random effect accounting for the ith individual's deviation from the typical value having zero mean and variance ω^2. The approximate CV% was reported as:

$$\%CV = \sqrt{\omega^2} \cdot 100\% \quad (2)$$

The multivariate vector of interindividual random effects (across parameters within each individual) has variance-covariance matrix Ω (OMEGA). The diagonal Ω matrix was applied first and other (unstructured) Ω block structures were also explored by examining the potential correlations among all the empirical Bayes estimates ("post-hoc") of the interindividual random effects (ηs) with the focus on the correlation of the central compartment parameters (e.g., between CL and V). The Ω block was built only if the correlation was observed.

Residual variability (ε) was modeled additively based on log-transformed observation data using thetarized variance-covariance matrix of the intraindividual random effects (σ, SIGMA):

$$\ln(Y_{ij}) = \ln(F_{ij}) + W \cdot \varepsilon_{ij} \quad (3)$$

where $\ln(Y_{ij})$ denotes the observed concentration for the ith patient at time t_j on logarithm scale, the $\ln(F_{ij})$ denotes the corresponding model-predicted concentration on logarithm scale, and ε_{ij} denotes the intraindividual random effect, assumed to have a mean of zero and variance σ^2 of 1. W was the estimated variance of the residual variability that was one of the θs to be estimated.

Adequacy of model fit was assessed through review of diagnostic plots. The result of this stage of model development was considered the final base model.

The only covariate considered in this analysis was the presence or absence of proton pump inhibitor, rabeprazole, on the absorption parameters. PPI was tested for significance in a stepwise manner with statistical criteria of $\alpha = 0.05$ for the forward inclusion step, which corresponds to an OFV change of 3.84 based on a χ^2 distribution with df = 1. The full model was then subjected to a backward elimination step with a statistical criterion of $\alpha = 0.001$, which corresponds to an OFV change of 10.83 based on a χ^2 distribution with df = 1. In order to obtain the most parsimonious and stable final model, the candidate covariate model resulting from the backward elimination step in SCM was subjected to a separate NONMEM run with a $COV step executed to examine any sign of model over parameterization and poorly estimated parameters.

Model adequacy, possible lack of fit, and the violation of assumptions were assessed at all stages of model development. Diagnostic plots of observations (OBS) versus Monte-Carlo-generated population predictions (EPRED) and OBS versus individual predictions (IPRED) were evaluated for randomness around the line of unity. Evaluation was also performed on the longitudinal profiles of PK concentration to compare observations and predictions. The plots of conditional weighted residuals (CWRES), individual weighted residuals (IWRES), and normalized prediction distribution errors (NPDE) versus

EPRED and time after dose were evaluated for randomness around the zero line. The distribution of ηs was checked to ensure approximately normal distribution.

In addition, the plots of ηs in the final model versus the presence or absence of PPI were compared to similar plots for the base model to demonstrate that the final model accounted for trends observed with the base model. The 95% CI around the parameter estimates were generated based on standard error (SE) generated from the NONMEM covariance step.

A comparison of the OFV statistics and parameter estimates for the base and final models was used to assess the degree of parsimony of the final model and to determine the statistical relevance of the covariate effects. A comparison of ω^2 between the models was made to assess the reduction in parameter variability by the inclusion of covariate effects.

Both η-shrinkage (1-SD[η]/w) and ε-shrinkage (1-SD[IWRES]) were evaluated to assess the validity of using post-hoc individual parameter estimates for model diagnosis [15].

The performance of the final model was evaluated by simulating data using the parameter estimates from the final model (fixed and random effects) and conducting a VPC. Simulations were performed using the patients' characteristics as well as the dosing and sampling history from the original dataset. From these simulations, concentration time data were summarized using median (50th), low (2.5th), and high (97.5th) percentiles. The concordance between individual observations and simulated values as well as the distribution of observed and simulated data were evaluated [16,17].

2.3. Absorption Models

The selected studies for this analysis were performed in healthy volunteer subjects under a well-controlled environment where no medications were allowed during the conduct of the trial, with the exception of rabeprazole, that could somehow interfere in the absorption or disposition of dacomitinib. Of note, rabeprazole is not known to impact the metabolism of dacomitinib; thus, the testing of the PPI effect on dacomitinib only occurred on absorption parameters.

Dacomitinib undergoes oxidative metabolism and glutathione conjugation. The oxidative metabolism of dacomitinib involves cytochrome P450 (CYP) 2D6 for the formation of O-desmethyl-dacomitinib and CYP3A for the formation of other minor oxidative metabolites [7,18]. The change in relative bioavailability (F) estimated in this study was the result of the relative change in absorption fraction, as the first pass metabolism should remain the same.

A two-compartment disposition model characterized well the disposition of dacomitinib and was implemented for this analysis [19]. Four different absorption models were tested:

First-order absorption: The disappearance of the drug from the gastrointestinal (GI) tract occurs by a first-order process characterized by an absorption rate constant, k_a. This model was tested with and without the addition of one more parameter: lag time (t_{lag}). T_{lag} often improves the model fit by shifting the time of dosing as if the drug were administered at a later time.

Transit compartment: This model helps with delayed absorption profiles describing drug absorption as a multiple step process represented by a chain of pre-systemic compartments:

$$\frac{da_n}{dt} = k_{tr} \cdot a_{(n-1)} - k_{tr} \cdot a_n \tag{4}$$

where da_n/dt is the rate of change of amount of drug on compartment n at time t, a_n is the drug amount in the nth compartment at time t, k_{tr} is the transit rate constant, and n is the number of transit compartments.

Using Stirling approximation to $n!$, the number of compartments to include can be estimated, avoiding stepwise addition of one compartment at a time.

$$a_n(t) = F \cdot Dose \cdot \frac{(k_{tr} \cdot t)^n}{n!} \cdot e^{-k_{tr} \cdot t} \tag{5}$$

The approximation of Stirling to $n!$:

$$n! \approx \sqrt{2\pi} \cdot n^{n+0.5} \cdot e^{-n} \tag{6}$$

The disappearance of drug from the absorption compartment (dA_a/dt) will be:

$$\frac{dA_a}{dt} = \text{Dose} \cdot F \cdot k_{tr} \cdot \frac{(k_{tr} \cdot t)^n \cdot e^{-k_{tr} \cdot t}}{\sqrt{2\pi} \cdot n^{n+0.5} \cdot e^{-n}} - k_a \cdot A_a \tag{7}$$

This model estimates a mean time of transit (MTT) parameter, which represents the average time spent by dacomitinib traveling from the first transit compartment to the absorption compartment [20]. The number of transit compartments was estimated in the base structural model and subsequently fixed for the characterization of the effect of rabeprazole effect on dacomitinib absorption.

<u>Sequential independent zero-order and first-order model:</u> It is assumed that two different kinetic absorption processes take place. First, a fraction of the dose, F2, is absorbed by zero-order kinetics during a given period of time (D2). The remaining fraction of the dose (1 − F2) is absorbed by first-order kinetics, characterized by ka. These two processes happen sequentially, first the zero-order, followed by the first-order absorption [21]. The database should include two records with the full dose (AMT), one with RATE = −2 and CMT = 2 (zero-order absorption kinetics to the central compartment) and another one with RATE = 0 and CMT = 1 (first-order absorption kinetics from the gastrointestinal (GI) compartment to the central compartment).

<u>Sequential but linked zero- and first-order absorption:</u> A more mechanistic model assumes that the initial absorption process follows zero-order kinetics and is limited by the solubility of dacomitinib in the GI tract fluid [21]. The database format should be similar, as indicated with sequential independent zero- and first-order kinetics. Zero-order kinetics assumes the volume of gut fluid is constant. The duration of this zero-order absorption (D2) ends when the dacomitinib dose has completely dissolved and all of the drug is in solution. The rest of the dose in the GI tract (1 − F2) follows a first-order absorption process characterized by an absorption rate constant k_a. By assuming a link between these two processes, the absorption constant, k_a, does not need to be estimated but rather is derived from F2 and D2 as follows:

$$\text{Absorption zero rate} = \frac{\text{F2} \cdot \text{Dose}}{\text{D2}} \tag{8}$$

Thus, the first order absorption rate constant will begin for all the remaining drug, which is no longer a saturated solution:

$$\text{Absorption zero rate} = \frac{\text{F2} \cdot \text{Dose}}{\text{D2}} = k_a \cdot (1 - \text{F2}) \cdot \text{Dose} \tag{9}$$

$$k_a = \frac{\text{F2}}{(1 - \text{F2}) \cdot \text{D2}} \tag{10}$$

As these analyses estimated changes in relative bioavailability, the bioavailability parameter was fixed to 1. In presence of rabeprazole, changes to the relative bioavailability as well as to the parameters involved in the absorption process (D2, k_a, and MTT) were screened via stepwise covariate modeling.

3. Results

Summary statistics for the different demographic factors: baseline body weight and age are shown in Table 2. The population comprised only male subjects with moderate variability in age and body weight. Figure 1 depicts the observed dacomitinib concentration time profiles using time after first dose by study.

Table 2. Demographic Characteristics for the Pooled Dataset of Dacomitinib Studies.

Study	n	Age (Years) Mean (SD)	Age (Years) Median (Min–Max)	Body Weight (kg) Mean (SD)	Body Weight (kg) Median (Min–Max)
1015	24	36.71 (9.60)	38.00 (21.00–54.00)	79.49 (8.80)	80.40 (65.05–97.80)
1021	14	41.00 (10.02)	43.50 (23.00–54.00)	84.78 (11.20)	84.25 (64.80–102.00)
1022	32	35.97 (10.27)	37.00 (20.00–54.00)	82.02 (10.20)	79.83 (66.10–103.00)
1039	14	39.29 (10.11)	40.00 (21.00–52.00)	79.93 (8.81)	78.00 (67.00–96.00)
1051	14	30.29 (6.67)	29.00 (21.00–43.00)	65.15 (6.26)	63.60 (56.20–73.60)
All Studies	98	36.53 (9.92)	37.00 (20.00–54.00)	79.09 (10.94)	78.35 (56.20–103.00)

Kg: kilogram; Max: maximum; Min: minimum; SD: standard deviation.

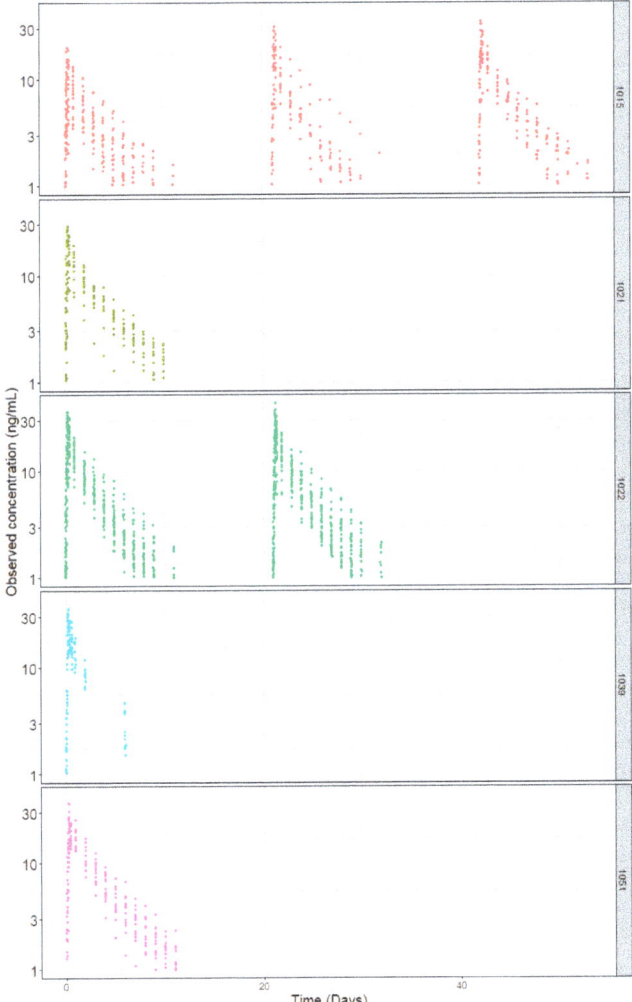

Figure 1. Dacomitinib Concentration-Time Profiles by Study.

The transit compartment model presented a significantly lower OFV than the first-order or combined zero- and first-order absorption models (Supplementary Material, Table S1). The condition number for the transit compartment model did not suggest ill conditioning and the VPC (Figure 2) captured the C_{max} better relative to the other base structural models. Table 3 summarizes the base model parameters for all 4 models tested.

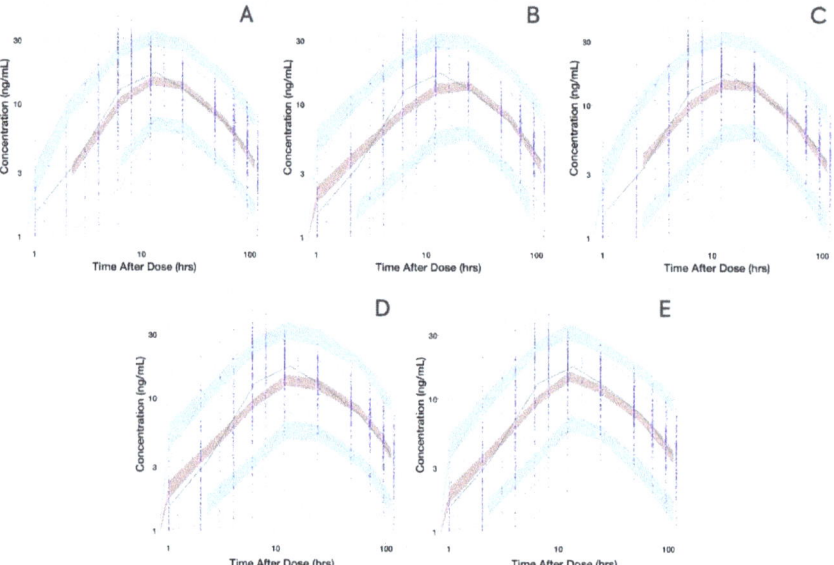

Figure 2. Visual Predictive Check for all Dacomitinib Base Models. (**A**): transit compartment model; (**B**): first-order absorption without lag time; (**C**): first-order absorption with lag time; (**D**): sequential but linked zero- and first-order absorption; (**E**): sequential independent zero- and first-order absorption. Time is presented in logarithmic scale to stretch the time around C_{max} and better appreciate how well the absorption phase is captured. Observed data are presented in blue circles with the 50th percentile of the observed data represented by the solid blue line and the 5th and 95th percentiles of the observed data represented by the dotted blue lines. Red shaded region represents the prediction interval for the 50th percentile. Blue shaded regions represent the prediction intervals at the 5th and 95th percentiles.

Table 3. Parameter Estimates for Dacomitinib Base Structural Models.

Parameter	Estimate (RSE%)				
	Transit	First-Order Absorption		Combined Zero- and First-Order Absorption	
		Without t_{lag}	With t_{lag}	Linked	Independent
CL (L/h)	29.2 (4.212)	30.5 (3.131)	31.0 (2.748)	26.1 (4.215)	28.4 (4.894)
V (L)	131 (10.840)	790 (0.796)	480 (20.833)	2260 (4.093)	1160 (4.052)
Q (L/h)	19.9 (16.583)	23.7 (4.641)	27.9 (18.961)	10.4 (8.135)	4.7 (45.106)
Vss (L)	2300 (16.783)	2300 (4.33)	2040 (3.250)	6000 (11.667)	6590 (9.347)
MTT (h)	6.91 (5.731)				
k_a (h^{-1})	0.0246 (12.48)	0.0419 (4.893)	0.0369 (23.55)		0.00966 (9.979)
F	1 FIX	1 FIX	1 FIX	1 FIX	1 FIX
t_{lag} (h)			0.749 (8.278)		
D2 (h)				9.78 (2.945)	10.4 (2.481)
* F1				0.455 (2.077)	0.0782 (15.729)
Residual error	0.331 (6.133)	0.403 (3.772)	0.346 (5.925)	0.378 (4.259)	0.362 (4.751)

* F1: Fraction absorbed by first order, F1 = 1 − F2.

The differences in PK parameter estimates obtained with the different models were more pronounced for the apparent distribution and clearance parameters, where F was fixed to 1 (CL, V, Q, and Vss) than for the absorption parameters (k_a, D2, and MTT), which are not associated to F. The estimated number of transit compartments for dacomitinib was 1.

Therefore, the transit model was carried forward for the characterization effect of rabeprazole on the dacomitinib absorption phase. The base model was then subjected to graphical examination (ηs versus PPI) to investigate whether the estimated parameters captured the PPI effect.

Figure 3 shows the distribution of the ηs in presence and absence of rabeprazole for each parameter. The presence and absence of rabeprazole was tested for significance in a stepwise manner with statistical criteria of $\alpha = 0.05$ for forward inclusion Using SCM, the full model was reached in three forward selection steps and included the effects of rabeprazole on F and ka. After one backward elimination step ($\alpha = 0.001$, removal of any of these covariates resulted in a more than 10.83 increase in OFV), the final model was achieved. None of the selected parameters identified in the full model were removed in the backward step. The final model, including the covariates, was further tested in NONMEM with a $COV step executed to examine any sign of model over parameterization and poorly estimated parameters. Figure 4 shows that the inclusion of rabeprazole on F and k_a in the final model corrected for the previously observed trend in plots of ηs on apparent CL and volume and k_a. Table 4 tabulates the final parameter estimates for the transit compartment model with the addition of PPI as a covariate on F and k_a.

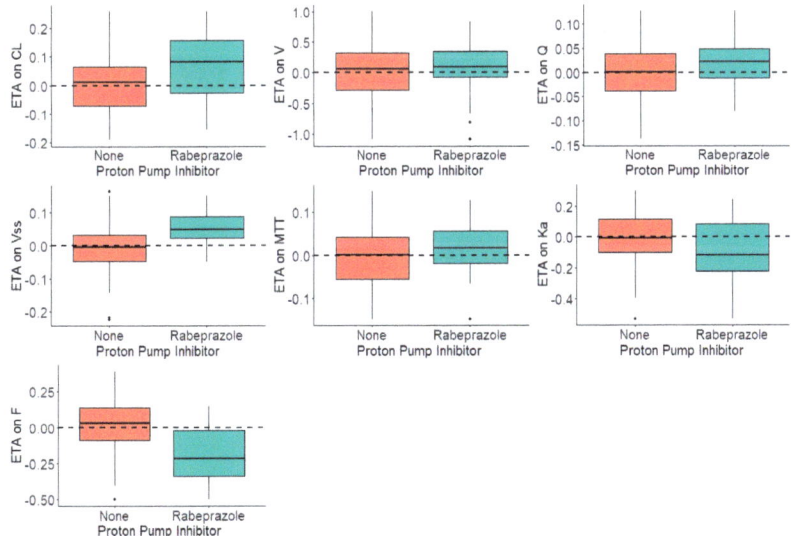

Figure 3. Distribution of ηs (ETAs) by the Presence and Absence of Proton Pump Inhibitor, Rabeprazole, in the Dacomitinib Base Model.

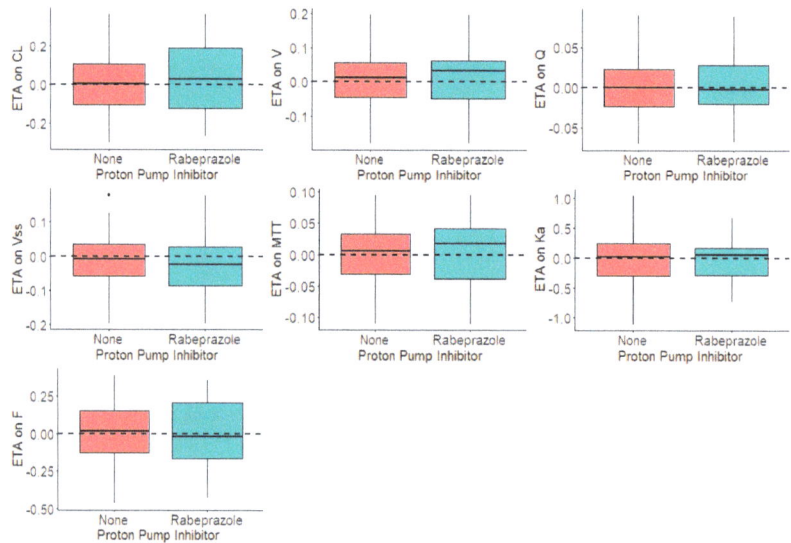

Figure 4. Distribution of ηs (ETAs) by the Presence and Absence of Proton Pump Inhibitor, Rabeprazole, in the Dacomitinib Final Model.

Table 4. Dacomitinib Final Model Pharmacokinetic Parameters Summary.

Parameter	Parameter Estimate	RSE (%)	IIV CV (%)	Shrinkage (%)
Clearance (CL, L/h)	29.893	3.03	18.475	21.56
Volume (V, L)	789.748	9.47	20.000	63.13
Inter-compartmental Clearance (Q, L/h)	76.796	7.62	15.811	77.94
Volume of Distribution at steady-state (Vss, L)	2276.46	3.48	15.811	51.68
Mean Transit Time (MTT, h)	12.033	6.00	15.811	70.55
Absorption Rate constant (k_a, h^{-1})	0.259	16.56	54.904	17.09
PPI on k_a	−0.524	−28.34	NA	NA
PPI on F	−0.487	−15.10	NA	NA
Relative Bioavailability (F)	1 (FIX)	-	23.275	17.17
Proportional Residual Error	0.289	5.23	NA	6.44

CV: coefficient of variation; h: hour; L: liter; NA: not applicable; RSE: relative standard error; IIV: inter-individual variability.

Prediction-based diagnostic plots (Figure 5) on the final model comparing OBS versus EPRED showed that the population prediction was a reasonable measure of central tendency of the data. Given that the ε-shrinkage was only 6.44% in the final model, the plot of OBS versus IPRED was informative and could be used to examine any model misspecification. The magnitude of the spread for OBS versus IPRED was small around the line of identity, indicating that the model predicted the observed concentrations well. Residual-based plots of IWRES, CWRES, and NPDE plotted against population predictions did not indicate any model misspecification of structural model or residual error model (Figure 6). In the plots of IWRES, CWRES, and NPDE versus time after dose, the majority of the data were evenly distributed across the x-axis, indicating no major deviation or trend over the entire observation time in the population (Figure 6).

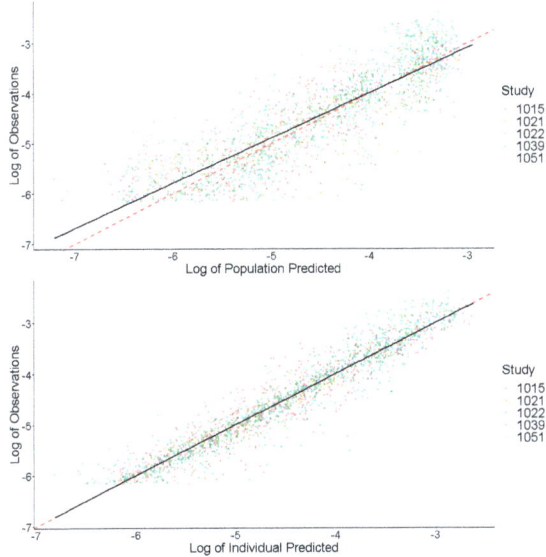

Figure 5. Prediction-Based Diagnostics for Dacomitinib Final Model. Observed concentrations (log transformed) are presented on the *y*-axis. Individual predicted concentrations (log transformed) are presented on the *x*-axis. The red dashed line represents a line of unity, and the black line represents a linear smooth line.

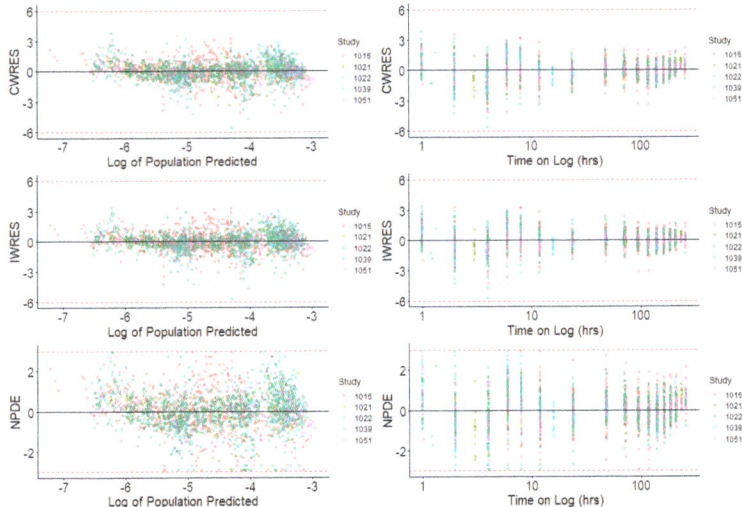

Figure 6. Residual-Based Diagnostics for Dacomitinib Final Model. Residual-based diagnostic plots of conditional weighted residuals (CWRES), individual weighted residuals (IWRES), and normalized prediction distribution errors (NPDE) versus population predicted concentrations (log transformed) on the left side, and time (on log scale) on the right side.

VPCs were performed for the final model, plotting the 5th, 50th, and 95th percentiles for observed data, and the 95% CIs around these percentiles for simulated data. The final model had good predictive performance, with the 5th, 50th, and 95th percentiles of the observed data lying within the 95%

prediction intervals of the simulated 5th, 50th, and 95th percentiles. The results are displayed in Figure 7.

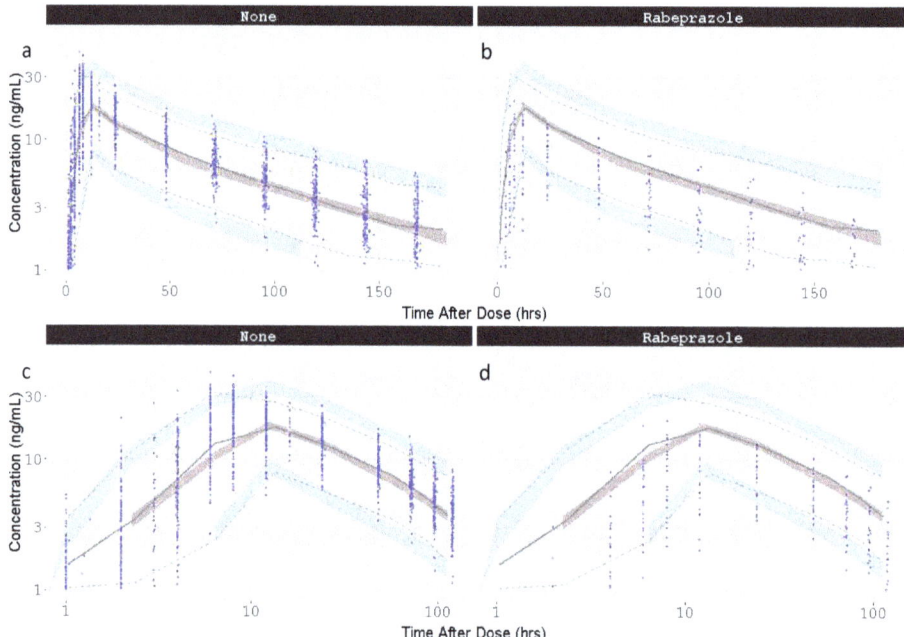

Figure 7. Visual Predictive Check for the Dacomitinib Final Model by Concomitant administration of Rabeprazole. Time is presented in linear and logarithmic scale to stretch the time around C_{max} and better appreciate how well the absorption phase is captured. (**a**) Dacomitinib without rabeprazole co-administation; (**b**) Dacomitinib with rabeprazole co-administration; (**c**) Dacomitinib without rabeprazole co-administation with time in the log scale; (**d**) Dacomitinib with rabeprazole co-administation with time in the log scale. Observed data are presented in blue circles with the 50th percentile of the observed data represented by the solid blue line and the 5th and 95th percentiles of the observed data represented by the dotted blue lines. Red shaded region represents the prediction interval for the 50th percentile. Blue shaded regions represent the prediction intervals at the 5th and 95th percentiles.

4. Discussion

Drug absorption is a complex process dependent on several variables, including pharmaceutical form (immediate release formulation, control release formulation, etc.), which determines the liberation of the drug from the formulation, physicochemical properties of the drug, and the physiological processes of the GI. Dissolution, solubility and permeability driven by the physicochemical properties of the active ingredient are the main factors affecting drug absorption, as reported by the Biopharmaceutical Classification System (BCS) [22–24]. Several physiological processes may affect drug absorption, including gut motility, pH, gastric emptying rate, and metabolism in the gut wall. The rate, extent, and length of time before the drug appears in the systemic circulation are often determined by a combination of these factors.

The use of physiology-based absorption models has been developed to account for physicochemical properties as well as many physiological processes. These mechanistic models require extensive prior knowledge not usually available, preventing the routine application of them in drug absorption estimation. The transit compartment model approximates to a physiological model as the presence of transit compartments describes the concentration-time profiles as a gradually increasing continuous function. Transit compartments describe a delay in absorption or a prolonged absorption phase as drug moves through a chain of identical compartments that are linked to the central compartment by a first-order absorption process explaining the delay in absorption in a smoother way than the lag time.

The parameter estimate D2, obtained with the base structural model for linked (9.78 h) and independent (10.4 h) combination kinetics, and the final MTT estimate (12 h) are all of similar magnitude, indicating that the absorption process takes place over at least 12 h, which is close to the observed T_{max} (see Figures 2 and 7). However, the estimated lag time was 0.749 h, which is close to the first concentration after dosing (1 h), suggesting that this parameter may be biased by the collection time of the first sampling.

This dacomitinib population pharmacokinetic analysis was based on pooled data from five clinical trials in healthy volunteer studies under well-controlled conditions. In these studies, dacomitinib was administered as a single dose under fasting conditions. Study 1015 concluded that there was no effect of food on dacomitinib PK; as such, the prescribing labels recommend dosing dacomitinib with or without food. This pooled population PK analysis demonstrated that a 2-compartment PK model with one transit compartment and a mean transit time of 12 h followed by a first-order constant rate of absorption accurately described the concentration time course of dacomitinib. Rabeprazole was a statistically significant predictor of relative bioavailability and ka variability. When rabeprazole is concomitantly administered with dacomitinib, the relative bioavailability and absorption rate constant of dacomitinib decreased by 52% and 49%, respectively.

For class II compounds, such as dacomitinib, for which solubility is pH dependent (the water solubility of dacomitinib dramatically decreases as pH exceeds 4.5), the administration of acid-reducing drugs may affect bioavailability (refer to Supplementary Material, Figure S1, for dacomitinib chemical structure and pKa). This is of particular concern in cancer patients, as concomitant use of acid-reducing agents such as PPIs is common, and several other small-molecule tyrosine kinase inhibitors (TKIs) undergo changes in drug exposure with use of these agents. The effects of the coadministration of a TKI with an acid-reducing agent have been reported with erlotinib [25,26], nilotinib [27], gefitinib [28], bosutinib [29], lapatinib [30], neratinib [31], nilotinib [32], and pazopanib [33], decreasing AUC by 46%, 34%, 44%, 26%, 26%, 65%, 34%, and 40%, respectively. Therefore, with anticancer agents, there is concern for a risk of not achieving therapeutic plasma concentrations.

5. Conclusions

Cancer patients are heavily medicated and may develop GERD as a result of anti-cancer treatment and progressive disease. Thus, patients often require acid-reducing agents for gastroprotection and symptom management. Based on the conclusions from Study 1015 and the population PK modeling, PPIs are not recommended to be used with dacomitinib treatment. Unlike the prolonged effect of PPIs, local antacids have a mild and short-acting acid-reducing effect. Patients treated with dacomitinib may be able to use shorter-acting acid-reducing agents, such as H_2-receptor antagonists and local antacids, and avoid treatment with PPIs.

Supplementary Materials: The following are available online at http://www.mdpi.com/1999-4923/12/4/330/s1, Figure S1: Assignment of pKa to the Dacomitinib Structure, Table S1: Dacomitinib Absorption Models: Base Structural Model Objective Function Value and Condition Number.

Author Contributions: Formal analysis, A.R.-G.; Supervision, W.T. and S.L.; Validation, J.L., M.H. and J.H.; Writing—original draft, A.R.-G.; Writing—review & editing, W.T., J.L., M.H., J.M., J.H. and S.L. All authors have read and agreed to the published version of the manuscript.

Funding: This research was funded by Pfizer Inc.

Conflicts of Interest: The authors declare no conflict of interest. W.T., J.L., M.H., J.M., J.H., and S.L. are current employees of Pfizer and A.R.-G. was a former employee of Pfizer. The company had no role in the design of the study; in the collection, analyses, or interpretation of data; in the writing of the manuscript, or in the decision to publish the results.

References

1. Vizimpro® (Dacomitinib) Tablet: Us Prescribing Information. Available online: https://www.Accessdata.Fda.Gov/Drugsatfda_Docs/Label/2018/211288s000lbl.Pdf (accessed on 21 February 2020).
2. Gonzales, A.J.; Hook, K.E.; Althaus, I.W.; Ellis, P.A.; Trachet, E.; Delaney, A.M.; Harvey, P.J.; Ellis, T.A.; Amato, D.M.; Nelson, J.M.; et al. Antitumor Activity and Pharmacokinetic Properties of Pf-00299804, a Second-Generation Irreversible Pan-Erbb Receptor Tyrosine Kinase Inhibitor. *Mol. Cancer Ther.* **2008**, *7*, 1880–1889. [CrossRef] [PubMed]
3. Engelman, J.A.; Zejnullahu, K.; Gale, C.M.; Lifshits, E.; Gonzales, A.J.; Shimamura, T.; Zhao, F.; Vincent, P.W.; Naumov, G.N.; Bradner, J.E.; et al. Pf00299804, an Irreversible Pan-Erbb Inhibitor, Is Effective in Lung Cancer Models with Egfr and Erbb2 Mutations That Are Resistant to Gefitinib. *Cancer Res.* **2007**, *67*, 11924–11932. [CrossRef] [PubMed]
4. Schwartz, P.A.; Kuzmic, P.; Solowiej, J.; Bergqvist, S.; Bolanos, B.; Almaden, C.; Nagata, A.; Ryan, K.; Feng, J.; Dalvie, D.; et al. Covalent EGFR Inhibitor Analysis Reveals Importance of Reversible Interactions to Potency and Mechanisms of Drug Resistance. *Proc. Natl. Acad. Sci. USA* **2014**, *111*, 173–178. [CrossRef] [PubMed]
5. Kalous, O.; Conklin, D.; Desai, A.J.; O'Brien, N.A.; Ginther, C.; Anderson, L.; Cohen, D.J.; Britten, C.D.; Taylor, I.; Christensen, J.G.; et al. Dacomitinib (PF-00299804), an Irreversible Pan-Her Inhibitor, Inhibits Proliferation of Her2-Amplified Breast Cancer Cell Lines Resistant to Trastuzumab and Lapatinib. *Mol. Cancer Ther.* **2012**, *11*, 1978–1987. [CrossRef]
6. Ruiz-Garcia, A.; Masters, J.C.; Mendes da Costa, L.; LaBadie, R.R.; Liang, Y.; Ni, G.; Ellery, C.A.; Boutros, T.; Goldberg, Z.; Bello, C.L. Effect of Food or Proton Pump Inhibitor Treatment on the Bioavailability of Dacomitinib in Healthy Volunteers. *J. Clin. Pharmacol.* **2016**, *56*, 223–230. [CrossRef]
7. Ruiz-Garcia, A.; Giri, N.; LaBadie, R.R.; Ni, G.; Boutros, T.; Richie, N.; Kocinsky, H.S.; Checchio, T.M.; Bello, C.L. A Phase I Open-Label Study to Investigate the Potential Drug–Drug Interaction between Single-Dose Dacomitinib and Steady-State Paroxetine in Healthy Volunteers. *J. Clin. Pharmacol.* **2014**, *54*, 555–562. [CrossRef]
8. A Bioequivalence (Be) Study Comparing the Commericializable and Clinical Formulations of Pf-00299804. Clinicaltrials.Gov Identifier: Nct01313793. Available online: https://Clinicaltrials.Gov/Ct2/Show/Nct01313793?Term=Pf-00299804%2c+Healthy+Volunteer&Draw=2&Rank=5 (accessed on 21 February 2020).
9. Bello, C.L.; LaBadie, R.R.; Ni, G.; Boutros, T.; McCormick, C.; Ndongo, M.N. The Effect of Dacomitinib (Pf-00299804) on Cyp2d6 Activity in Healthy Volunteers Who Are Extensive or Intermediate Metabolizers. *Cancer Chemother. Pharmacol.* **2012**, *69*, 991–997. [CrossRef]
10. Chen, X.; Jiang, J.; Giri, N.; Hu, P. Phase 1 Study to Investigate the Pharmacokinetic Properties of Dacomitinib in Healthy Adult Chinese Subjects Genotyped for Cyp2d6. *Xenobiotica* **2018**, *48*, 459–466. [CrossRef]
11. Harling, K.; Hooker, A.; Ueckert, S.; Jonsson, E.; Karlsson, M.O. Perl speaks Nonmem (PsN) and Xpose. In Proceedings of the Population Approach Group in Europe (PAGE), Berlin, Germany, 9–11 June 2010.
12. R Development Core Team. *2014 R: A Language and Environment for Statistical Computing*; R Foundation for Statistical Computing: Vienna, Austria, 2014.
13. Bauer, R.J. Nonmem Users Guide Introduction to Nonmem 7.5.0. Available online: https://Nonmem.Iconplc.Com/Nonmem75b3/Intro7.Pdf?Token=E2911eb1-54d0-11ea-A325-005056911489&Html (accessed on 28 February 2020).
14. Bonate, P.L.; Strougo, A.; Desai, A.; Roy, M.; Yassen, A.; van der Walt, J.S.; Kaibara, A.; Tannenbaum, S. Guidelines for the Quality Control of Population Pharmacokinetic-Pharmacodynamic Analyses: An Industry Perspective. *AAPS J.* **2012**, *14*, 749–758. [CrossRef]
15. Savic, R.M.; Karlsson, M.O. Importance of Shrinkage in Empirical Bayes Estimates for Diagnostics: Problems and Solutions. *AAPS J.* **2009**, *11*, 558–569. [CrossRef]
16. Holford, N.H. An Introduction to Visual Predictive Checks. Available online: https://130.216.88.98/Docs/Vpc-Tutorial-and-Datatop.Pdf (accessed on 28 February 2020).
17. Bergstrand, M.; Hooker, A.C.; Wallin, J.E.; Karlsson, M.O. Prediction-Corrected Visual Predictive Checks for Diagnosing Nonlinear Mixed-Effects Models. *AAPS J.* **2011**, *13*, 143–151. [CrossRef] [PubMed]

18. Bello, C.L.; Smith, E.; Ruiz-Garcia, A.; Ni, G.; Alvey, C.; Loi, C.M. A Phase I, Open-Label, Mass Balance Study of [^{14}C] Dacomitinib (PF-00299804) in Healthy Male Volunteers. *Cancer Chemother. Pharmacol.* **2013**, *72*, 379–385. [CrossRef] [PubMed]
19. Giri, N.; Upton, R.; Mould, D.R.; Bello, C.L.; Amantea, M.A. Population Pharmacokinetic Model (Poppk) for Dacomitinib and Its Metabolite in Healthy Volunteers (HV) and Patients with Advanced Solid Tumors. *J. Pharmacokinet. Pharmacodyn.* **2015**, *42*, S29–S30.
20. Savic, R.M.; Jonker, D.M.; Kerbusch, T.; Karlsson, M.O. Implementation of a Transit Compartment Model for Describing Drug Absorption in Pharmacokinetic Studies. *J. Pharmacokinet. Pharmacodyn.* **2007**, *34*, 711–726. [CrossRef]
21. Holford, N.H.; Ambros, R.J.; Stoeckel, K. Models for Describing Absorption Rate and Estimating Extent of Bioavailability: Application to Cefetamet Pivoxil. *J. Pharmacokinet. Biopharm.* **1992**, *20*, 421–442. [CrossRef] [PubMed]
22. Amidon, G.L.; Lennernas, H.; Shah, V.P.; Crison, J.R. A Theoretical Basis for a Biopharmaceutic Drug Classification: The Correlation of in Vitro Drug Product Dissolution and in Vivo Bioavailability. *Pharm. Res.* **1995**, *12*, 413–420. [CrossRef]
23. Yu, L.X.; Amidon, G.L.; Polli, J.E.; Zhao, H.; Mehta, M.U.; Conner, D.P.; Shah, V.P.; Lesko, L.J.; Chen, M.L.; Lee, V.H.; et al. Biopharmaceutics Classification System: The Scientific Basis for Biowaiver Extensions. *Pharm. Res.* **2002**, *19*, 921–925. [CrossRef]
24. Guidance for Industry: Immediate Release Solid Oral Dosage Forms. Available online: https://www.Fda.Gov/Media/70949/Download (accessed on 28 February 2020).
25. Grunwald, V.; Hidalgo, M. Development of the Epidermal Growth Factor Receptor Inhibitor Tarceva (Osi-774). *Adv. Exp. Med. Biol.* **2003**, *532*, 235–246.
26. Shepherd, F.A.; Rodrigues Pereira, J.; Ciuleanu, T.; Tan, E.H.; Hirsh, V.; Thongprasert, S.; Campos, D.; Maoleekoonpiroj, S.; Smylie, M.; Martins, R.; et al. Erlotinib in Previously Treated Non-Small-Cell Lung Cancer. *N. Engl. J. Med.* **2005**, *353*, 123–132. [CrossRef]
27. Tasigna® (Nilotinib) Capsules: Us Prescribing Information. Available online: https://www.Accessdata.Fda.Gov/Drugsatfda_Docs/Label/2019/022068s031lbl.Pdf (accessed on 21 February 2020).
28. Iressa® (Gefitinib) Tablets: Us Prescribing Information. Available online: https://www.Accessdata.Fda.Gov/Drugsatfda_Docs/Label/2018/206995s003lbl.Pdf (accessed on 21 February 2020).
29. Abbas, R.; Leister, C.; Sonnichsen, D. A Clinical Study to Examine the Potential Effect of Lansoprazole on the Pharmacokinetics of Bosutinib When Administered Concomitantly to Healthy Subjects. *Clin. Drug Investig.* **2013**, *33*, 589–595. [CrossRef]
30. Koch, K.M.; Im, Y.H.; Kim, S.B.; Urruticoechea Ribate, A.; Stephenson, J.; Botbyl, J.; Cartee, L.; Holshouser, J.; Ridgway, D. Effects of Esomeprazole on the Pharmacokinetics of Lapatinib in Breast Cancer Patients. *Clin. Pharmacol. Drug Dev.* **2013**, *2*, 336–341. [CrossRef] [PubMed]
31. Keyvanjah, K.; DiPrimeo, D.; Li, A.; Obaidi, M.; Swearingen, D.; Wong, A. Pharmacokinetics of Neratinib During Coadministration with Lansoprazole in Healthy Subjects. *Br. J. Clin. Pharmacol.* **2017**, *83*, 554–561. [CrossRef] [PubMed]
32. Yin, O.Q.; Gallagher, N.; Fischer, D.; Demirhan, E.; Zhou, W.; Golor, G.; Schran, H. Effect of the Proton Pump Inhibitor Esomeprazole on the Oral Absorption and Pharmacokinetics of Nilotinib. *J. Clin. Pharmacol.* **2010**, *50*, 960–967. [CrossRef] [PubMed]
33. Tan, A.R.; Gibbon, D.G.; Stein, M.N.; Lindquist, D.; Edenfield, J.W.; Martin, J.C.; Gregory, C.; Suttle, A.B.; Tada, H.; Botbyl, J.; et al. Effects of Ketoconazole and Esomeprazole on the Pharmacokinetics of Pazopanib in Patients with Solid Tumors. *Cancer Chemother. Pharmacol.* **2013**, *71*, 1635–1643. [CrossRef] [PubMed]

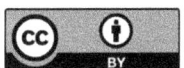

© 2020 by the authors. Licensee MDPI, Basel, Switzerland. This article is an open access article distributed under the terms and conditions of the Creative Commons Attribution (CC BY) license (http://creativecommons.org/licenses/by/4.0/).

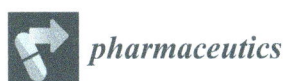

Article

Regional Intestinal Drug Permeability and Effects of Permeation Enhancers in Rat

David Dahlgren [1], Maria-Jose Cano-Cebrián [2], Tobias Olander [1], Mikael Hedeland [3,4], Markus Sjöblom [5] and Hans Lennernäs [1,*]

[1] Department of Pharmacy, Division of Biopharmaceutics, Uppsala University, 752 36 Uppsala, Sweden; david.dahlgren@farmaci.uu.se (D.D.); olander92@hotmail.com (T.O.)
[2] Department of Pharmacy and Pharmaceutical Technology and Parasitology, University of Valencia, 46010 València, Spain; Maria.Jose.Cano@uv.es
[3] Department of Medicinal Chemistry, Analytical Pharmaceutical Chemistry, Uppsala University, 752 36 Uppsala, Sweden; mikael.hedeland@ilk.uu.se
[4] Department of Chemistry, Environment and Feed Hygiene, National Veterinary Institute (SVA), 751 89 Uppsala, Sweden
[5] Department of Neuroscience, Division of Physiology, Uppsala University, 752 36 Uppsala, Sweden; Markus.Sjoblom@neuro.uu.se
* Correspondence: hans.lennernas@farmaci.uu.se

Received: 23 January 2020; Accepted: 3 March 2020; Published: 8 March 2020

Abstract: Sufficient colonic absorption is necessary for all systemically acting drugs in dosage forms that release the drug in the large intestine. Preclinically, colonic absorption is often investigated using the rat single-pass intestinal perfusion model. This model can determine intestinal permeability based on luminal drug disappearance, as well as the effect of permeation enhancers on drug permeability. However, it is uncertain how accurate the rat single-pass intestinal perfusion model predicts regional intestinal permeability and absorption in human. There is also a shortage of systematic in vivo investigations of the direct effect of permeation enhancers in the small and large intestine. In this rat single-pass intestinal perfusion study, the jejunal and colonic permeability of two low permeability drugs (atenolol and enalaprilat) and two high-permeability ones (ketoprofen and metoprolol) was determined based on plasma appearance. These values were compared to already available corresponding human data from a study conducted in our lab. The colonic effect of four permeation enhancers—sodium dodecyl sulfate, chitosan, ethylenediaminetetraacetic acid (EDTA), and caprate—on drug permeability and transport of chromium EDTA (an established clinical marker for intestinal barrier integrity) was determined. There was no difference in jejunal and colonic permeability determined from plasma appearance data of any of the four model drugs. This questions the validity of the rat single-pass intestinal perfusion model for predicting human regional intestinal permeability. It was also shown that the effect of permeation enhancers on drug permeability in the colon was similar to previously reported data from the rat jejunum, whereas the transport of chromium EDTA was significantly higher ($p < 0.05$) in the colon than in jejunum. Therefore, the use of permeation enhancers for increasing colonic drug permeability has greater risks than potential medical rewards, as indicated by the higher permeation of chromium EDTA compared to the drugs.

Keywords: regional intestinal permeability; permeation enhancers; absorption-modifying excipients; oral peptide delivery; intestinal perfusion; pharmaceutical development

1. Introduction

The rat single-pass intestinal perfusion (SPIP) model investigates epithelial membrane permeability, a key biopharmaceutical variable in drug absorption following oral intake [1]. The model is therefore frequently used in pharmaceutical development to evaluate the potential success of a drug, for instance with oral modified-release (MR) dosage forms. In MR dosage forms, the drug is released throughout the gastrointestinal (GI) tract prior to absorption so the regional intestinal permeability needs to be sufficiently high in both the small and large intestine. The rat and human small intestine have similar drug intestinal absorption profiles and transporter expression patterns, but differ in their enzymatic metabolism [2]. Differences in absorption from the rat and human colon have not been extensively compared, but a recent meta-analysis of rat SPIP data reports regional differences in drug permeability for 42 drugs in this species [3].

How relevant for humans are the regional intestinal drug permeability values determined in the rat SPIP model? It is difficult to answer this because of the limited amount of human reference permeability data from the lower GI tract (colon), and inter-laboratory variability in permeability determinations using the rat SPIP model [3,4]. Foremost, it is inherently difficult to accurately determine the luminal disappearance of medium-to-low permeability drugs in the SPIP model. Permeability is often overestimated for drugs with a low permeability because differences in the perfusate concentrations entering and leaving the perfused segment may be too small for accurate quantification. To circumvent this problem for low-permeation compounds, the drug permeability can be determined on the basis of plasma appearance data of intact drug (corrected for first-pass extraction) [5]. For instance, a recent study in the rat jejunum showed that the permeability value of the low permeability drugs atenolol and enalaprilat was >10 times higher in the same rat when determined from luminal disappearance, compared to plasma appearance [5]. In the same rat study, as well as in a human study, there were no differences for the high-permeability compounds metoprolol and ketoprofen. Thus, the choice of determination method seems to be important only for low-permeation compounds [4]. Accordingly, there is need for an evaluation of the human in vivo predictive relevance of regional intestinal drug permeability values determined from plasma appearance in the rat SPIP model.

The rat SPIP model may also be used to investigate regional intestinal differences in how pharmaceutical excipient(s) affect drug permeation and overall absorption rate. This is especially relevant because of the renewed interest in permeation enhancers (PE), also called absorption-modifying excipients (AME), for enabling oral administration of low-permeation compounds, for example, peptides [6,7]. Some advocates of this formulation approach propose the colon as a potential target for PEs, because the colon has a longer residence time, its mucosa may be more easily affected, and it does not have the higher peptidase activity of the upper GI tract [8,9].

However, few comparisons of the small and large intestine in rat have been made on the direct permeability effects of PEs in the same laboratory. Even fewer comparisons have used in vivo models, which are substantially more resilient to intestinal PE effects than in vitro models such as cell- and tissue-based systems [10]. Accordingly, there is a need for a systematic evaluation of PE effects in the small and large intestine in the more relevant in vivo permeability models, such as SPIP.

The primary objective of this rat SPIP study was to investigate the regional intestinal differences (jejunum vs colon) in lumen-to-blood drug permeability, as determined from plasma appearance data. Permeability values were determined at both pH 6.5 and 7.4 for two low permeability model drugs (atenolol and enalaprilat) and for two high-permeation ones (ketoprofen and metoprolol). The second objective was to evaluate the relevance of the rat model, by comparing the regional intestinal permeability values with reported values of three model drugs (not enalaprilat) in human, as determined from plasma drug appearance. The third objective was to investigate the effect in the rat colon of four PEs with different mechanisms of action: sodium dodecyl sulfate (SDS), chitosan, ethylenediaminetetraacetic acid (EDTA), and sodium caprate. These four PEs have previous rat jejunal reference values at the same luminal concentrations determined at our laboratory [11,12]. The PE effects were evaluated based on changes in permeability of the four model drugs, and in blood-to-lumen clearance of ^{51}chromium-labeled ethylenediaminetetraacetate ($CL_{Cr\text{-}EDTA}$), an established clinical marker for mucosal barrier integrity [13].

2. Materials and Methods

2.1. Active Pharmaceutical Ingredients, Pharmaceutical Excipients and Other Chemicals

Four model compounds were selected: atenolol, enalaprilat, ketoprofen, and metoprolol. Biopharmaceutical classification (BCS) and some physicochemical properties for the four drugs are summarized in Table 1. Four PEs with different mechanisms of action were selected: SDS (anionic surfactant), sodium caprate (fatty acid), chitosan (polysaccharide), and EDTA (chelating agent). Atenolol and metoprolol tartrate were provided by AstraZeneca AB (Mölndal, Sweden). Enalaprilat, ketoprofen, sodium caprate, SDS, bovine albumin (A2153), EDTA, and inactin (thiobutabarbital) were purchased from Sigma-Aldrich (St. Louis, MO, USA). Sodium phosphate dibasic dihydrate ($Na_2HPO_4 \cdot 2H_2O$), potassium dihydrogen phosphate (KH_2PO_4), sodium hydroxide (NaOH), and sodium chloride (NaCl) were purchased from Merck KGaA (Darmstadt, Germany). ^{51}Cr-EDTA was purchased from PerkinElmer Life Sciences (Boston, MA, USA). Chitosan hydrochloride (molecular mass 40-300 kDa, degree of acetylation 8.8%) was purchased from Kraeber and Co GmbH (Ellerbek, Germany). Parecoxib (dynastat) was obtained from Apoteket AB, Uppsala, Sweden.

Table 1. Some physicochemical properties and Biopharmaceutics Classification System (BCS) classification of the four model drugs [14].

Compounds (BCS Class)	MM (g/mol)	pK_a	PSA	HBA/HBD	Log P	Log $D_{7.4}$	Log $D_{6.5}$
Atenolol (III)	266	9.6 [b]	88.1	4/4	0.18	−2.0	<−2.0
Enalaprilat (III)	348	3.17 [b]/7.84 [a]	102.1	6/3	−0.13	−1.0	−1.0
Metoprolol (I)	267	9.6 [b]	57.8	4/2	2.07	0.0	−0.5
Ketoprofen (II)	254	3.89 [a]	54.2	3/1	3.37	0.1	0.8

[a] acid, [b] base, HBA/HBD—hydrogen bond acceptor/donor, Log $D_{7.4/6.5}$—n-octanol–water partition coefficient at pH 7.4/6.5, Log P—n-octanol–water coefficient, MM—molar mass, pKa—dissociation constant, PSA—polar surface area.

2.2. Study Formulations

Eight isotonic (290 mOsm) phosphate-buffered perfusates were prepared, each containing all four drugs atenolol, enalaprilat, ketoprofen, and metoprolol at 100 µM. There were two control solutions at pH 6.5 and 7.4 containing no PEs, and six test formulations containing PEs. The phosphate buffer strength was 8 mM at pH 6.5, and 80 mM at pH 7.4 to avoid a reduction in pH during the perfusion. Five of the test formulations were perfused at pH 6.5 and contained one of the following PEs in solution: SDS at 1 and 5 mg/mL (3.5 and 17.3 mM), EDTA at 1 and 5 mg/mL (3.4 and 17.1 mM), and chitosan at 5 mg/mL (≈30 µM). One of test formulations was perfused at pH 7.4 and contained a suspension of sodium caprate at 10 mg/mL (51 mM). The higher pH in the perfusate was used for caprate as it has no permeation enhancing effect at pH 6.5 in either the rat or human SPIP models, as its solubility is higher at pH 7.4 (2 vs. 5 mg/mL) [11,15]. The PE concentrations of 1, 5, and 10 mg/mL correspond to oral doses of 0.2, 1.0, and 2.0 g administered with 200 mL water, as these values are previously shown to affect the intestinal permeability of low-permeation model compounds in the rat SPIP model [11,12].

The preparation procedure of the perfusion formulations (100 mL) is described in detail earlier [12]. No incompatibility, degradation, or apparent binding to glass/plastic of the study compounds in solution (pH 6.5, 37 °C) was observed during 4 h. Osmolarity was determined (after addition of all perfusate constituents, e.g., salt, PE, water) by freezing-point depression using a Micro Osmometer (Model 3MO; Advanced Instruments, Needham Heights, MA, USA).

2.3. Animals and Study Design

The surgical procedure and experimental setup of the rat SPIP experiment has been previously described [12]. The study was approved by the local ethics committee for animal research (no: C64/16) in Uppsala, Sweden. In short, male Han Wistar rats (strain 273) from Charles River Co. (Cologne, Germany), weight 270–420 g, were used. On the study day, the rats were anesthetized using an intraperitoneal injection of a 5% *w/v* inactin solution (180 mg/kg). Body temperature was maintained at 37.5 ± 0.5 °C. Systemic arterial blood pressure was continuously recorded to validate the condition of the animal. This was done by connecting an arterial catheter to a transducer operating a PowerLab system (AD Instruments, Hastings, UK).

At the SPIP experiment, the abdomen was opened along the midline and a jejunal (10–12 cm) or colonic (6–12 cm) segment was cannulated, covered with polyethylene wrap, and placed outside the abdomen [5]. The bile duct was cannulated to avoid pancreaticobiliary secretion into the duodenum at the jejunal perfusion. After completion of surgery, ^{51}Cr-EDTA was administered intravenously (iv) as a bolus of 75 µCi (0.4 mL), followed by a continuous iv infusion at a rate of 50 µCi per hour (1 mL/h) for the duration of the experiment. During the first 30 min following surgery, each small and large intestinal segment was single-passed perfused with 37 °C, phosphate-buffered saline (6 mM) at pH 6.5 or 7.4. This stabilized cardiovascular, respiratory, and intestinal functions and the ^{51}Cr-EDTA levels in the blood (plasma). The length and wet tissue weight of each intestinal segment was determined after the experiment. The single-pass perfusion rate was at all times 0.2 mL/min (peristaltic pump, Gilson Minipuls 3, Le Bel, France).

Each of the six PE experiments was performed in the colon and was divided into two parts. In the first part, the segment was perfused with the control buffer solution (containing model compounds but no PE) for 60 min. In the second part, the segment was perfused for 75 min with one of the six test formulations, containing model compounds and one of the following PEs: SDS at 1 or 5 mg/mL, EDTA at 1 or 5 mg/mL, chitosan at 5 mg/mL (pH 6.5), and caprate at 10 mg/mL (pH 7.4). The six PE experiments were designed so that each rat was its own control. For regional intestinal comparisons, all the above PE concentrations and pH values were previously evaluated in the jejunum, at our laboratory and using the same experimental design.

To evaluate regional intestinal differences in basal permeability values of the four model drugs, two perfusions were also performed in the jejunum using only the control solutions (no PE) for 60 min, at pH 6.5 and 7.4. This established a basal permeability value for comparison with the values determined in the control period of the PE experiments in the colon.

All experimental periods started with a rapid filling (<30 s) of the whole segment with the perfusate (about 1.5 mL for a 10-cm segment). The intestinal segment and perfusates were kept at 37 °C and all outgoing perfusate was quantitatively collected and weighed at 15-min intervals.

Blood samples of <0.3 mL were collected from the femoral artery for a maximum volume of 4 mL during each experiment. All sampled blood volumes were replaced by an equivalent volume of saline (0.9% NaCl) solution with 70 mg/mL bovine serum albumin. Blood was sampled at 15-min intervals for 135 min (9 samples) in each of the six PE experiments, and for 60 min (4 samples) in the jejunal controls. The blood samples were put on ice and centrifuged (5000× *g*, 3 min at 4 °C) within 10 min. 100 µL of the plasma was transferred to 500 µL microtubes and stored at −20 °C until analysis.

2.4. Determination of Blood-to-Lumen Jejunal ^{51}Cr-EDTA Clearance ($CL_{Cr\text{-}EDTA}$)

In the six PE experiments, all luminal perfusates and blood plasma were analyzed at 0 and 135 min for ^{51}Cr activity (cpm) in a gamma counter (1282 Compugamma CS, Pharmacia AB, Uppsala, Sweden). A linear regression analysis of the plasma samples was made to obtain a corresponding plasma value for each perfusate sample. The blood-to-lumen $CL_{Cr\text{-}EDTA}$ was calculated using Equation (1) [16].

$$CL_{Cr-EDTA} = \frac{C_{perfusate} \times Q_{in}}{C_{plasma} \times tissue\ weight} \times 100 \quad (1)$$

where $C_{perfusate}$ and C_{plasma} is the activity in the perfusate and plasma (cpm/mL), and Q_{in} is the flow rate (mL/min). $CL_{Cr\text{-}EDTA}$ was determined during the last 45 min for the control solution and during the last 60 min for the test solutions, of which the first 15 min of each period were for equilibration.

The mean CL$_{Cr\text{-}EDTA}$ value of the two perfusion periods was regarded as representative for each individual rat.

2.5. Bioanalysis

The plasma concentrations of atenolol, metoprolol, enalaprilat and ketoprofen were determined using Ultra-High Performance Liquid Chromatography coupled to Tandem Mass Spectrometry. The method used has been previously published [17]. The only modification was that the lower limit of quantification for ketoprofen was decreased to 52 nM in this study.

2.6. Intestinal Effective Permeability (P_{eff}) Calculation

Jejunal and colonic lumen-to-blood effective permeability (P_{eff}) of the four model compounds was determined based on a modification of the method described by Sjögren et al., 2015 [18]. This method has been successfully implemented in human, dog and rat [4,18–21]. In short, an input rate was acquired by deconvolution of the plasma concentration–time profiles following the intestinal perfusion using Phoenix software version 8.2 (Certara USA, Princeton, NJ, USA). Previous intravenous pharmacokinetic data from a two-compartment analysis of the model drugs in Han Wistar rats was used as impulse response in the deconvolution [12]. An absorption rate was then calculated by compensating for first-pass extraction ($F_{firstpass}$) of each compound in the rat intestine and liver. The $F_{firstpass}$ values for atenolol (1.0), enalaprilat (0.99), ketoprofen (0.99), and metoprolol (0.22) were based on literature data for the fraction of the model compound as follows: (i) the amount metabolized/excreted in the rat liver; (ii) plasma CL values derived from the two-compartment analysis of the intravenous plasma data; and (iii) an assumed rat-liver blood flow of 47 mL/min/kg [22–24]. The P_{eff} (cm/s) was then calculated by relating the absorption rate to the intestinal luminal area using Equation (2):

$$P_{eff} = \frac{\text{absorption rate}}{A \times C} \quad (2)$$

where A is the area of the exposed intestinal segment described as a smooth cylinder with a radius of 0.2 cm, and C is the concentration entering the luminal segment.

In the six colonic PE experiments, P_{eff} was evaluated from 0 to 135 min and the mean P_{eff} value of the two perfusion periods (60-min control and 75-min test) was regarded as representative for each individual rat. In the control experiments performed in jejunum, P_{eff} was evaluated from 0 to 60 min and the mean P_{eff} value was regarded as representative for each individual rat.

2.7. Statistical Analysis

The sample size in each study group was six rats, on the basis of power analysis and previous perfusion studies [12,25]. Plasma concentration, P_{eff}, and CL$_{Cr\text{-}EDTA}$ values are expressed as mean ± standard deviation (SD) or standard error of the mean (SEM). The jejunal vs colonic P_{eff} ratio, is presented as well as the P_{eff} and CL$_{Cr\text{-}EDTA}$ ratio between the 45-min control and 60-min test period in the six colonic PE perfusions (Equation (3)).

$$\text{Ratio}\left(CL_{Cr-EDTA} \text{ or } P_{eff}\right) = \frac{\text{mean value (jejunum or test period)}}{\text{mean value (colon or control period)}} \quad (3)$$

The ratio was compared using the paired student's t-test with the Benjamini–Hochberg multiple t-test correction. Multiple comparisons between groups were performed using a two-way ANOVA with a post-hoc Holm–Sidak multiple comparison test. Log transformation of values was performed when the original measured data were heteroscedastic and not normally distributed; this was investigated using the Bartlett test. Differences were considered to be statistically significant for p-values < than 0.05.

3. Results

3.1. Plasma Profiles

The mean (±SEM) plasma concentration–time profiles are presented in Figure 1a–d for atenolol, enalaprilat, ketoprofen, and metoprolol following the jejunal and colonic perfusions (first 60 min) of the control solutions at pH 6.5 and 7.4. These plasma concentration–time data for the selected model drugs were used to determine regional intestinal basal P_{eff} values using Equation (2).

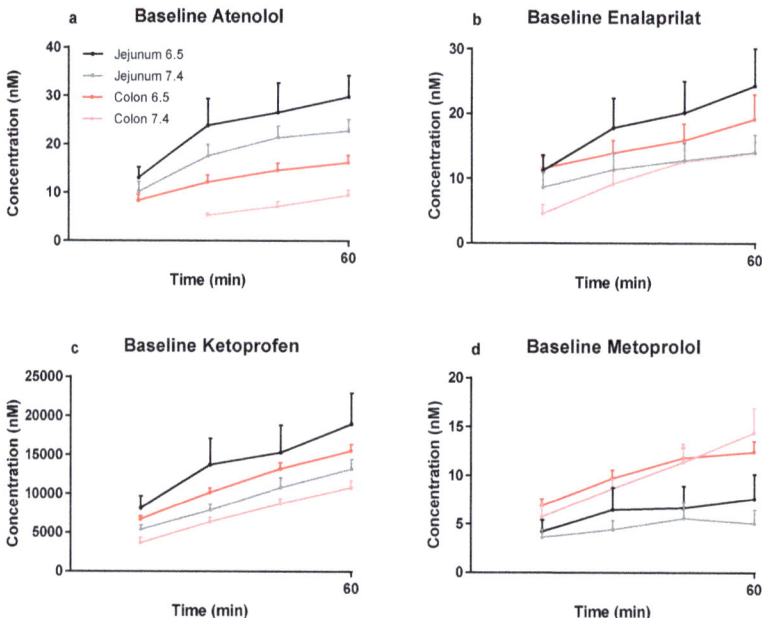

Figure 1. The mean ±SEM rat plasma concentration–time profiles (n = 30 for colon at pH 7.4, and n = 6 for the other three groups) of: (**a**) atenolol, (**b**) enalaprilat, (**c**) ketoprofen, and (**d**) metoprolol following single-pass jejunal and colonic perfusions of the pH 6.5 and 7.4 control solutions (0–60 min). These plasma data were used to determine regional intestinal basal P_{eff} values using Equation (2) (Table 2).

The mean (±SEM) plasma concentration–time profiles are presented in Figure 2a–d for atenolol, enalaprilat, ketoprofen, and metoprolol after: (i) the colonic perfusions of the control solutions (0–60 min), and (ii) then followed by the six PE-containing test formulations (60–135 min). These plasma concentration–time data were used to determine the PE-induced increase in P_{eff} ratio (test/control period) using Equation (3).

3.2. Lumen-to-Blood Effective Permeability (P_{eff}) of Model Drugs

The mean (±SEM) basal jejunal and colonic P_{eff} at pH 6.5 and pH 7.4 are presented in Table 2 for atenolol, enalaprilat, ketoprofen, and metoprolol. There were no statistical ($p < 0.05$) differences in basal permeability for any of the model drugs at either pH or in any intestinal segment.

The mean P_{eff} ratio between the jejunum and colon of atenolol (1.5), enalaprilat (0.6), ketoprofen (1.3), and metoprolol (0.7) at pH 6.5 are presented in Figure 3. For species comparison, Figure 3 also contains the previously published human/dog P_{eff} ratio between the jejunum and colon for atenolol (35/5), enalaprilat (not available/8), ketoprofen (2.6/1.0), and metoprolol (1.3/1.5) at pH 6.5 (plasma appearance data) [4,19].

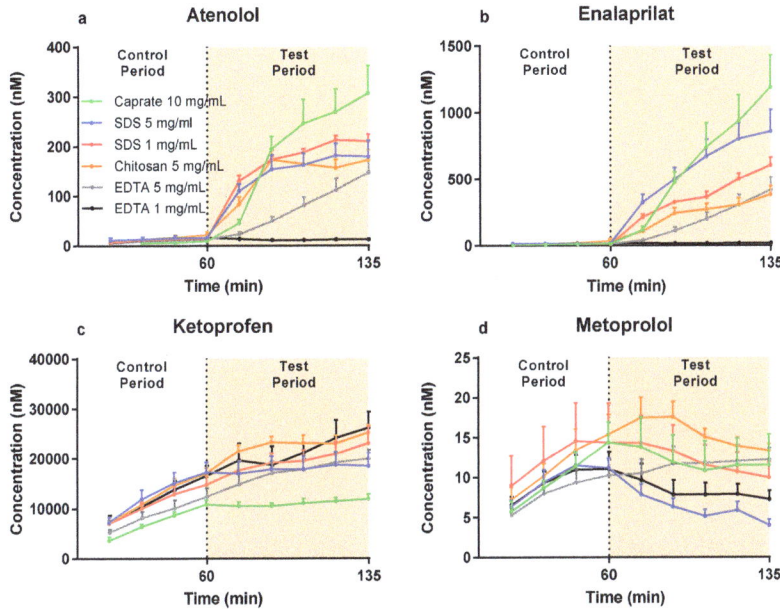

Figure 2. The mean ±SEM rat colonic plasma concentration–time profiles ($n = 6$) of: (**a**) atenolol, (**b**) enalaprilat, (**c**) ketoprofen, and (**d**) metoprolol following single-pass intestinal perfusions of a control solution for 60 min, followed by a 75-min perfusion of any of six test formulations containing a permeation enhancer (PE). The control solution and all test formulations contained 100 µM atenolol, enalaprilat, ketoprofen, and metoprolol. The control and test formulation perfusate pH was 6.5 for the PEs: sodium dodecyl sulfate (SDS) at 1 and 5 mg/mL, chitosan at 5 mg/mL, and ethylenediaminetetraacetic acid (EDTA) at 1 and 5 mg/mL. The control and test formulation perfusate pH was 7.4 for caprate at 10 mg/mL. All formulations were solutions, except caprate which was a suspension (its solubility at pH 7.4 is 5 mg/mL).

Table 2. The mean ±SD rat permeability (P_{eff}) values for the four model compounds determined in the jejunum and colon at pH 6.5 and 7.4 ($n = 6$).

Conditions	Plasma Appearance P_{eff} (×10^{-4} cm/s)			
	Atenolol	Enalaprilat	Ketoprofen	Metoprolol
Jejunum pH 6.5	0.022 ± 0.01	0.005 ± 0.004	1.5 ± 1.1	0.28 ± 0.24
Jejunum pH 7.4	0.016 ± 0.005	0.004 ± 0.001	0.64 ± 0.15	0.17 ± 0.095
Colon pH 6.5	0.015 ± 0.007	0.009 ± 0.007	1.1 ± 0.3	0.41 ± 0.19
Colon pH 7.4	0.011 ± 0.005	0.006 ± 0.004	0.73 ± 0.14	0.38 ± 0.15

The mean (±SEM) P_{eff} ratio of the test and control periods for the six test formulations in the colon are shown in Figure 4a–d for atenolol, enalaprilat, ketoprofen, and metoprolol. Figure 4a–d (blue symbols) also contains previous jejunal P_{eff} ratio data of atenolol, enalaprilat, and ketoprofen for chitosan at 5 mg/mL, and for SDS at 1 and 5 mg/mL (and for enalaprilat with caprate at 10 mg/mL) [11,12]. The colon seems to be more sensitive than the jejunum to caprate at 10 mg/mL, as the P_{eff} ratio of enalaprilat was significantly ($p < 0.05$) higher in the colon. There were no statistical differences between intestinal segments for any of the other model drugs and PEs.

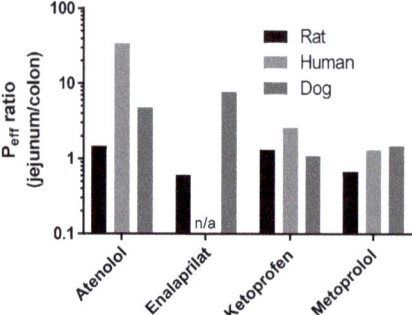

Figure 3. The P_{eff} ratio between the jejunum and colon at pH 6.5 in rat of atenolol, enalaprilat, ketoprofen, and metoprolol (Table 2). The historical human and dog P_{eff} ratios between the jejunum and colon at pH 6.5 of atenolol, enalaprilat (not human), ketoprofen, and metoprolol are also presented for species comparison [4,19].

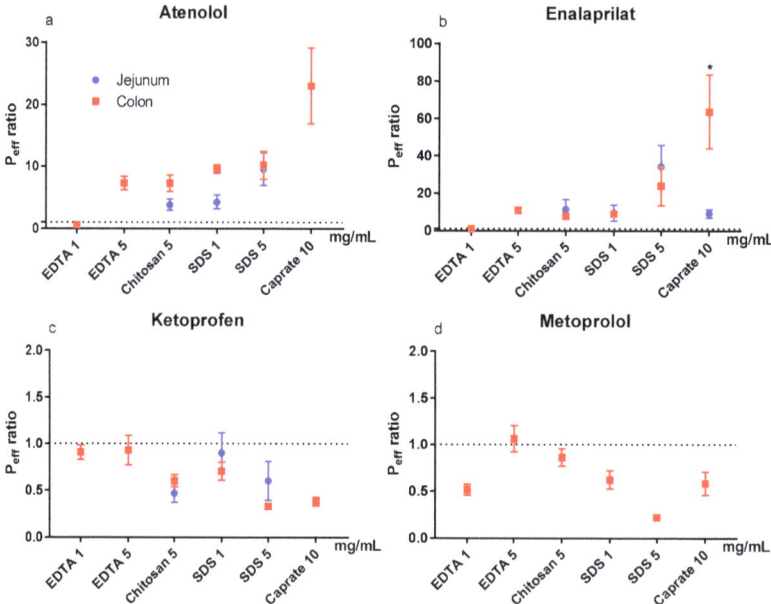

Figure 4. The mean ±SEM rat jejunal (historical data) and colonic lumen-to-blood intestinal effective permeability (P_{eff}) ratio ($n = 6$) of: (**a**) atenolol, (**b**) enalaprilat, (**c**) ketoprofen, and (**d**) metoprolol, after intestinal perfusions of a control solution for 60 min, followed by a 75-min perfusion of any of six permeation enhancing (PE) test formulations [11,12]. The control and test formulation perfusate pH was 6.5 for the PEs: sodium dodecyl sulfate (SDS) at 1 and 5 mg/mL, chitosan at 5 mg/mL, and ethylenediaminetetraacetic acid (EDTA) at 1 and 5 mg/mL. The control and test formulation perfusate pH was 7.4 for caprate at 10 mg/mL. All formulations were solutions, except caprate which was a suspension (its solubility at pH 7.4 is 5 mg/mL). There is no jejunal historical data for metoprolol and only jejunal historical data for EDTA and caprate for enalaprilat. A * represents a significant difference in jejunal and colonic P_{eff} (two-way ANOVA, Holm–Sidak).

3.3. Blood-to-Lumen $CL_{Cr\text{-}EDTA}$ Ratio

The mean (±SD) colonic $CL_{Cr\text{-}EDTA}$ for the control solutions ($n = 38$) was 0.038 ± 0.050 mL/min/100 g. The mean (±SEM) $CL_{Cr\text{-}EDTA}$ ratios between the control and test period for the six test formulations in the colon (and for previously reported jejunal data, blue symbols) are shown in Figure 5. Unlike the P_{eff} ratios, there was a significant PE-induced increase in $CL_{Cr\text{-}EDTA}$ ratio in the colon compared to the control for all test formulations, except EDTA at 1 mg/mL. The increases were also significantly higher in the colon than in the jejunum for all test formulations.

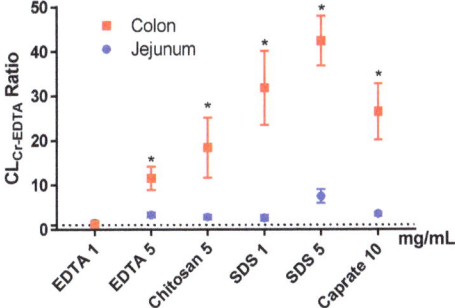

Figure 5. The mean ±SEM rat jejunal (historical data) and colonic blood-to-lumen ^{51}Cr-EDTA clearance ($CL_{Cr\text{-}EDTA}$) ratio ($n = 6$), after intestinal perfusions of a control solution for 60 min, followed by a 75-min perfusion of any of six permeation enhancing (PE) test formulations. The control and test formulation perfusate pH was 6.5 for the PEs: sodium dodecyl sulfate (SDS) at 1 and 5 mg/mL, chitosan at 5 mg/mL, and ethylenediaminetetraacetic acid (EDTA) at 1 and 5 mg/mL. The control and test formulation perfusate pH was 7.4 for caprate at 10 mg/mL. All formulations were solutions, except caprate which was a suspension (its solubility at pH 7.4 is 5 mg/mL). A * represents a significant difference in jejunal and colonic $CL_{Cr\text{-}EDTA}$ ratio (two-way ANOVA, Holm–Sidak).

4. Discussion

This rat single-pass intestinal perfusion (SPIP) study is part of a sequence of mechanistic studies to evaluate regional intestinal differences in drug absorption in different species and models. The study also evaluates the in vivo effect of permeation enhancers (PEs) on intestinal transport of model drugs/peptides and marker compounds [12,25–27]. The primary objective was to investigate the regional intestinal differences in lumen-to-blood effective drug permeability (P_{eff})—as determined from plasma appearance data in the rat SPIP model—and to compare it to corresponding historical human data [4]. P_{eff} was determined for two low-permeation model drugs, atenolol and enalaprilat, and for two high-permeation drugs, ketoprofen and metoprolol.

The secondary objective was to evaluate the effect of PEs on drug permeability in the rat colon, compared to previous jejunal data. The effects were evaluated based on model drug P_{eff} and blood-to-lumen clearance of ^{51}Cr-EDTA ($CL_{Cr\text{-}EDTA}$), an established clinical marker for mucosal barrier integrity.

A modified-release (MR) dosage form can be used to optimize plasma pharmacokinetics, dosage regimens, and improve clinical performance. MRs enable once-per-day drug administration, reduce side effects, and increase patient compliance [28]. Successful development of such a dosage form requires that the drug be absorbed in all parts of the intestines, as drug release needs to be substantially longer than the typical human small intestinal transit time of 3–5 h [29]. Reliable preclinical data on regional intestinal permeability is therefore needed early in the development of any novel MR dosage form. The rat SPIP model is commonly used to determine regional permeability data on the basis of luminal drug disappearance. However, a recent meta-analysis shows wide variability in regional intestinal permeability data between studies and between laboratories. This raises the question how relevant individual studies on rats are for in vivo predictions in humans [3]. The lack of a correlation may be related to the method of drug permeability determination. A recent rat SPIP study demonstrated that the permeability values of the low permeability drugs, atenolol and enalaprilat, is 9 to 59 times higher when determined on the basis of luminal disappearance compared to plasma appearance [5]. Therefore, the primary aim of this study was to evaluate the suitability of the rat SPIP model for measurements of human regional intestinal drug permeability on the basis of plasma appearance data [4,30].

In our study, there were only small differences in jejunal and colonic rat P_{eff} at pH 6.5 for the high-permeability compounds, ketoprofen and metoprolol, when determined from plasma appearance. This is in good agreement with regional intestinal permeability data based on luminal disappearance in the rat SPIP model, as well as with human regional intestinal permeability data based on plasma appearance [4,20,31]. Our results show that the rat SPIP model accurately predicted regional differences (jejunum vs colon) in the permeability of high-permeability drugs, regardless whether these were determined by luminal disappearance or plasma appearance.

For the low permeability drugs, atenolol and enalaprilat, plasma appearance data showed no differences in jejunal and colonic P_{eff}. In contrast, the jejunal permeability of atenolol in human was 35 times higher than in colon. There is no reference value in human for enalaprilat, but in dog the corresponding jejunal value is eight-fold higher than the colonic permeability based on plasma appearance data [19]. Since the dog is well-known to have a colon that is much more permeable to drugs than that of human, presumably any reference value in human would result in a jejunal vs colonic ratio at least within the same order of magnitude as observed in dog [32]. Consequently, the plasma appearance of these two drugs suggests that the rat SPIP model is unable to accurately predict regional intestinal permeability of medium-to-low permeability drugs in human, which is also reported by others [33]. However, it should be emphasized that the rat SPIP model is still useful for evaluating a range of other biopharmaceutical, physiological, and biochemical processes. For instance, the rat jejunum is representative of human jejunal P_{eff} values determined from plasma appearance [4,5]. Therefore, the permeability data from the SPIP model will be useful for boundary BCS classification of permeability and for investigation of the potential effect of different concentrations of pharmaceutical excipients on local intestinal permeability [34].

There was a trend for a slightly higher (1.1- to 2.3-fold) jejunal and colonic permeability of all four model drugs at pH 6.5 compared to 7.4. On the basis of the pH-partitioning hypothesis, this was expected for the acid, ketoprofen, but not for the bases, atenolol and metoprolol [35]. These conflicting results indicate that parameters other than molecular charge dominate. For instance, passive membrane transport is also affected by paracellular pore selectivity, molecular elongation, and intramolecular hydrogen bonding, which might be better understood using complex molecular dynamic simulations [36]. Consequently, any pH-dependent permeability values determined in the rat SPIP model should be interpreted with care, and a linear pH-permeability relationship should not be used to predict intestinal drug transport and absorption.

Peptide drugs with a very low intestinal stability and/or permeability are, with a few exceptions, not administered orally because of their low intestinal absorption. Their low stability can be related to stomach pH denaturation, the high concentrations of luminal gastric and pancreatic peptidases and proteinases, and the high peptidase activity in the brush border membrane of the enterocytes [7]. These issues can be partly circumvented by the formulation approaches. For instance, (1) enteric coating can prevent gastric chemical instability and peptide degradation; the (2) proteinase/peptidase inhibitors in the formulation can increase the local luminal stability of the drug; and (3) drug release may be targeted to the colon where peptidase activity tends to be lower than in the small intestine [9,37,38].

The low intestinal permeability of most peptides is related to their large size, low lipophilicity, and extensive hydrogen binding, all of which are physicochemical properties that predict low passive membrane transport [39]. A strategy to circumvent low intestinal permeability was recently approved for the first time in an oral product, for which a PE increased the intestinal membrane transport of semaglutide, a pharmaceutical peptide containing 31 amino acids, even though the bioavailability in dog is as low as 0.29% of the oral dose (data from patent: wo2012080471) [6]. The use of PEs has also been proposed in the colon, as the low luminal volumes and long transit time allow for high local mucosal PE concentrations at extended exposure times. Together these increase the likelihood of a positive effect on peptide membrane permeation. Accordingly, rat luminal instillation studies report a generally higher effect of PE in the colon than the jejunum on the plasma exposure of various molecular probes and peptides [8,40–44]. However, the rat luminal instillation model does not differentiate between PE effects on membrane permeability, and on transit/motility, dilution, and hydrodynamics in the luminal segment. This is in contrast to the SPIP model in which luminal and experimental conditions are controlled [10]. Therefore, our study performed a systematic evaluation of the effect of four permeation enhancers with different mechanisms of action at different luminal concentrations in colon.

In our rat SPIP study, all PEs (except EDTA at 1 mg/mL) increased the P_{eff} of the two low permeability drugs, atenolol and enalaprilat. However, for the vast majority of the PEs in this study, the increase in P_{eff} ratio was not different from what we have previously observed in the jejunum in our laboratory [11,12]. This is in stark contrast to the significantly higher effect of all PEs in this study on $CL_{Cr-EDTA}$ ratio in the colon compared to the jejunum. The substantially higher effect on the transport of the clinical marker for mucosal integrity and damage, compared to drug absorption, indicates a greater risk for tissue damage than medical benefit in using PE for increasing colonic drug absorption. On the basis of the data from our study, we agree with other reports that the rationale is weak for colonic targeting of systemically acting drugs/peptides in combination with PEs [45].

In conclusion, this rat SPIP study showed no difference in jejunal and colonic permeability determined from plasma appearance data of two low permeability model compounds (atenolol and enalaprilat) and two high-permeability ones (ketoprofen and metoprolol). Comparison of these data with previous human data challenges ability of the rat SPIP model for predicting differences in human regional intestinal permeability of low-to-medium permeability drugs. The effect of PEs on drug permeability in the colon was similar to previously reported data from the rat jejunum. In contrast, their effect on the transport of Cr-EDTA—a clinical marker for mucosal barrier integrity—was significantly higher in the colon than in jejunum. These results indicate that the risk of using PE for increasing colonic drug permeability is higher than the potential medical reward.

Author Contributions: Conceptualization, D.D., M.-J.C.-C., M.H., M.S. and H.L.; Data curation, D.D., M.-J.C.-C., T.O., M.H., M.S. and H.L.; Formal analysis, D.D., M.H. and H.L.; Funding acquisition, M.S. and H.L.; Investigation, D.D., M.-J.C.-C., T.O. and M.S.; Methodology, D.D., M.-J.C.-C., T.O., M.S. and H.L.; Project administration, M.H.; Resources, H.L.; Supervision, D.D.; Writing—original draft, D.D.; Writing—review & editing, D.D., M.-J.C.-C., T.O., M.H., M.S. and H.L. All authors have read and agreed to the published version of the manuscript.

Funding: This research received no external funding.

Acknowledgments: We thank Margareta Sprycha at the National Veterinary Institute (SVA) for her hard work with the bioanalysis.

Conflicts of Interest: The authors declare no conflicts of interest.

Abbreviations

AME—absorption-modifying excipient, $CL_{Cr-EDTA}$—clearance of ^{51}Cr-EDTA, P_{eff}—intestinal effective permeability, PE—permeation enhancer, SDS—sodium dodecyl sulfate, SPIP—single-pass intestinal perfusion

References

1. Amidon, G.L.; Sinko, P.J.; Fleisher, D. Estimating human oral fraction dose absorbed: A correlation using rat intestinal membrane permeability for passive and carrier-mediated compounds. *Pharm. Res.* **1988**, *5*, 651–654. [CrossRef]

2. Cao, X.; Gibbs, S.T.; Fang, L.; Miller, H.A.; Landowski, C.P.; Shin, H.-C.; Lennernas, H.; Zhong, Y.; Amidon, G.L.; Lawrence, X.Y. Why is it challenging to predict intestinal drug absorption and oral bioavailability in human using rat model. *Pharm. Res.* **2006**, *23*, 1675–1686. [CrossRef]
3. Dubbelboer, I.; Dahlgren, D.; Sjögren, E.; Lennernäs, H. Rat intestinal drug permeability: A status report and summary of repeated determinations. *Eur. J. Pharm. Biopharm.* **2019**, *142*, 364–376. [CrossRef]
4. Dahlgren, D.; Roos, C.; Lundqvist, A.; Abrahamsson, B.; Tannergren, C.; Hellström, P.M.; Sjögren, E.; Lennernäs, H. Regional intestinal permeability of three model drugs in human. *Mol. Pharm.* **2016**, *13*, 3013–3021. [CrossRef]
5. Dahlgren, D.; Roos, C.; Peters, K.; Lundqvist, A.; Tannergren, C.; Sjögren, E.; Sjöblom, M.; Lennernäs, H. Evaluation of drug permeability calculation based on luminal disappearance and plasma appearance in the rat single-pass intestinal perfusion model. *Eur. J. Pharm. Biopharm.* **2019**, *142*, 31–37. [CrossRef] [PubMed]
6. Buckley, S.T.; Bækdal, T.A.; Vegge, A.; Maarbjerg, S.J.; Pyke, C.; Ahnfelt-Rønne, J.; Madsen, K.G.; Schéele, S.G.; Alanentalo, T.; Kirk, R.K. Transcellular stomach absorption of a derivatized glucagon-like peptide-1 receptor agonist. *Sci. Transl. Med.* **2018**, *10*, eaar7047. [CrossRef] [PubMed]
7. Tyagi, P.; Pechenov, S.; Subramony, J.A. Oral peptide delivery: Translational challenges due to physiological effects. *J. Control. Release* **2018**, *287*, 167–176. [CrossRef] [PubMed]
8. Petersen, S.B.; Nielsen, L.G.; Rahbek, U.L.; Guldbrandt, M.; Brayden, D.J. Colonic absorption of salmon calcitonin using tetradecyl maltoside (TDM) as a permeation enhancer. *Eur. J. Pharm. Sci.* **2013**, *48*, 726–734. [CrossRef] [PubMed]
9. Rubinstein, A.; Tirosh, B.; Baluom, M.; Nassar, T.; David, A.; Radai, R.; Gliko-Kabir, I.; Friedman, M. The rationale for peptide drug delivery to the colon and the potential of polymeric carriers as effective tools. *J. Control. Release* **1997**, *46*, 59–73. [CrossRef]
10. Dahlgren, D.; Sjöblom, M.; Lennernäs, H. Intestinal absorption-modifying excipients: A current update on preclinical in vivo evaluations. *Eur. J. Pharm. Biopharm.* **2019**, *142*, 411–420. [CrossRef]
11. Dahlgren, D.; Sjöblom, M.; Hedeland, M.; Lennernäs, H. The in vivo effect of transcellular permeation enhancers on the intestinal permeability of two peptide drugs enalaprilat and hexarelin. *Pharmaceutics* **2020**, *2*, 99. [CrossRef] [PubMed]
12. Dahlgren, D.; Roos, C.; Lundqvist, A.; Langguth, P.; Tannergren, C.; Sjöblom, M.; Sjögren, E.; Lennernas, H. Preclinical effect of absorption modifying excipients on rat intestinal transport of five model compounds and the intestinal barrier marker 51Cr-EDTA. *Mol. Pharm.* **2017**, *14*, 4243–4251. [CrossRef] [PubMed]
13. Nylander, O.; Sababi, M.; Bark, J. Characterization of 51Cr-EDTA as a marker of duodenal mucosal permeability. *Acta Physiologica* **1991**, *143*, 117–126. [CrossRef] [PubMed]
14. Winiwarter, S.; Bonham, N.M.; Ax, F.; Hallberg, A.; Lennernäs, H.; Karlén, A. Correlation of human jejunal permeability (in vivo) of drugs with experimentally and theoretically derived parameters. A multivariate data analysis approach. *J. Med. Chem.* **1998**, *41*, 4939–4949. [CrossRef] [PubMed]
15. Lennernäs, H.; Gjellan, K.; Hällgren, R.; Graffner, C. The influence of caprate on rectal absorption of phenoxymethylpenicillin: Experience from an in-vivo perfusion in humans. *J. Pharm. Pharmacol.* **2002**, *54*, 499–508. [CrossRef]
16. Nylander, O.; Kvietys, P.; Granger, D.N. Effects of hydrochloric acid on duodenal and jejunal mucosal permeability in the rat. *Am. J. Physiol. Gastrointest. Liver Physiol.* **1989**, *257*, G653–G660. [CrossRef]
17. Roos, C.; Dahlgren, D.; Sjögren, E.; Sjöblom, M.; Hedeland, M.; Lennernäs, H. Effects of absorption-modifying excipients on jejunal drug absorption in simulated fasted and fed luminal conditions. *Eur. J. Pharm. Biopharm.* **2019**, *142*, 387–395. [CrossRef]
18. Sjögren, E.; Dahlgren, D.; Roos, C.; Lennernas, H. Human in vivo regional intestinal permeability: Quantitation using site-specific drug absorption data. *Mol. Pharm.* **2015**, *12*, 2026–2039. [CrossRef]
19. Dahlgren, D.; Roos, C.; Johansson, P.; Lundqvist, A.; Tannergren, C.; Abrahamsson, B.; Sjögren, E.; Lennernäs, H. Regional intestinal permeability in dogs: Biopharmaceutical aspects for development of oral modified-release dosage forms. *Mol. Pharm.* **2016**, *13*, 3022–3033. [CrossRef]
20. Roos, C.; Dahlgren, D.; Tannergren, C.; Abrahamsson, B.; Sjögren, E.; Lennernas, H. Regional intestinal permeability in rats: A comparison of methods. *Mol. Pharm.* **2017**, *14*, 4252–4261. [CrossRef] [PubMed]
21. Roos, C.; Dahlgren, D.; Berg, S.; Westergren, J.; Abrahamsson, B.; Tannergren, C.; Sjögren, E.; Lennernäs, H. In Vivo Mechanisms of Intestinal Drug Absorption from Aprepitant Nanoformulations. *Mol. Pharm.* **2017**, *14*, 4233–4242. [CrossRef] [PubMed]

22. Davies, B.; Morris, T. Physiological parameters in laboratory animals and humans. *Pharm. Res.* **1993**, *10*, 1093–1095. [CrossRef] [PubMed]
23. de Lannoy, I.A.; Barker III, F.; Pang, K.S. Formed and preformed metabolite excretion clearances in liver, a metabolite formation organ: Studies on enalapril and enalaprilat in the single-pass and recirculating perfused rat liver. *J. Pharm. Biopharm.* **1993**, *21*, 395–422. [CrossRef] [PubMed]
24. Roumi, M.; Marleau, S.; du Souich, P.; Maggi, T.; Deghenghi, R.; Ong, H. Kinetics and disposition of hexarelin, a peptidic growth hormone secretagogue, in rats. *Drug Metab. Dispos.* **2000**, *28*, 44–50.
25. Dahlgren, D.; Roos, C.; Lundqvist, A.; Tannergren, C.; Sjöblom, M.; Sjögren, E.; Lennernas, H. Effect of absorption-modifying excipients, hypotonicity, and enteric neural activity in an in vivo model for small intestinal transport. *Int. J. Pharm.* **2018**, *549*, 239–248. [CrossRef]
26. Dahlgren, D.; Roos, C.; Johansson, P.; Tannergren, C.; Lundqvist, A.; Langguth, P.; Sjöblom, M.; Sjögren, E.; Lennernas, H. The effects of three absorption-modifying critical excipients on the in vivo intestinal absorption of six model compounds in rats and dogs. *Int. J. Pharm.* **2018**, *547*, 158–168. [CrossRef]
27. Dahlgren, D.; Roos, C.; Lundqvist, A.; Tannergren, C.; Sjöblom, M.; Sjögren, E.; Lennernäs, H. Time-dependent effects on small intestinal transport by absorption-modifying excipients. *Eur. J. Pharm. Biopharm.* **2018**, *132*, 19–28. [CrossRef]
28. Paradissis, G.N.; Garegnani, J.A.; Whaley, R.S. Extended Release Pharmaceutical Formulations. U.S. Patent 5,133,974, 28 July 1992.
29. Wang, Y.T.; Mohammed, S.D.; Farmer, A.D.; Wang, D.; Zarate, N.; Hobson, A.R.; Hellström, P.M.; Semler, J.R.; Kuo, B.; Rao, S.S. Regional gastrointestinal transit and pH studied in 215 healthy volunteers using the wireless motility capsule: Influence of age, gender, study country and testing protocol. *Aliment. Pharmacol. Ther.* **2015**, *42*, 761–772. [CrossRef]
30. Dahlgren, D.; Roos, C.; Sjögren, E.; Lennernäs, H. Direct In Vivo Human Intestinal Permeability (Peff) Determined with Different Clinical Perfusion and Intubation Methods. *J. Pharm. Sci.* **2014**, *104*, 2702–2726. [CrossRef]
31. Fagerholm, U.; Lindahl, A.; Lennernäs, H. Regional intestinal permeability in rats of compounds with different physicochemical properties and transport mechanisms. *J. Pharm. Pharmacol.* **1997**, *49*, 687–690. [CrossRef]
32. Sutton, S.C.; Evans, L.A.; Fortner, J.H.; McCarthy, J.M.; Sweeney, K. Dog colonoscopy model for predicting human colon absorption. *Pharm. Res.* **2006**, *23*, 1554–1563. [CrossRef] [PubMed]
33. Lozoya-Agullo, I.; González-Álvarez, I.; González-Álvarez, M.; Merino-Sanjuán, M.; Bermejo, M. In situ perfusion model in rat colon for drug absorption studies: Comparison with small intestine and Caco-2 cell model. *J. Pharm. Sci.* **2015**, *104*, 3136–3145. [CrossRef] [PubMed]
34. Bransford, P.; Cook, J.; Gupta, M.; Haertter, S.; He, H.; Ju, R.; Kanodia, J.; Lennernäs, H.; Lindley, D.; Polli, J.E. ICH M9 Guideline in development on Biopharmaceutics Classification System-based biowaivers: An Industrial Perspective from the IQ Consortium. *Mol. Pharm.* **2019**, *17*, 361–372. [CrossRef] [PubMed]
35. Thomae, A.V.; Wunderli-Allenspach, H.; Krämer, S.D. Permeation of aromatic carboxylic acids across lipid bilayers: The pH-partition hypothesis revisited. *Biophys. J.* **2005**, *89*, 1802–1811. [CrossRef]
36. Dahlgren, D.; Lennernäs, H. Intestinal Permeability and Drug Absorption: Predictive Experimental, Computational and In Vivo Approaches. *Pharmaceutics* **2019**, *11*, 411. [CrossRef]
37. Yamamoto, A.; Taniguchi, T.; Rikyuu, K.; Tsuji, T.; Fujita, T.; Murakami, M.; Muranishi, S. Effects of various protease inhibitors on the intestinal absorption and degradation of insulin in rats. *Pharm. Res.* **1994**, *11*, 1496–1500. [CrossRef]
38. Wu, L.; Zhang, G.; Lu, Q.; Sun, Q.; Wang, M.; Li, N.; Gao, Z.; Sun, Y.; Li, T.; Han, D. Evaluation of salmon calcitonin (sCT) enteric-coated capsule for enhanced absorption and GI tolerability in rats. *Drug Dev. Ind. Pharm.* **2010**, *36*, 362–370. [CrossRef]
39. Lipinski, C.A.; Lombardo, F.; Dominy, B.W.; Feeney, P.J. Experimental and computational approaches to estimate solubility and permeability in drug discovery and development settings. *Adv. Drug Deliv. Rev.* **1997**, *23*, 3–25. [CrossRef]
40. Fetih, G.; Lindberg, S.; Itoh, K.; Okada, N.; Fujita, T.; Habib, F.; Artersson, P.; Attia, M.; Yamamoto, A. Improvement of absorption enhancing effects of n-dodecyl-β-D-maltopyranoside by its colon-specific delivery using chitosan capsules. *Int. J. Pharm.* **2005**, *293*, 127–135. [CrossRef]

41. Ishizawa, T.; Hayashi, M.; Awazu, S. Enhancement of jejunal and colonic absorption of fosfomycin by promoters in the rat. *J. Pharm. Pharmacol.* **1987**, *39*, 892–895. [CrossRef]
42. Maher, S.; Wang, X.; Bzik, V.; McClean, S.; Brayden, D.J. Evaluation of intestinal absorption and mucosal toxicity using two promoters. II. Rat instillation and perfusion studies. *Eur. J. Pharm. Sci.* **2009**, *38*, 301–311. [CrossRef] [PubMed]
43. Murakami, M.; Kusanoi, Y.; Takada, K.; Muranishi, S. Assessment of enhancing ability of medium-chain alkyl saccharides as new absorption enhancers in rat rectum. *Int. J. Pharm* **1992**, *79*, 159–169.
44. Muranushi, N.; Mack, E.; Kim, S. The effects of fatty acids and their derivatives on the intestinal absorption of insulin in rat. *Drug Dev. Ind. Pharm.* **1993**, *19*, 929–941. [CrossRef]
45. Maher, S.; Mrsny, R.J.; Brayden, D.J. Intestinal permeation enhancers for oral peptide delivery. *Adv. Drug Deliv. Rev.* **2016**, *106*, 277–319. [CrossRef]

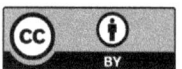

© 2020 by the authors. Licensee MDPI, Basel, Switzerland. This article is an open access article distributed under the terms and conditions of the Creative Commons Attribution (CC BY) license (http://creativecommons.org/licenses/by/4.0/).

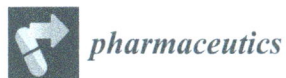

Article

Enteric Hard Capsules for Targeting the Small Intestine: Positive Correlation between In Vitro Disintegration and Dissolution Times

Maoqi Fu [†], Jozef Al-Gousous [†], Johannes Andreas Blechar and Peter Langguth *

Department of Biopharmaceutics and Pharmaceutical Technology, Johannes Gutenberg University Mainz, D-55099 Mainz, Germany; maoqifu1@uni-mainz.de (M.F.); joalgous@uni-mainz.de (J.A.-G.); jblechar@uni-mainz.de (J.A.B.)
* Correspondence: langguth@uni-mainz.de
† These authors contributed equally.

Received: 10 December 2019; Accepted: 31 January 2020; Published: 3 February 2020

Abstract: In this study, the potential for correlation between disintegration and dissolution performance of enteric-coated (EC) dosage forms was investigated. Different enteric hard shell capsule formulations containing caffeine as model drug were tested for disintegration (in a compendial disintegration tester) and for dissolution in both USP type I (basket) and type II (paddle) apparatuses using different media. Overall, good correlations were obtained. This was observed for both the basket and the paddle apparatus, indicating that the use of disintegration testing as a surrogate for dissolution testing (allowed by International Conference on Harmonization (ICH) for immediate release dosage forms in case, in addition to other conditions, a correlation between disintegration and dissolution is proven) could be extended to include delayed release dosage forms.

Keywords: disintegration; dissolution; enteric-coated; ICH; quality control

1. Introduction

Disintegration tests have been used to evaluate dosage form performance since the early 20th century, with the current compendial disintegration tester being available since the 1950s [1]. Despite the limitation of the released amount of the active pharmaceutical ingredient (API) not being measured, these tests are still widely used in pharmaceutical practice owing to their simplicity and speediness compared to dissolution tests. This contributed to the International Conference on Harmonization (ICH) allowing disintegration tests to be used as dissolution test surrogates if (among other conditions) a correlation between disintegration and dissolution is proven [2].

In this regard, it appears from the literature data that the likelihood of obtaining a disintegration–dissolution correlation varies greatly from formulation to formulation, with Gupta et al. [3] testing a 12 different verapamil hydrochloride formulations and finding that only one of them gave a satisfactory correlation. Radwan et al. [4] investigated different trospium chloride formulations under different conditions and found that a correlation is possible when the disintegration is not too rapid. Nickerson et al. [5] on the other hand found good correlations for several immediate formulations of an unnamed API. However, the focus has generally been restricted to immediate release dosage forms, most probably because of the ICH guidance restricting the possibility of employing disintegration test as a dissolution test surrogate to non-modified release dosage forms.

However, one class of modified release dosage forms, namely enteric-coated (EC) formulations, offers at least a theoretical possibility for obtaining good disintegration dissolution correlations. For, in the presence of a rapidly disintegrating and dissolving core, having a situation where the disintegration of the enteric coat strongly influences the overall release performance is likely. Therefore, this work is going to investigate the correlation between disintegration and dissolution of enteric-coated hard shell capsules in order to explore the feasibility of employing the disintegration test as a dissolution test surrogate for EC dosage forms.

2. Materials and Methods

2.1. Materials

Hydroxypropyl methylcellulose size 0 capsules (ACG Nature Caps Plus) were received form ACG Associated Capsules Pvt Ltd (Mumbai, India). DRcaps® (nutraceutical capsules with inherent enteric properties of the capsule shell) were obtained from Neue Lebensqualität (Badendorf, Germany). Caffeine (median particle size 48 µm) and magnesium stearate were purchased from Caesar & Loretz GmbH (Hilden, Germany). Fumed silica was purchased from Fagron GmbH & CO.KG (Glinde, Germany). Hypromellose phthalate (HP-50), hypromellose acetate succinate (HPMCAS-HG, AQOAT) and low substituted hydroxypropyl cellulose (L-HPC) were received as a gift from Shin-Etsu (Wiesbaden, Germany). Lactose (FlowLac® 90) was received from Molkerei Meggle (Wasserburg, Germany). Triethyl citrate (TEC) was purchased from Sigma-Aldrich (Overijse, Belgium). Talc was purchased from Imerys (Luzenac, France). All other materials were of analytical grade.

2.2. Capsule Filling

The HPMC capsules and DRcaps® were filled manually (aponorm® Kapselfüllgerät, WEPA Apothekenbedarf GmbH & CO.KG, Hillscheid, Germany) with a powder formulation. The powder formulation was prepared using a 1.6 L Turbula mixer (Willy A. Bachofen GmbH, Muttenz, Switzerland) at 49 rpm (batch size 600 g), and its composition is described in Table 1. The capsules were filled with 375 mg of the powder (i.e., 75 mg of caffeine). The filled capsules complied with the content uniformity requirements of the European Pharmacopoeia 9.0.

Table 1. Formulation of the capsule filling. All values (%) are based on the total weight (m/m).

Substance	% (m/m)	Weights of the Components per Capsule (mg)
Caffeine	20	75
L-HPC	15	56.25
Lactose	63.75	239.06
Silica	0.25	0.94
Magnesium stearate	1	3.75
Total	100	375

2.3. Capsule Coating

The ACG Nature Caps Plus were coated. Two different batches of coated capsules were prepared from them. The coating formulations are described in Table 2. First, the ethanol–water solution was prepared. The polymer was dissolved in 80% of the solvent and the remaining 20% of the solvent were used to disperse the talc. Afterwards, the polymer solution is combined with the talc dispersion. Last, triethyl citrate is added to the formulation (in case of the HPMCAS-HG formulation). Before coating, the polymer solution is filtered using a sieve with a pore size of 0.2–0.4 mm. The coating levels of the capsules coated with HP-50 and HPMCAS-HG are 10 mg polymer/cm^2 and 9 mg polymer/cm^2 (30% and 27% weight gain), respectively. A Solidlab 1 drum coater (Robert Bosch Packaging Technology GmbH, Waiblingen, Germany) was used for coating with the following parameters: 230 g of capsules/batch preheated to 30 °C; spray rate of 6.5–7 g/min and a atomizing pressure of 2.0 bar; nozzle diameter of

0.5 mm; the inlet air was heated to 58–60 °C and had a flow rate of 55 m^3/h; product temperature of 35–38 °C.

Table 2. Coating formulation. All values (%) are based on the total solution.

Substance	HP-50 Formulation		HPMCAS-HG Formulation	
	% (m/m)	Weights of the Components (g)	% (m/m)	Weights of the Components (g)
Polymer	6	60	5	40
Talc	7.5	75	7.5	60
TEC	-	-	2	16
Ethanol	69.2	747.7	68.4	591.25
Water	17.3	117.3	17.1	92.75

2.4. Disintegration Test

The capsule disintegration was performed with disks using a DT2 Disintegration Tester (Sotax AG, Aesh, Switzerland) complying with the European Pharmacopoeia specifications for a type A disintegration testing apparatus. All capsules were first exposed to 700 mL of 0.1 M HCl for one hour followed by one hour testing in 700 mL of buffer. The temperature was maintained at 37.0 ± 0.5 °C There were three different buffers tested, namely the 50 mM USP phosphate buffer pH 6.8, blank FaSSIF buffer (28.4 mM) pH 6.5 and a 15 mM phosphate buffer pH 6.5 that showed to be biopredictive in previous studies (henceforth referred to as the "Al-Gousous et al. medium" [6]). The disintegration times recorded are the times at which the capsules ruptured, which helps reduce the uncertainty associated with determining the disintegration times based on "complete disintegration" [7]. Accordingly, these times are defined as the times at which first visible cracks in the capsule shell appear. In order to avoid observer bias, disintegration tests were performed before dissolution tests.

2.5. Acid Uptake Test

Six capsules were individually weighed and then tested in a disintegration tester as outlined above (the Disintegration Test subsection) but without disks, and only in HCl (0.1 and 0.01 M) for one and two hours. Sinkers (Japanese Pharmacopoeia Standard, Pharma Test, Hainburg, Germany) were used to prevent the capsules from floating. At the end of the test the capsules were removed, blotted and the %weight gain was calculated as follows:

$$\% \text{ weight gain in acid} = \frac{\text{mass after acid exposure} - \text{mass before acid exposure}}{\text{mass before acid exposure}} \times 100\%$$

2.6. Dissolution Test

The drug release was tested with a DT6R dissolution tester (Erweka GmbH & CO.KG, Langen, Germany). The device was used as a USP type I dissolution tester at 100 rpm as well as a USP type II dissolution tester with sinkers (same as in previous subsection) at 50 rpm. The use of sinkers prevented the capsules from floating in the paddle apparatus. In accordance with the disintegration test, the capsules were studied for one hour in 0.1 M HCl followed by a media change to either one of the buffers described previously. The volume of the dissolution media was 700 mL. The temperature was maintained at 37.0 ± 0.2 °C. The 5 mL samples were filtered through a 0.8 μm cellulose acetate nitrate filter (Rotilab Spritzenfilter CME, Carl Roth, Karlsruhe, Germany). The first 1 mL of the filtrate was discarded to saturate the membrane. Blank buffer was used to replace the sample volume. Caffeine was quantified spectrophotometrically at λ = 275 nm.

2.7. Correlation between Disintegration and Dissolution Results

Disintegration times were correlated with the times required to achieve 10%, 50% and 80% release (t10%, t50% and t80% respectively) representing the early, middle and late portions of the dissolution profiles. The aforementioned times were calculated using linear interpolation. The correlation was done using simple linear regression performed by Microsoft Excel (Microsoft Office 2013, Microsoft Corporation, Redmond, WA, USA). Hypothesis testing was performed on the slope using a one-sided t-test (With the null hypothesis being slope = 0). One-sided p-values were calculated since a positive correlation is expected. The hypothesis testing was performed using the vassarstats website [8].

3. Results and Discussion

3.1. Disintegration and Acid Uptake

As shown in Figure 1, DRcaps®Enteric gave the fastest disintegration while HPMCAS-HG gave the slowest. Disintegration tended to be fastest in the USP dissolution testing medium and slowest in the Al-Gousous et al. medium as would be expected based on the buffer molarities of the media. The fast disintegration of DRcaps®Enteric, however, seems to be associated with poor resistance to acid as evidenced by the acid uptake values shown in Table 3 and by the deformation exhibited by those capsules (Figure 2). This indicates that it is rather the weakened capsule shell structure that results in rapid disintegration in buffer. This is rather in line with the findings of Al-Tabakha et al. [7], where even rupture of such capsule shells was observed in simulated gastric fluid.

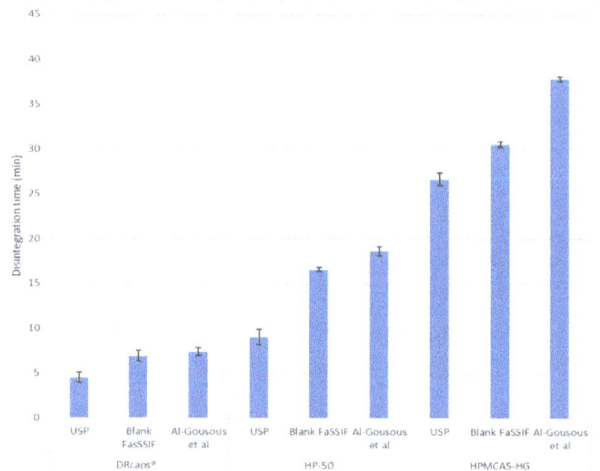

Figure 1. Disintegration times (mean ± SD) of the tested formulations (n = 6).

Table 3. Weight gain (mean ± SD) of the tested formulations (n = 6) after 1 h in acidic media.

Formulation	% Weight gain in 0.1 M HCl		% Weight gain in 0.01 M HCl	
	After 1 h	After 2 h	After 1 h	After 2 h
DRcaps®	6.5 ± 0.7	7.4 ± 0.3	11.2 ± 0.2	13.5 ± 0.6
HP-50	3.4 ± 0.6	4.2 ± 0.3	3.8 ± 0.1	6.1 ± 0.7
HPMCAS-HG	2.5 ± 0.4	Ruptured	2.8 ± 0.6	Ruptured

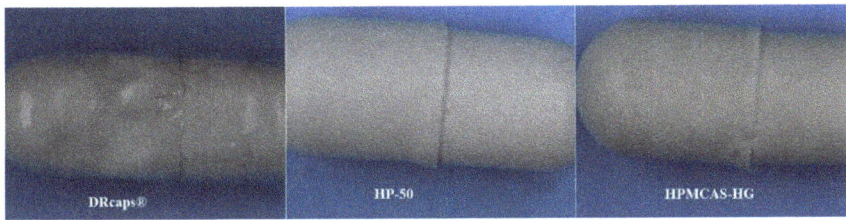

Figure 2. Appearance of DRcaps® and coated capsules after 1 h in 0.1 M HCl.

It is interesting that despite showing the lowest acid uptake at one hour, the HPMCAS-HG capsules ruptured in acid within roughly 1.5–2 h during the acid uptake tests. This might be related to mechanical instability. Figure 2 shows that while the DRCaps® show extensive deformation, HP-50-coated ones show only some wear at the gap between the body and the cap. HPMCAS-HG-coated capsules behave in a manner similar to the HP-50-coated ones but the wear at the gap seems to be a bit more extensive, which may impart mechanical instability to the capsule. The causes behind this need to be further investigated.

As shown in Figure 1, after 1 h in acid, the capsules coated with HPMCAS-HG still show the longest disintegration times. Only the high buffer capacity USP medium [6] showed large acceleration in disintegration compared to the situation where testing in acid was continued for one further hour (in the acid uptake tests with sinkers and without disks). This further supports the mechanical instability hypothesis. As for why the presence of disks in the disintegration test (compared to their absence in the acid uptake test) does not seem to have a dramatic effect, this might be related to the disk impacting the capsule from above rather than tearing it apart. Other factors could be the force generated on contact between the capsules and the sinkers in the disk-free setup as well as the tilted orientation of the capsules in the disintegration tester tubes when inside sinkers and its potential effects on hydrodynamics. Further investigation is needed regarding this issue, which is outside the scope of this manuscript.

3.2. Dissolution

As shown in Figure 3, the dissolution results followed the trends exhibited by the disintegration times. The disintegration times are lesser even than the t10% values, which is most probably associated with the capsule rupture being a pre-requisite for significant drug release and with the greater mechanical stresses in the disintegration tester [9]. Dissolution tended to be slower in the basket apparatus. This may be associated with the lower fluid velocities in the central and upper regions of the basket (at 100 rpm) where the capsule tends to be located owing to its buoyancy compared to the bottom of the vessel in a paddle apparatus (at 50 rpm) [10]. This implies that hydrodynamic differences between the different apparatuses play an important role in the obtained correlations.

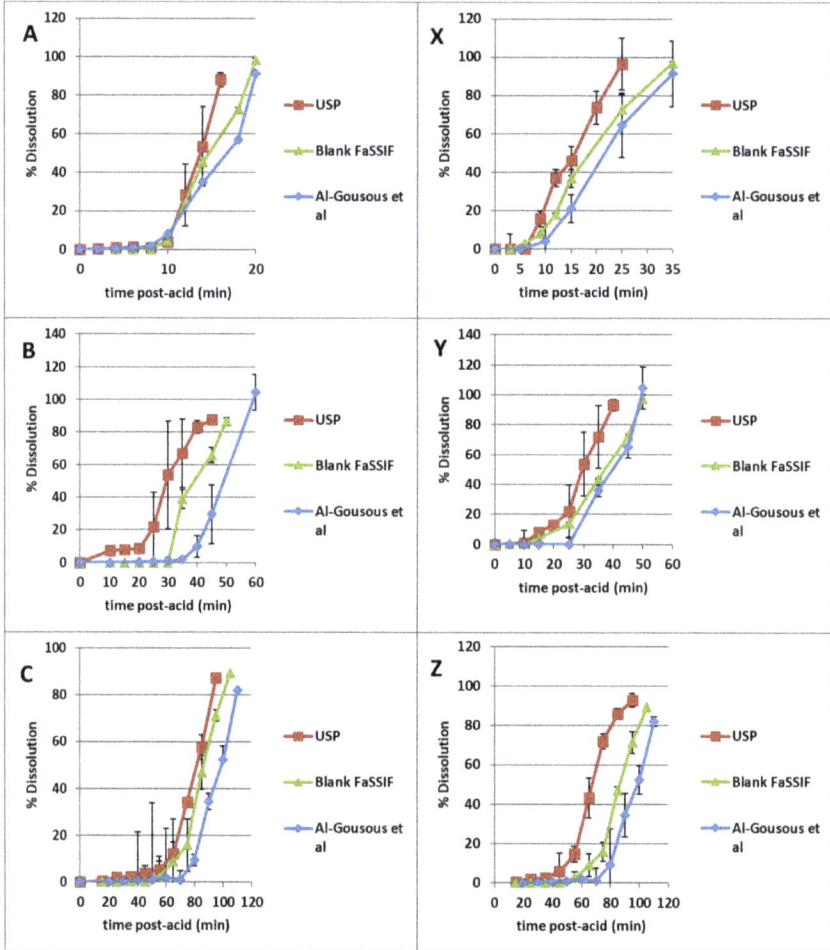

Figure 3. Dissolution test results (mean ± SD) of the tested formulations (n = 6). Panels (**A–C**) represent DRcaps®, HP-50 and HPMCAS-H respectively in basket apparatus, while panels **X**, **Y** and **Z** represent DRcaps®, HP-50 and HPMCAS-H respectively in paddle apparatus.

3.3. Correlation between Disintegration and Dissolution Results

Disintegration times were correlated with the times required to achieve 10, 50 and 80% release (t10%, t50% and t80% respectively) representing the early, middle and late portions of the dissolution profiles. When all the dissolution times were correlated with their respective disintegration times, good overall correlations were obtained for all dissolution profile portions (Figure 4).

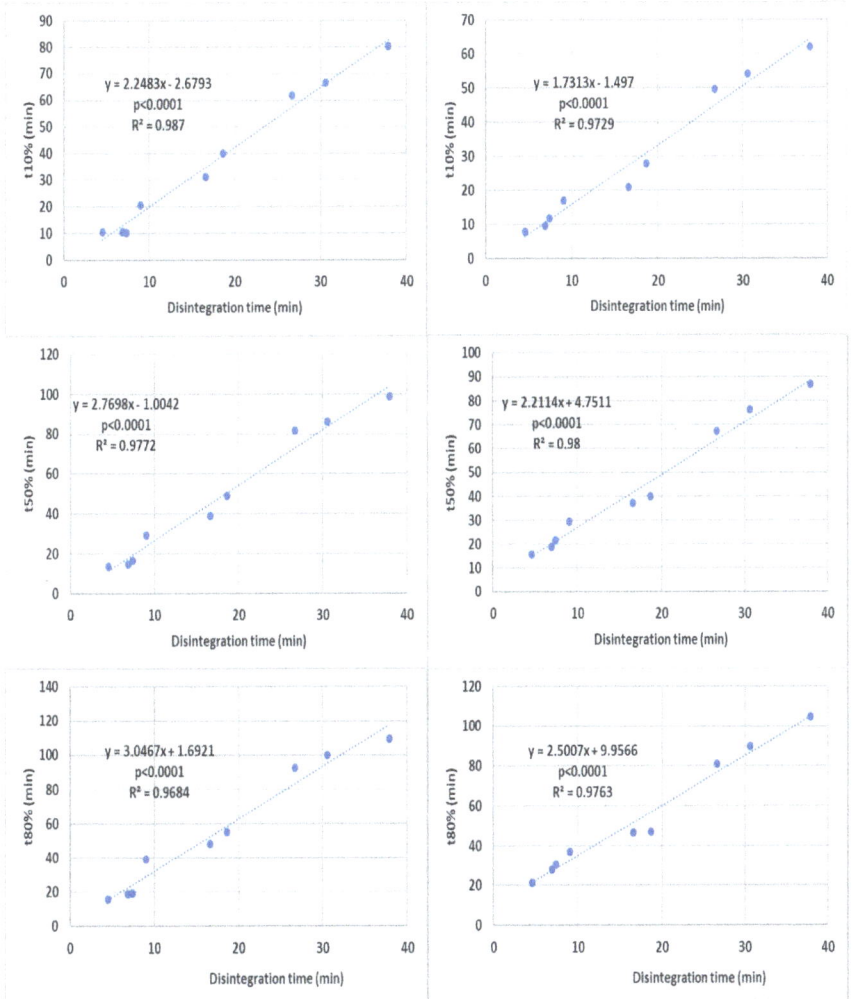

Figure 4. Overall correlation of all the disintegration results with their respective dissolution results (all formulations in all media are present in each graph) in the basket apparatus (right-hand side) and the paddle apparatus (left-hand-side). The *p*-value is a one-sided value for a *t*-test applied to the slope.

A more detailed analysis was performed by making three point correlations for formulation effects (Figures 5 and 6) and medium effects (Figures 7 and 8). When the results of different formulations tested in the same medium were correlated, good r^2 and p-values were almost invariably obtained. However, the situation was different when correlating results of the same formulation in different media (Figures 8 and 9), where the differences tended to be smaller than the inter-formulation differences.

Poor correlations were generally obtained for DRcaps® (with the notable exception of the t80% case). A possible explanation for that could be that the weakened capsule shell structure made the initial rupture more associated with random mechanical events and less with the enteric-polymer dissolution promoting capabilities of the buffer. The complete process of shell dissolution/disintegration was less confounded by such random effects resulting in better correlations for t80%. As for the weak correlations obtained for the t10% and t80% parameters for the HP-50-coated capsules, they seem to be caused by the close disintegration times in the blank FaSSIF and Al-Gousous et al. media. This is most probably related to the different discriminative abilities of the disintegration tester vs. paddle and basket apparatuses (owing to the different hydrodynamics). HPMCAS-HG gave the best correlations likely due to the slow capsule shell disintegration relative to drug dissolution. Anyway, despite multiple instances of weak correlations, when correlating the results of one formulation in different media, each formulation shows at least one instance with $p < 0.05$.

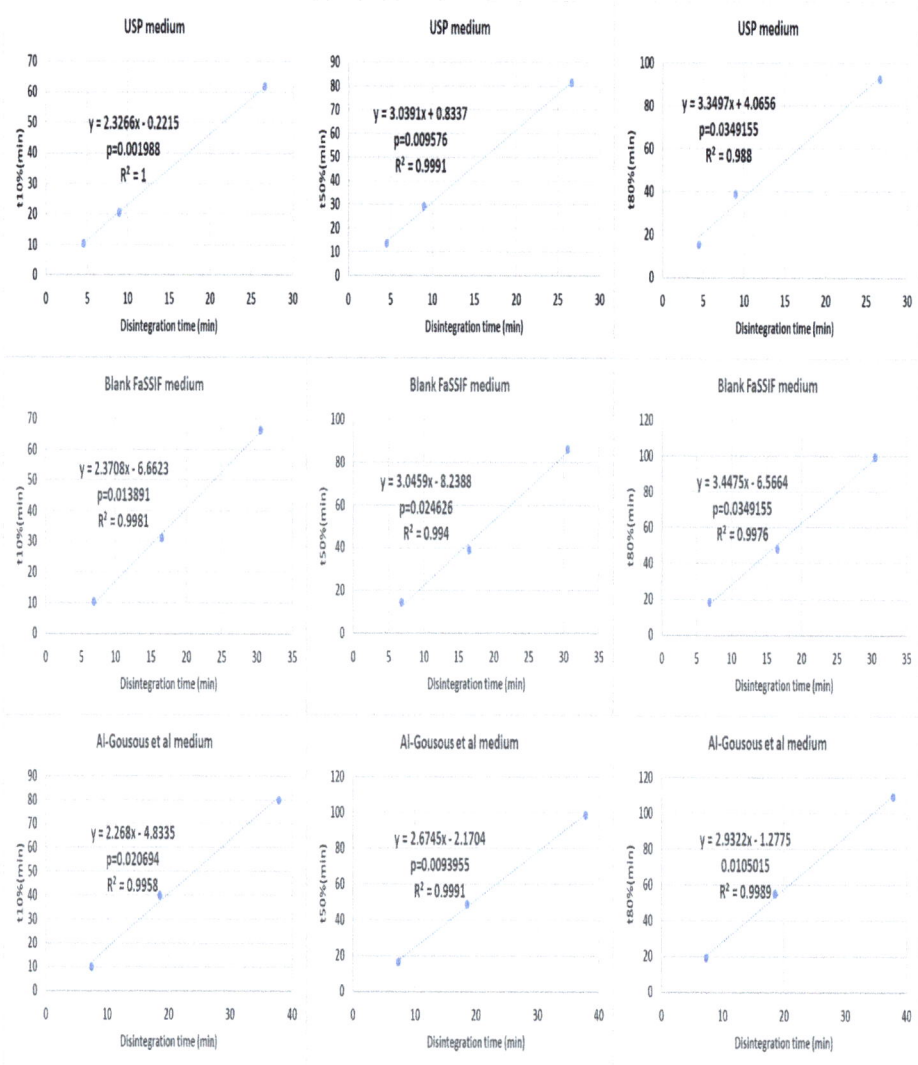

Figure 5. Correlating disintegration times with different dissolution parameters (basket apparatus) for different formulations tested in one medium. The p-value is a one-sided value for a t-test applied to the slope.

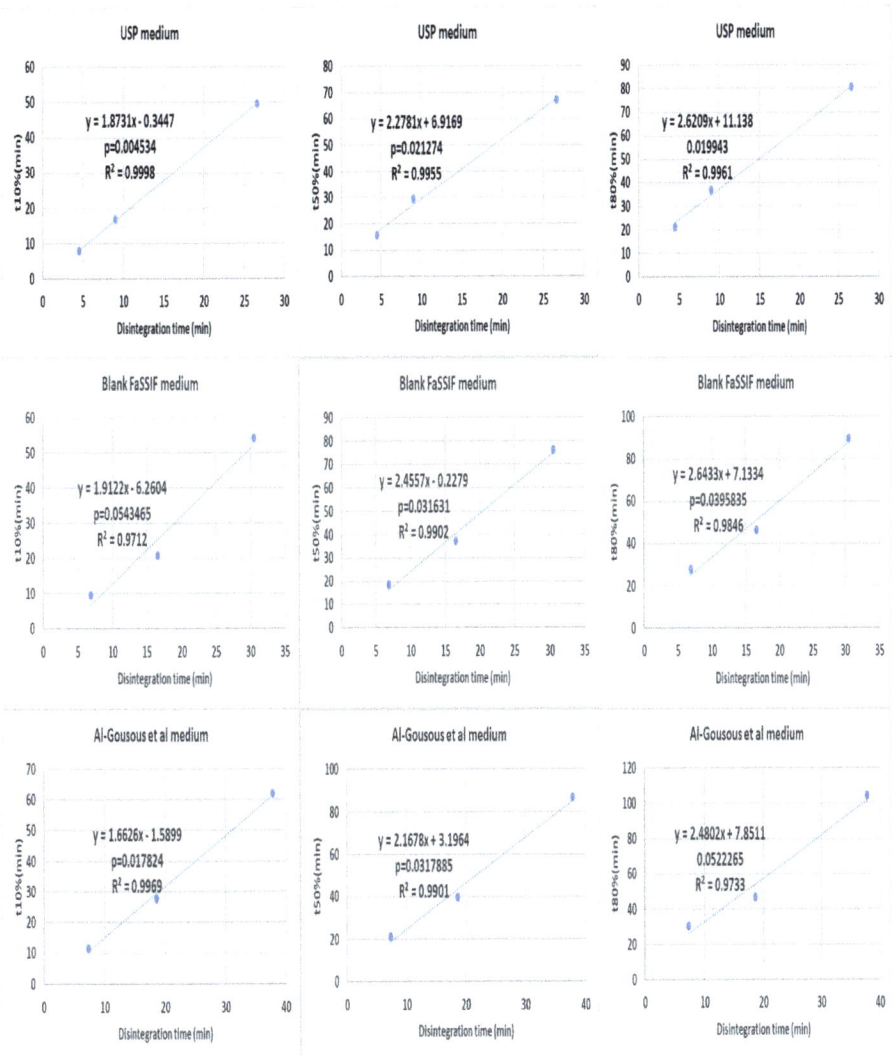

Figure 6. Correlating disintegration times with different dissolution (paddle apparatus) parameters for different formulations tested in one medium. The *p*-value is a one-sided value for a *t*-test applied to the slope.

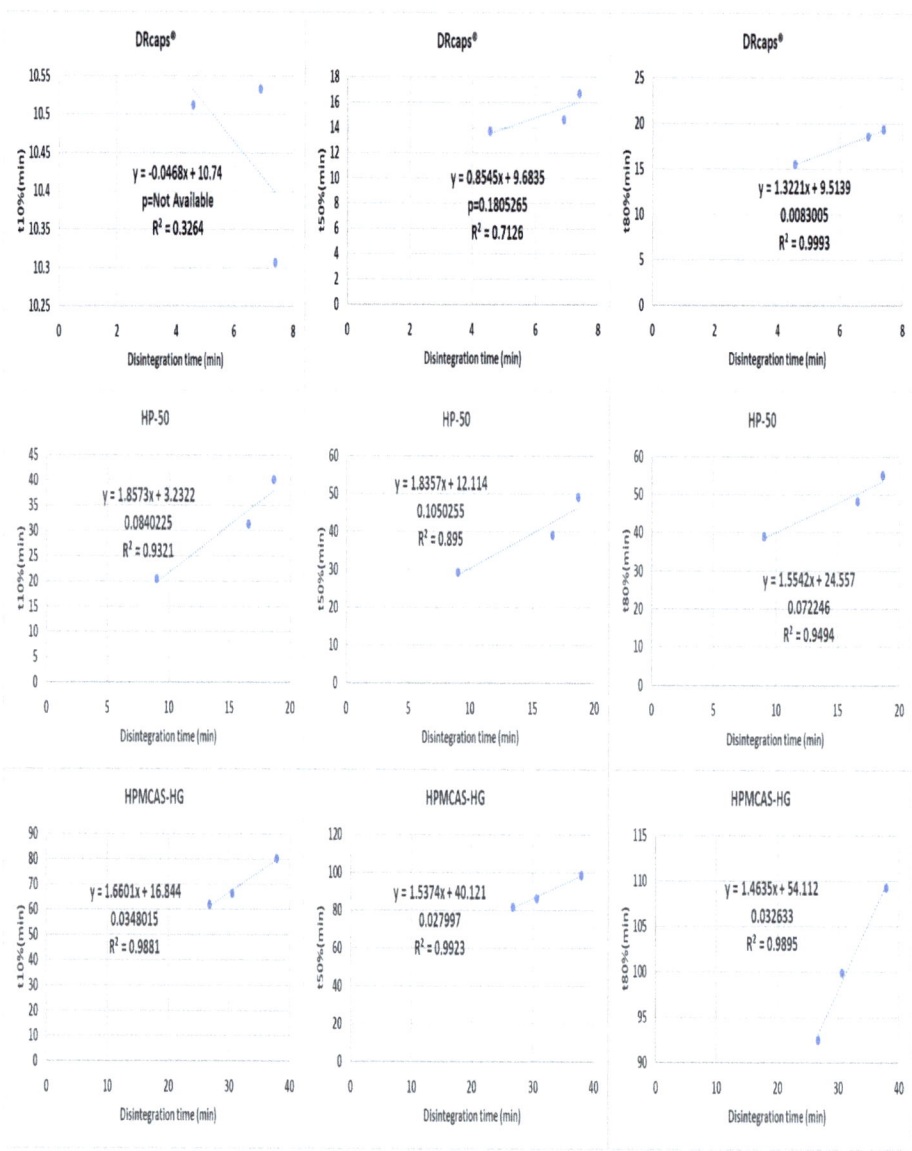

Figure 7. Correlating disintegration times with different dissolution (basket apparatus) parameters for one formulation in different media. The *p*-value is a one-sided value for a *t*-test applied to the slope.

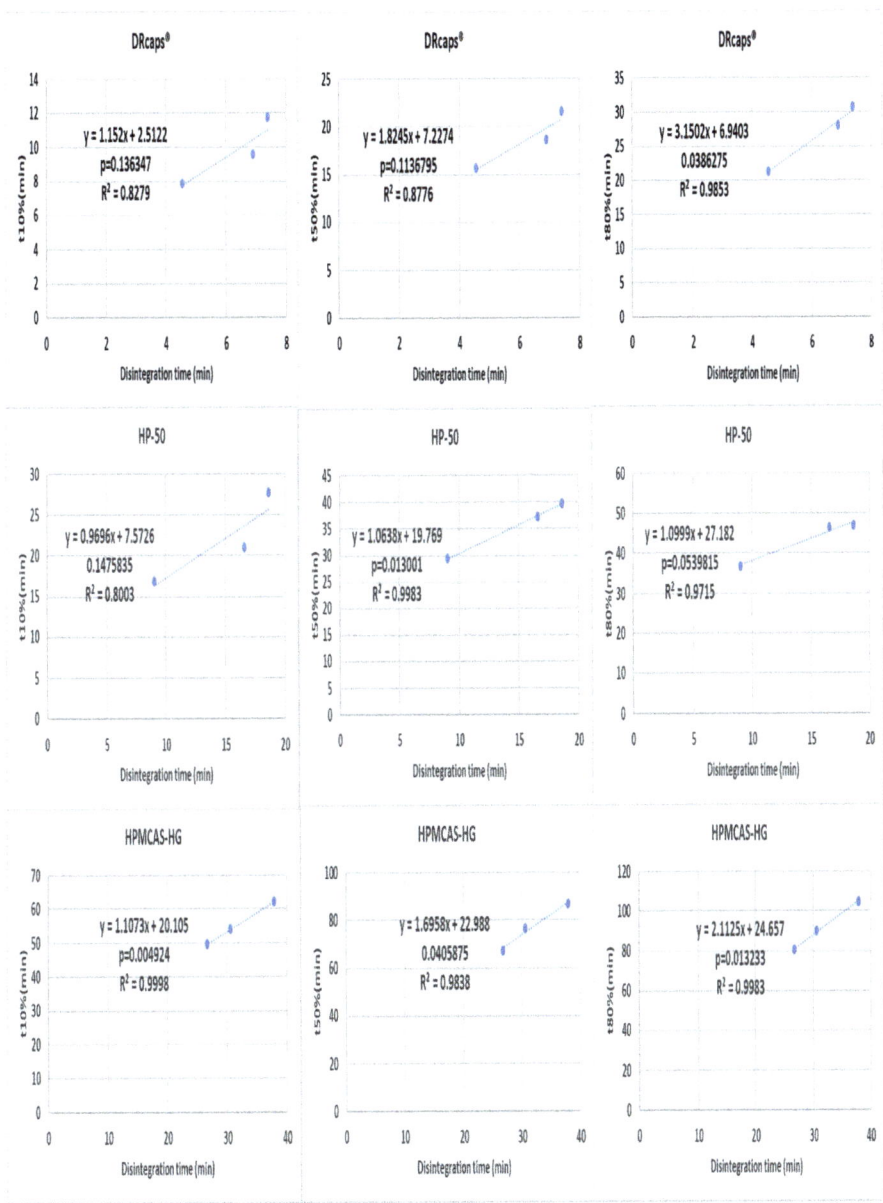

Figure 8. Correlation of disintegration times with different dissolution (paddle apparatus) parameters for one formulation in different media. The *p*-value is a one-sided value for a *t*-test applied to the slope.

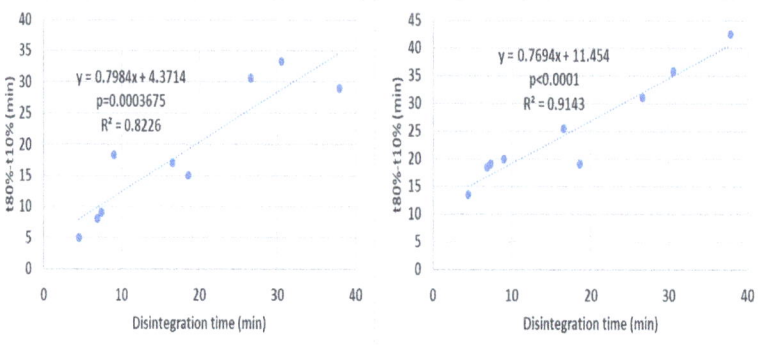

Figure 9. Overall correlation of all the disintegration times with their (t80%–t10%) values results (all formulations in all media are present in each graph) in the basket apparatus (right-hand side) and the paddle apparatus (left-hand-side). The *p*-value is a one-sided value for a *t*-test applied to the slope.

An additional observation is that the correlations for different dissolution time points show not only different intercepts but also different slopes. This indicates that the disintegration times do not correlate with the different dissolution times solely because of the profiles being shifted because of different coat rupture times, but also because of the influence of the disintegration on the overall post-capsule rupture release kinetics. This is shown by the fair to strong overall correlations obtained for the difference between t80% and t10% (corresponding to the time required for % release to rise from 10% to 80%).

Figure 9 shows stronger correlation for the paddle apparatus. A possible reason could be that variation in the floating capsule orientation inside the basket, together with the more variable fluid velocities in the upper region of the basket [10], leads to the greater data point scatter observed for the basket apparatus.

All in all, the obtained set of correlations shows that enteric-coated formulations seem promising with regard to using disintegration tests as dissolution surrogates. This shows that the use of disintegration testing as dissolution testing surrogate might not have to be restricted only to immediate release dosage forms. However, further investigations on further EC dosage forms need to be performed before making a definitive judgment on this matter.

4. Conclusions

Obtaining good correlations between the dissolution and disintegration results of EC dosage forms is possible. This opens the way for more rigorous research that could help in expanding the dissolution test waiver concept beyond immediate release dosage forms. Further investigations on additional EC formulations could help to establish regulatory criteria regarding this matter. However, extrapolating these findings to the in vivo situation should be done with extreme caution since many factors like (among others) possible transporter saturation effects [11], interplay with food and gastric emptying effects [12,13] as well as different hydrodynamics and mechanical stresses [9] complicate the correlation between disintegration and bioavailability. These issues need to be taken into account when considering an expanded role for disintegration testing in product evaluation.

Author Contributions: Data curation, J.A.-G.; Formal analysis, P.L.; Investigation, M.F. and J.A.B.; Project administration, P.L.; Resources, P.L.; Supervision, P.L.; Writing—original draft, J.A.-G. and P.L. All authors have read and agreed to the published version of the manuscript.

Funding: This research received no external funding.

Acknowledgments: This work was supported by a scholarship from China government (China Scholarship Council, CSC). We are grateful to Shin-Etsu Tylose GmbH & Co. (Wiesbaden, Germany) for the use of drum coater and the scanning electron microscope and supplying Aqoat®AS-LG, MG, HG, HPMCP coating polymers. Special appreciation is expressed to Andreas Sauer for the advice in the whole processing and to Ilja. Lesser and Tobias Eggers for their technical assistance and support. We would also like to thank ACG Associated Capsules (Mumbai, India) for supplying the ACG Nature Caps Plus.

Conflicts of Interest: The authors declare no conflict of interest.

References

1. Al-Gousous, J.; Langguth, P. Oral Solid Dosage Form Disintegration Testing-The Forgotten Test. *J. Pharm. Sci.* **2015**, *104*, 2664–2675. [CrossRef] [PubMed]
2. International Conference on Harmonization. Available online: https://database.ich.org/sites/default/files/Q6A_Guideline.pdf (accessed on 28 November 2019).
3. Gupta, A.; Hunt, R.L.; Shah, R.B.; Sayeed, V.A.; Khan, M.A. Disintegration of highly soluble immediate release tablets: A surrogate for dissolution. *Aaps Pharm. Sci. Tech.* **2009**, *10*, 495–499. [CrossRef] [PubMed]
4. Radwan, A.; Amidon, G.L.; Langguth, P. Mechanistic investigation of food effect on disintegration and dissolution of BCS class III compound solid formulations: The importance of viscosity. *Biopharm. Drug Dispos.* **2012**, *33*, 403–416. [CrossRef] [PubMed]
5. Nickerson, B.; Kong, A.; Gerst, P.; Kao, S. Correlation of dissolution and disintegration results for an immediate-release tablet. *J. Pharm. Biomed. Anal.* **2018**, *150*, 333–340. [CrossRef] [PubMed]
6. Al-Gousous, J.; Amidon, G.L.; Langguth, P. Toward Biopredictive Dissolution for Enteric Coated Dosage Forms. *Mol. Pharmaceutics.* **2016**, *13*, 1927–1936. [CrossRef] [PubMed]
7. Al-Tabakha, M.M.; Arida, A.I.; Fahelelbom, K.M.S.; Sadek, B.; Jarad, R.A.A. Performances of New Generation of Delayed Release Capsules. *J. Young Pharm.* **2015**, *7*, 36–44. [CrossRef]
8. VassarStats. Available online: http://vassarstats.net/ (accessed on 1 December 2019).
9. Kamba, M.; Seta, Y.; Takeda, N.; Hamaura, T.; Kusai, A.; Nakane, H.; Nishimura, K. Measurement of agitation force in dissolution test and mechanical destructive force in disintegration test. *Int. J. Pharm.* **2003**, *250*, 99–109. [CrossRef]
10. D'Arcy, D.M.; Corrigan, O.I.; Healy, A.M. Evaluation of hydrodynamics in the basket dissolution apparatus using computational fluid dynamics–Dissolution rate implications. *Eur. J. Pharm. Sci.* **2006**, *27*, 259–267. [CrossRef] [PubMed]
11. Bhagavan, H.N.; Wolkoff, B.I. Correlation between the disintegration time and the bioavailability of vitamin C tablets. *Pharm. Res.* **1993**, *10*, 239–242. [CrossRef] [PubMed]
12. Brouwers, J.; Tack, J.; Augustijns, P. Parallel monitoring of plasma and intraluminal drug concentrations in man after oral administration of fosamprenavir in the fasted and fed state. *Pharm. Res.* **2007**, *24*, 1862–1869. [CrossRef] [PubMed]
13. Brouwers, J.; Anneveld, B.; Goudappel, G.J.; Duchateau, G.; Annaert, P.; Augustijns, P.; Zeijdner, E. Food-dependent disintegration of immediate release fosamprenavir tablets: In vitro evaluation using magnetic resonance imaging and a dynamic gastrointestinal system. *Eur. J. Pharm. Biopharm.* **2011**, *77*, 313–319. [CrossRef] [PubMed]

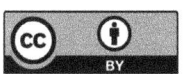

© 2020 by the authors. Licensee MDPI, Basel, Switzerland. This article is an open access article distributed under the terms and conditions of the Creative Commons Attribution (CC BY) license (http://creativecommons.org/licenses/by/4.0/).

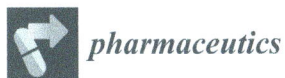

Article

Segmental-Dependent Solubility and Permeability as Key Factors Guiding Controlled Release Drug Product Development

Milica Markovic [1,†], Moran Zur [1,†], Noa Fine-Shamir [1], Ester Haimov [1], Isabel González-Álvarez [2] and Arik Dahan [1,*]

1. Department of Clinical Pharmacology, School of Pharmacy, Faculty of Health Sciences, Ben-Gurion University of the Negev, Beer-Sheva 8410501, Israel
2. Department of Pharmacokinetics and Pharmaceutical Technology, Miguel Hernandez University, 03550 San Juan de Alicante, Spain
* Correspondence: arikd@bgu.ac.il; Tel.: +972-8-6479483; Fax: +972-8-6479303
† These authors contributed equally to the article.

Received: 23 January 2020; Accepted: 20 March 2020; Published: 24 March 2020

Abstract: The main factors influencing the absorption of orally administered drugs are solubility and permeability, which are location-dependent and may vary along the gastrointestinal tract (GIT). The purpose of this work was to investigate segmental-dependent intestinal absorption and its role in controlled-release (CR) drug product development. The solubility/dissolution and permeability of carvedilol (vs. metoprolol) were thoroughly studied, in vitro/in vivo (Octanol-buffer distribution coefficients (Log D), parallel artificial membrane permeability assay (PAMPA), rat intestinal perfusion), focusing on location-dependent effects. Carvedilol exhibits changing solubility in different conditions throughout the GIT, attributable to its zwitterionic nature. A biorelevant pH-dilution dissolution study for carvedilol immediate release (IR) vs. CR scenario elucidates that while the IR dose (25 mg) may dissolve in the GIT luminal conditions, higher doses used in CR products would precipitate if administered at once, highlighting the advantage of CR from the solubility/dissolution point of view. Likewise, segmental-dependent permeability was evident, with higher permeability of carvedilol vs. the low/high P_{eff} marker metoprolol throughout the GIT, confirming it as a biopharmaceutical classification system (BCS) class II drug. Theoretical analysis of relevant physicochemical properties confirmed these results as well. A CR product may shift the carvedilol's solubility behavior from class II to I since only a small dose portion needs to be solubilized at a given time point. The permeability of carvedilol surpasses the threshold of metoprolol jejunal permeability throughout the entire GIT, including the colon, establishing it as a suitable candidate for CR product development. Altogether, this work may serve as an analysis model in the decision process of CR formulation development and may increase our biopharmaceutical understanding of a successful CR drug product.

Keywords: controlled release drug product; biopharmaceutics classification system; drug solubility; drug permeability; location-dependent absorption

---

1. Introduction

Oral drug absorption depends on various parameters: physicochemical (e.g., ionization, pKa, solubility, physicochemical stability, lipophilic nature, polar surface area (PSA), molecular weight,), physiological (e.g., gastrointestinal pH, surface area available for absorption, transit time, expression of certain transporters, enzymes), and parameters associated with the dosage form [1–3]. However, keeping this complexity in mind, it was determined that the drug permeability and solubility/dissolution in the gastrointestinal aqueous milieu are the two essential variables that guide absorption in the gastrointestinal tract (GIT) [4].

These two key factors, the solubility and the permeability, are location-dependent and can vary along the GIT. Change in pH or presence of bile salts can modify drug solubility/dissolution in a given intestinal segment; for a drug to be considered as a high solubility compound as per the biopharmaceutical classification system (BCS), it needs to be dissolved in an aqueous media (250 mL or less) with the different pH values relevant to the GIT lumen (1.0–6.8) [5–7]. Likewise, intestinal permeability is also location-dependent, and pertains in each region of the GIT [1,3,8,9]. Therefore, in different scenarios, e.g., drug discovery, drug and formulation development, and regulatory considerations, assigning the BSC class membership founded only on physicochemical drug features may lead to the incorrect decision [2,10–13]. Thus, regional-dependent permeability factors also need to be considered, for instance, expression of membrane transporters (influx/efflux) along the intestinal tract [11,14–16], luminal pH that influences the changes in the drug ionization [1,3,8,13], local water absorption [10], and others.

Segmental-dependent biopharmaceutical considerations are particularly important for controlled-release (CR) drug products; the drug is continuously released throughout the entire GI; therefore, it is not sufficient for a drug moiety to have suitable solubility/permeability in only one particular intestinal segment [17–19].

Carvedilol is a third-generation β-blocker, and is commonly used for treating hypertension, heart failure, and left ventricular dysfunction (LVD) [20,21]. The pharmacokinetics and pharmacodynamics of carvedilol from controlled release (CR) and immediate release (IR) products were compared in two clinical studies [22,23]. The data from these studies demonstrated that once-daily CR carvedilol is clinically correspondent to the IR carvedilol drug product administered two times a day, in patients with heart failure and asymptomatic post-myocardial infarction [23]. In addition, carvedilol CR maintains steady β_1-adrenergic blockade with a dose administered once every 24 h [22]. Metoprolol is a passively transported drug which is not affected by the P-glycoprotein (P-gp) efflux transport [24], while carvedilol is a substrate of P-gp [25]. Carvedilol inhibits the activity of P-glycoprotein (P-gp) transporter [26,27]. It also undergoes extensive stereoselective first-pass metabolism; the main cytochrome P450 enzymes responsible for the metabolism of both R(+) and S(−)-carvedilol are CYP2D6 and CYP2C9, with some of the resulting metabolites having pharmacological activity. Despite its extensive first-pass metabolism, marketed carvedilol CR capsules have a bioavailability of 85% relative to IR tablets, with good clinical efficacy [23]. Hence, carvedilol was shown as a successful candidate for development as a controlled-release drug product, despite the fact that the pH variations along the GIT may significantly alter both the solubility and the permeability of this ionizable (basic) drug [28,29]. This raises the question of carvedilol's location-dependent intestinal solubility and permeability and its successful use as a CR product.

This work aimed to study the segmental-dependent biopharmaceutical consideration of carvedilol as a model basic drug, analyzed in view of CR scenario, allowing to pinpoint the rational for a successful CR drug product. Carvedilol solubility/dissolution and permeability were systematically investigated, through in vitro/in vivo (Octanol-buffer distribution coefficients (Log D), parallel artificial membrane permeability assay (PAMPA), rat intestinal perfusion) techniques, focusing on location-dependent variations, as well as theoretical physicochemical properties analysis of the drug. As a Food and Drug Administration (FDA) recommended standard for the low-high permeability class boundary, we used metoprolol, which also served as an accompanying model compound, since it is also marketed as a CR drug product. This study offers a deeper understanding of the factors that could influence segmental-dependent permeability and solubility in a controlled-release setting, and their contribution to a successful controlled-release drug product.

2. Materials and Methods

2.1. Materials

Carvedilol, metoprolol, sodium chloride, potassium phosphate monobasic, and sodium phosphate dibasic, hexadecane, octanol, and trifluoroacetic acid (TFA) were purchased from Sigma Chemical Co. (St. Louis, MO, USA). Water and acetonitrile (Merck KGaA, Darmstadt, Germany) were ultra-performance liquid chromatography (UPLC) purity grade. All other substances were of analytical reagent grade.

2.2. Solubility

The pH-dependent solubility, as well as carvedilol solubility BCS classification, was evaluated by the shake-flask method, as previously reported [8,30]. Briefly, the equilibrium solubility of carvedilol was studied at 37 °C, at pH 7.5 with phosphate buffer (potassium phosphate monobasic and sodium phosphate dibasic), pH 4.5 acetate buffer (sodium acetate and acetic acid), and pH 1.0 maleate buffer (maleic acid). Five hundred microliters of buffer was added to glass vials, and excess carvedilol quantities were added to buffer-containing glass vials, until the solution was no longer clear. Equilibrium was verified by comparison of 48- and 72-h samples. The pH of each solution was measured following the drug's addition to the buffer solution. The vial caps were firmly sealed, and the vials were placed in a shaking incubator (100 rpm, 37 °C). Before the drug concentration was analyzed, the vials were centrifuged at 10,000 rpm (10,621 rcf) for 10 min, and the supernatant was removed, followed by drug quantification with UPLC. For dose number (D_0) calculations, the highest dose of carvedilol immediate-release (IR) oral drug product was taken to be 25 mg [22].

2.3. Octanol-Buffer Distribution Coefficients

Octanol-buffer distribution coefficients (Log D) for carvedilol and metoprolol were determined at pH 6.5, 7.0, and 7.5 using the shake-flask method [12,30]. This pH range represents the physiological pH relevant for the intestinal tract (naturally, permeability from the stomach is considered not significant). Carvedilol and metoprolol solutions were prepared in a phosphate buffer saturated with octanol (pH 6.5, 7.0, and 7.5.), and consequently equilibrated at 37 °C, 48 h with an equal volume of buffer saturated with octanol of corresponding pH. The aqueous and octanol phase were parted by centrifugation, and the concentration of the drug in the aqueous phase was quantified by UPLC; the drug in the octanol phase was determined by mass balance.

2.4. Biorelevant pH-Dilution Dissolution Studies

An in vitro biorelevant pH-dilution dissolution study was performed (n = 5 each) as we have previously published [31–33], to simulate drug dose dissolution while traveling along the GIT, in two scenarios: carvedilol concentrations of 100 µg/mL vs. 320 µg/mL, simulating the highest IR dose (25 mg; COREG™) and CR dose (80 mg; COREG CR™) on the market, taken with 250 mL of water. An aqueous suspension of the drug dose was first diluted into HCl 0.1M to obtain a pH of 1.2 (dilution factor 1:0.66) and agitated for 15 min (100 rpm at 37 °C), to mimic the stomach compartment, as we have previously reported. Then, samples were further diluted with fasted state simulated intestinal fluid (FaSSIF) (Biorelevant.Com Ltd., London, UK) with a dilution factor (1:1) for 30 min, followed by a dilution factor of 1:1.5, agitated for 30 min, and consequently 2 other dilutions of 1:1 with agitation time of 1 h each, to closely mimic the conditions throughout the small intestinal travel; the complete time of the study was 3 hours and 15 min (with samples taken at time points 0, 15, 45, 75, 105, 135, 195 min). During the course of the study, samples were centrifuged, filtrated, and the drug concentration was instantly quantified by UPLC. The solubilized drug amount, quantified by UPLC, was compared to the total amount of drug, which was calculated using the initial drug dose and consequent dilutions. This comparison enabled evaluation of the fraction of dose dissolved vs. precipitated for the IR vs.

CR simulated experiments. The pH gradient throughout the experiment was designed to mimic the physiological conditions along the GIT, with a final pH of 7.6.

2.5. Parallel Artificial Membrane Permeability Assay Studies

In vitro permeability studies through an artificial membrane were carried out in the hexadecane-based parallel artificial membrane permeability assay (PAMPA) using Millipore (Danvers, MA) 96-well MultiScreen-Permeability filter plates with 0.3 cm^2 polycarbonate filter support (0.45 µm). The filter supports in every well were impregnated with 15 µL of a 5% solution (v/v) of hexadecane in hexanes and were then permitted to dry for 1 h. This time frame allowed the hexanes to be entirely evaporated, producing a consistent hexadecane layer. The permeability studies using hexadecane layer were carried out according to the standard protocol, with minor modifications [13]. Briefly, both carvedilol and metoprolol solutions (n = 4) were prepared in phosphate buffer solution (pH 6.5, 7.0, and 7.5) with comparable ionic strength and osmolality (290 mOsm/L). PAMPA sandwich plates were composed of donor wells containing various drug solutions (200 µL), and the receiver wells containing blank buffers (300 µL). The plate was incubated at room temperature, and samples were taken from the receiver plates every hour for a total of 4 h. Apparent permeability coefficient (P_{app}) was calculated from the linear plot of drug collected in the acceptor side vs. time with the following equation:

$$P_{app} = \frac{dQ/dT}{A \times C_0}$$

where dQ/dt is the appearance rate in the steady-state of carvedilol/metoprolol from the receiver side, C_0 is the starting drug concentration in the donor side (0.02 mM for carvedilol, and 0.1 mM for metoprolol), and A is the membrane surface area (0.048 cm^2). Linear regression was used to acquire the steady-state appearance rate of the drug on the receiver side.

2.6. Rat Single-Pass Intestinal Perfusion (SPIP)

The rat effective permeability coefficient (P_{eff}) of carvedilol and metoprolol in different intestinal regions was evaluated using the single-pass intestinal perfusion (SPIP) model. This experimental model was designed and validated to account for the complex physiological background of drug absorption along the GIT: the living animal, intact and viable GIT including tissue composition, membrane morphology, expression/distribution of functional transporters/enzymes, and the composition of the luminal milieu of the different segments, are all part of the high biorelevance of this model [34–36]. All animal experiments were performed according to the protocols accepted by the Ben-Gurion University of the Negev Animal Use and Care Committee (Protocol IL-07-01-2015). The animals (male Wistar rats weighing 230–260 g, Harlan, Israel) were housed and handled in agreement with the Ben-Gurion University of the Negev Unit for Laboratory Animal Medicine Guidelines.

The experimental procedure used for the in situ experiments in rats was previously described [3,12,13,30]. Prior to the experiment, the rats were fasted overnight. Namely, rats were anesthetized and positioned on a 37 °C surface (Harvard Apparatus Inc., Holliston, MA, USA), and a 3 cm midline abdominal incision was performed. Considering the complexity behind each of the intestinal segments, permeability was simultaneously measured through 3 separate intestinal regions (length of 10 cm each); a proximal segment of the jejunum at pH 6.5 (beginning at 2 cm under the ligament of the Treitz), a distal segment of the ileum at pH 7.5 (finishing 2 cm above the cecum), and the colonic segment at pH 6.5 (approximately 6 cm); the pH values through each region corresponded to the physiological pH of that region [1,3]. Each intestinal segment was cannulated at both sides and was rinsed with the relevant blank perfusion buffer. Phosphate buffers containing carvedilol and metoprolol were prepared at pH 6.5 and 7.5, while maintaining similar ionic strength and osmolality (290 mOsm/L) in all buffers. All solutions were incubated in a water bath at 37 °C. The steady-state conditions were established by perfusing the drug-containing buffer solution (0.02 mM) for 1 h, and an additional hour of perfusion followed, with sample collection every 10 min. The pH value was determined in the outlet samples to ensure the there was no pH variation during the course of perfusion. At the end of the perfusion study, the drug concentration in the outlet samples was determined by UPLC, and the length of the intestinal segment used for perfusion was measured for further permeability calculations. The effective permeability (P_{eff}; cm/s) through the gut wall was calculated through to the following equation:

$$P_{eff} = \frac{-Q \ln(C'_{out}/C'_{in})}{2\pi RL}$$

Q being the perfusion buffer flow rate (0.2 mL/min), C'_{out}/C'_{in} is the ratio of the outlet and the inlet drug concentration that has been adjusted for water transport by the gravimetric method [37–39], R is the radius of the intestinal segment (conventionally used as 0.2 cm), and L is the length of the perfused intestinal segment.

2.7. Physicochemical Analysis

The theoretical fraction extracted into octanol (f_e) was calculated using the following equation [40,41]:

$$f_e = \frac{f_u P}{1 + f_u P}$$

where P stands for the octanol–water distribution coefficient of the unionized drug form and f_u is the drug fraction unionized at a certain pH. The f_u vs. pH was plotted according to the Henderson–Hasselbalch equation, using the following literature pKa values: 9.7 for metoprolol [42] and 7.8 for carvedilol [28].

2.8. Ultra-Performance Liquid Chromatography

An ultra-performance liquid chromatography (UPLC) instrument Waters (Milford, MA, USA) Acquity UPLC H-Class was equipped with a photodiode array detector and Empower software. The instantaneous determination of carvedilol and metoprolol was accomplished using a Waters Acquity UPLC XTerra C_{18} 3.5-μm 4.6 × 250 mm column. The gradient mobile phase consisted of 90:10 going to 30:70 (v/v) water:acetonitrile (containing 0.1% TFA) at a flow rate of 0.5 mL/min during 4 min. The wavelength of detection and retention times for carvedilol and metoprolol were 230 and 275 nm and 2.5, 3.1 min, respectively. UPLC injection volumes for all analyses were in a range from 2 to 50 μL. The limit of quantitation was termed as the lowest drug concentration that could be measured with an accuracy and precision of <20%, as per US Food and Drug Administration Guidelines. Precision was stated as the intra- and inter-day relative standard deviation (RSD). Intra-day accuracy and precision were determined by analyzing six replicates of control samples on the same day (samples of known concentration), while the inter-day accuracy and precision were evaluated by measuring six replicates of control samples on three different days. The carvedilol limit of quantification was 5 ng/mL, and for metoprolol 25 ng/mL, and the inter- and intra-day coefficients of variations were <1.0% and 0.5%, respectively.

2.9. Statistical Analysis

Log D studies and PAMPA assays were replicated with n = 6 and n = 4, respectively. Animal studies were replicated with n = 6. All values are stated as means ± standard deviation (SD). Statistically significant differences between the experimental groups were evaluated by the nonparametric Kruskal–Wallis test for multiple comparisons, and the two-tailed nonparametric Mann–Whitney U test for two-group comparison. A $p < 0.05$ was considered statistically significant.

3. Results

3.1. Solubility

The solubility data for carvedilol in the three pH values (1.0, 4.0, and 7.5) at 37 °C are presented in Table 1. The solubility data presents a complex picture: from pH 1.0 to 4.0, the solubility was rising, and again decreased towards pH 7.5, where the solubility was very low. The dose number was calculated using the subsequent equation: $D_0 = M/V_0/C_s$, where M is the highest single-unit dose strength of carvedilol (25 mg) [22], V_0 is the initial volume of water (250 mL), and C_s is the solubility at each pH; drug molecules with $D_0 \leq 1$ are considered highly soluble. At a pH of 1.0 and 7.5, the dose number for carvedilol was higher than 1, indicating low BCS solubility class membership. The chemical structure of carvedilol is presented in Table 2.

Table 1. Carvedilol solubility values (mg/mL) in the tree pH values 1.0, 4.0, and 7.5, at 37 °C, and the corresponding dose number (D_0) for a 25 mg dose. Data presented as mean ± SD; n = 6.

pH	Solubility (mg/mL)	Corresponding D_0
1.0	0.021 (±0.004)	4.720
4.0	2.320 (±1.090)	0.043
7.5	0.035 (±0.002)	2.880

Table 2. Carvedilol and metoprolol molecular structures and relevant physicochemical parameters.

Drug	Molecular Structure	pKa	Log P	PSA
Carvedilol	(structure)	7.8 [43]	3.8 [43]	75.7 [44]
Metoprolol	(structure)	9.7 [42]	2.2 [45]	50.7 [46]

3.2. Biorelevant pH-Dilution Dissolution Studies

We have studied the ability of the two highest marketed dosages for both IR (25 mg) and CR (80 mg) carvedilol drug products to accomplish and maintain complete dissolution of the carvedilol dose in the dynamic GIT environment using the pH-dilution method we have previously developed [31]. The dissolution results are presented in Figure 1, where it can be observed that a significant difference between the dissolution behavior of the 25 mg and 80 mg drug product was detected. The results indicate what may happen if these doses were to be orally administered at once; while the 80 mg dose would quickly precipitate, the 25 mg dose was completely dissolved (with ~15 min delay) and maintained dissolved throughout the GIT travel.

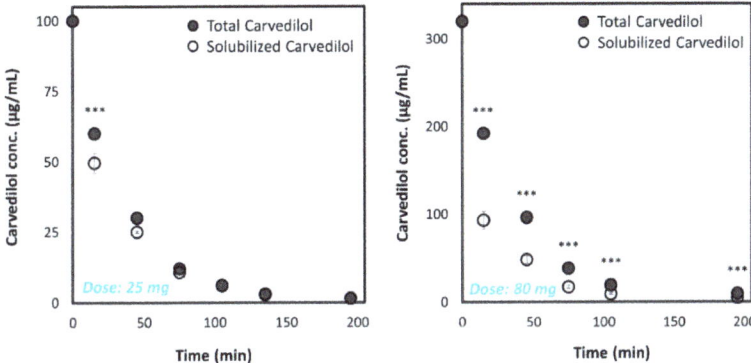

Figure 1. Dissolution of the highest carvedilol dose for IR and CR drug products on the market (25 mg and 80 mg, respectively) in the dynamic GIT environment, using the pH-dilution dissolution method. Values are presented as means ± SD; *** $p < 0.001$; n = 5. The pH at each time point for IR: 1.4 at 15 min; 1.9 at 45 min; 5.8 at 75 min; 6.9 at 105 min; 7.2 at 135 min; 7.3 at 195 min; and for CR drug product: 1.6 at 15 min; 2.9 at 45 min; 7.0 at 75 min; 7.4 at 105 min; 7.6 at 195 min.

3.3. Log D

The octanol–water distribution coefficients (Log D) for carvedilol and metoprolol were measured at the three pH values of 6.5, 7.0, and 7.5, representative of the environment of the small intestine (Figure 2). It can be seen that both carvedilol and metoprolol have evident pH-dependent upward Log D in the investigated pH range (6.5–7.5), however, while the Log D of metoprolol ranged from 0.8 (pH 6.5) to −0.2 (pH 7.5), carvedilol Log D was positive and ranged from 2.7 (pH 6.5) to 3.7 (pH 7.5).

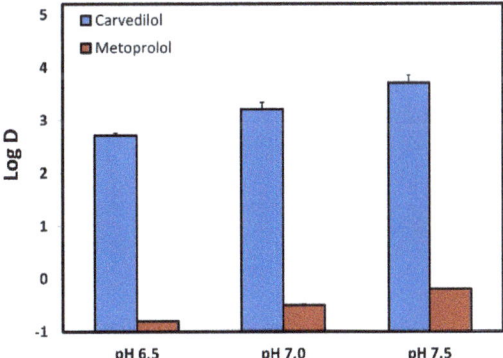

Figure 2. The octanol-buffer distribution coefficients for carvedilol vs. metoprolol at pH values of 6.5, 7.0, and 7.5. Values are presented as means ± SD; n = 6.

3.4. Physicochemical Analysis

The theoretical fraction unionized (f_u) and fraction extracted into octanol (f_e) as a function of pH for carvedilol vs. metoprolol are presented in Figure 3. The f_u of the basic drugs carvedilol and metoprolol was negligible at low pH, and rose as the pH increased, producing a standard sigmoidal shape. It can be seen that the f_e vs. pH plot of both drugs shows a similar pattern, but with a shift to the left at the lower pH values. The shift degree equals to Log (P − 1) at the midpoint of the f_e and f_u sigmoidal curves [40]. Experimental octanol-buffer distribution of the drugs at the three pH values of 6.5, 7.0, and 7.5 are also presented in Figure 3 and are in excellent correlation with the theoretical plots.

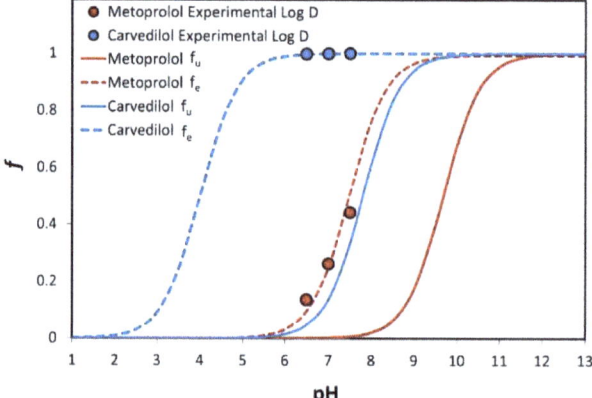

Figure 3. The theoretical fraction unionized (f_u) and fraction extracted into octanol (f_e) plots are presented as a function of pH for carvedilol and metoprolol. Log D values for both drugs are presented as circles; n = 6.

3.5. PAMPA Assay

The transported amounts vs. time in the PAMPA experiment for carvedilol and metoprolol are presented in Figure 4, with their matching P_{app} values. Compatibly to the log D results, the same pH-dependent upward permeability trend was found for both drugs; carvedilol showed considerably higher log D than metoprolol in the studied pH range, and the PAMPA permeability values confirmed this trend, as can be seen in Figure 4.

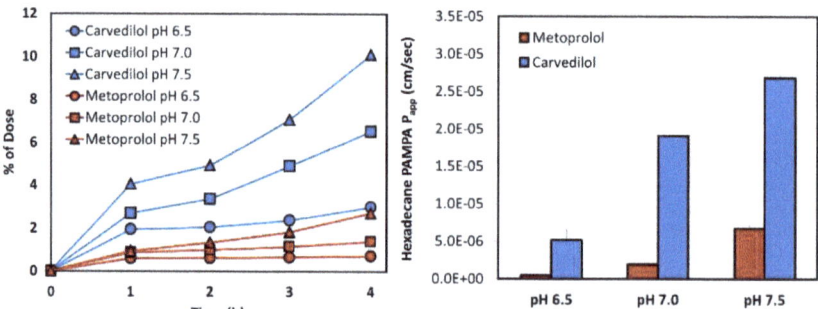

Figure 4. The hexadecane-based parallel artificial membrane permeability assay (PAMPA) permeability studies for carvedilol vs. metoprolol in the different pH conditions along the small intestine: amounts transported (mmol) as a function of time (left panel), and the corresponding P_{app} values (right panel; cm/s). Mean ± SD; n = 4.

3.6. Rat Intestinal Perfusion Studies

The values of carvedilol vs. metoprolol effective permeability coefficient (P_{eff}) determined using the rat SPIP model, through the three intestinal segments: the proximal jejunum (pH 6.5), the distal ileum (pH 7.5), and the colon (pH 6.5), are presented in Figure 5. It can be observed that all of the permeability studies revealed a similar trend: higher pH led to higher permeability values, and as a result, the permeability of carvedilol and metoprolol in the ileum was significantly higher than in the jejunum. Furthermore, at any given intestinal segment/pH, the permeability of carvedilol was higher than that of metoprolol. In addition, when looking at the colon, the permeability value of carvedilol was higher than that of metoprolol in the jejunum (marked as a dashed line in Figure 5).

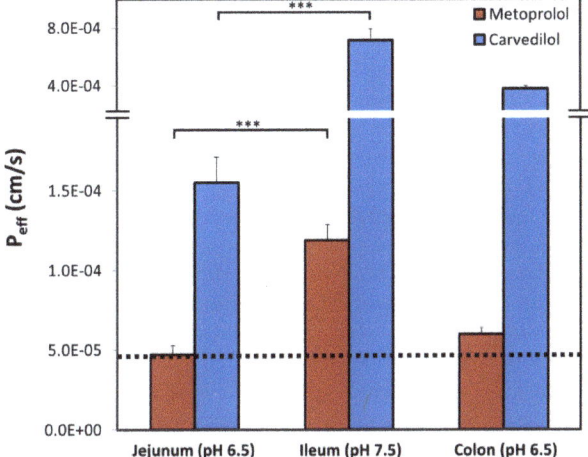

Figure 5. Effective permeability coefficient (P_{eff}; cm/s) obtained for carvedilol vs. metoprolol in three rat intestinal segments, the upper jejunum (pH 6.5), terminal ileum (pH 7.5), and the colon (pH 6.5). The black dashed line represents the permeability of metoprolol in the jejunum (pH 6.5), which is the low/high P_{eff} class boundary standard. Data are presented as means ± SD; *** $p < 0.001$ between jejunum and ileum for both carvedilol and metoprolol; n = 6.

4. Discussion

The variable physiological conditions throughout the GIT can greatly influence the rate and degree of oral drug absorption [10]. It was previously shown that there is a high level of correlation between the drug jejunal permeability and the fraction of dose absorbed from an IR drug product [11,47,48]. Conversely, for CR formulations, to obtain an optimal dissolution, intestinal permeability, and hence, acceptable bioavailability, a larger part of the GIT has to be accounted for in comparison to IR drug product, highlighting the crucial importance of regional variation among absorption factors. Both metoprolol and carvedilol are marketed as controlled-release products (metoprolol extended-release tablets of 25, 50, 100, or 200 mg; and carvedilol CR of 10, 20, 40, or 80 mg) which allows us to use them as model drugs in predicting important parameters that may dictate the development of a successful CR product [49,50].

Carvedilol is an alkaline drug that exhibits poor solubility in different conditions throughout the GIT [29]. However, the solubility studies revealed a high solubility at pH 4.0 (Table 1). In different studies, using simulated/aspirated media, it was shown that depending upon the experimental technique, some discrepancies are noticed [51,52], however, an apparent rise in solubility in the simulated intestinal fluid in the fed state (FeSSIF; pH = 5) is evident. This could be explained by the carvedilol chemical structure, where the aliphatic -NH group is more basic than the carbazole -NH group, which could lead to protonation, creating a soluble salt with the anionic form of the buffer, causing an increase in solubility [28,53]; in acidic media, the aliphatic -NH is ionized forming a cationic center, while in basic media, the carbazole -NH is ionized forming a anionic center. This zwitterionic nature is responsible for the unique solubility pattern presented in Table 1. At any rate, the low solubility values of carvedilol at acidic and neutral environment indicate a low-solubility BCS classification, as in the case of IR carvedilol product, a maximal single unit dose is 25 mg [23], leading to a dose number higher than 1 in different GIT locations. Alongside the high permeability values throughout the GIT, it was confirmed that carvedilol is indeed a BCS class II compound.

Under such solubility limitations, developing carvedilol as a CR drug product may, in a way, help to avoid solubility limitations. By definition, a CR product releases the drug gradually from the formulation while traveling along the GIT, and so, in place of requiring the solubilization the entire dose at once, only a small fraction of the dose needs to be solubilized at a given time point, which may allow overcoming solubility limitations. On the other hand, at each point throughout the intestinal tract, the aqueous volume is lower than the 250 mL initially taken with the drug dose. In particular, it was reported that when simulating the fate of low-solubility drugs after oral administration, the small intestinal water volume that allowed the best fits with in vivo data was about 130 mL (ranging 10–150 mL in the fasted state), and 10 mL in the colon (with estimations as large as 125 mL in the fasted state) [54]. Nevertheless, if there is sufficient fluid in the lumen at each point, it may be possible to obtain adequate drug solubility throughout the digestive system.

The pH-dilution dissolution experimental method mimics the passage and fate of the drug dose through the different GIT segments over time and hence, allows revealing whether the drug can be solubilized, and remain dissolved, while in the GIT. Our results elucidate that generally the highest IR dose (25 mg) has the ability to be dissolved, and remain such throughout the GIT travel, which explains why this formulation is an efficient marketed drug product. On the other hand, if the CR dose of carvedilol (80 mg) were to be administered at once as a simple IR formulation, rapid precipitation would take place (Figure 1), preventing the success of such drug products. Formulating this carvedilol dose as a CR product allows overcoming this solubility/dissolution limitation by distributing small portions of the dose at each stage throughout the GIT. This model analysis illustrates the application of biopharmaceutical aspects in the decision process of successful CR formulation development.

A literature search showed that carvedilol in vitro absorption was studied in a model called the Boehringer–Mannheim ring model using porcine intestine [55]. According to this study, the main route of absorption for carvedilol was transcellular, and the optimal absorption was obtained in the neutral pH of 6.8. In situ intestinal perfusion with mesenteric blood sampling in rats using human intestinal fluids and biorelevant media was used to study the food effect on the intestinal solubility and permeability of carvedilol [52]; however, the use of biorelevant media that contain high lecithin concentration would also affect the solubility aspect of carvedilol in comparison to our SPIP study. Therefore, we used the buffers for the perfusion study instead. This study also did not account for the segmental-dependency of the solubility/permeability of carvedilol.

Prior to evaluating intestinal permeability (P_{eff}) results, the threshold for the low/high permeability class membership must be set, since it reflects the penetration degree that allows complete absorption. For this purpose, metoprolol is a widely used and accepted standard compound [56,57]. Metoprolol exhibits significant segmental-dependent intestinal permeability with increasing P_{eff} towards the distal parts of the small intestine. Therefore, the question is raised, which permeability should be taken as the class boundary: jejunal ($\sim 5 \times 10^{-5}$ cm/s) or the much higher ileal value ($\sim 1.2 \times 10^{-4}$ cm/s), presented in Figure 5. Absorption data obtained from humans revealed that 80% of metoprolol dose from IR product occurs already in the upper 50 cm of the small intestine (duodenum and proximal jejunum), leaving no drug for absorption in the ileum [58]. This was later shown in rats as well [59]. Therefore, ileal permeability values of metoprolol are not physiologically relevant for an IR drug product; it can be claimed that from an IR metoprolol product, no drug arrives into the ileum, as the entire dose gets absorbed much earlier. Hence, the jejunum permeability of metoprolol allows its complete absorption, and this value should be taken as the low/high threshold for permeability classification. Similarly, carvedilol demonstrated segmental-dependent permeability that matched the trend of metoprolol (the permeability in the ileum was significantly higher than in the jejunum, as demonstrated in Figure 5). However, the P_{eff} values of carvedilol were significantly higher than that of metoprolol in each intestinal segment. Importantly, colonic permeability values for both carvedilol and metoprolol were higher than that of metoprolol in the jejunum (illustrated as a dashed black line in Figure 5), validating the biopharmaceutical suitability of carvedilol, and metoprolol, to be developed as CR drug products. Typically, a CR drug product releases the drug continuously over 12–24, and since the transit time throughout the small intestine is 3-4 hours [60], the majority of the dose is released in the colon. This explains why high colonic drug permeability is a key biopharmaceutical factor in the decision process of CR drug product development. This permeability analysis of both model drugs (carvedilol and metoprolol) demonstrated the decision process required for successful CR dosage form development.

Permeability studies both in vitro and in vivo (Log D, PAMPA, SPIP) resulted in higher permeability of carvedilol vs. metoprolol in all of the investigated segments/pHs. Both PAMPA and SPIP methods (Figures 4 and 5) showed the same upward trend. The in vitro permeability models used in this work account for simple passive diffusion, without taking into account intestinal transporters, however, the in vivo SPIP model accounts for all permeability mechanisms, including active transport. When looking at the in vivo results (Figure 5), it can be seen that throughout the entire intestinal tract, carvedilol's permeability was higher than that of metoprolol's in the jejunum. In the colon (Figure 5), carvedilol's permeability was higher than both metoprolol's high/low permeability benchmark and permeability of carvedilol in the jejunum. The permeability of carvedilol in the colon was lower than in the ileum, likely due to a shift in the ionization state. This correlation between artificial and animal permeability studies depicts the main mechanism of carvedilol's permeability as passive absorption. Furthermore, the octanol-buffer distribution coefficient of carvedilol was tremendously higher than that of metoprolol at different pH values (Figure 2). Even though Log P and Log D values are widely used as a replacement for passive intestinal permeability, relying solely on physicochemical drug properties when assessing drug permeation may lead to incorrect conclusions. For instance, the polar surface area (PSA) of carvedilol and metoprolol is 75.7 A^2 and 50.7 A^2 (Table 2), respectively [44,46]; lower PSA is usually associated with higher permeability, and hence, judging merely based on this characteristic would lead to the wrong conclusion. Therefore, prior to assigning a BCS classification, the many relevant aspects need to be thoroughly considered, to circumvent misconception in drug research, development, and regulation.

The solubility–permeability interplay is an important part of evaluating a novel drug formulation. By merely looking at the solubility improvement that the formulation allows can be ambiguous in terms of predicting the consequent oral drug absorption, and vice versa, this interplay must be accounted for when aiming to optimize the solubility–permeability balance, and the overall drug absorption. Carvedilol is a low solubility compound whose solubility enhancement when developing a CR drug product relied on using a phosphate salt in the CR formulation. This increase in solubility might be responsible for a slight decrease in overall bioavailability. However, in the case of this drug product, it did not affect the clinical efficacy of carvedilol.

Carvedilol is both a substrate [26,61] and inhibitor [62] of the efflux transporter P-glycoprotein (P-gp). The involvement of intestinal transporters in general, and specifically P-gp, in the absorption process following oral administration is more biorelevant for low-permeability drugs, and the regional-dependent expression of the relevant transporters should be considered in these cases [63,64]. However, for high-permeability compounds, neither active uptake nor efflux transporters are expected to be rate-limiting [65,66]. Given that carvedilol has very high passive intestinal permeability throughout the entire GIT (Figure 5), the fact that it is a P-gp substrate would not be significant in the in vivo conditions. In addition, as mentioned before, carvedilol undergoes extensive stereoselective first-pass (CYP2D6 and CYP2C9). Similarly to transporters, intestinal enzymes may also exhibit regional-dependent expression, which needs to be accounted for when developing oral CR formulation [67]. Extensive knowledge of intestinal/hepatic transport and enzymatic metabolism is essential in the development process of a CR product.

5. Conclusions

Altogether, the analysis of carvedilol/metoprolol presented in this work serves as a model for a suitable candidate for a CR product development, from both the permeability and solubility/dissolution point of view. This work may increase our biopharmaceutical understanding of a successful CR drug product.

Regional-dependent drug permeability and solubility/dissolution, and the effects of these factors on CR drug product development is often overlooked, and in this article, we aimed to emphasize these important issues; yet, additional data, including pharmacokinetics, metabolism, and pharmacotherapy considerations, are essential for the thorough prediction of a CR candidate.

Author Contributions: M.M., M.Z., N.F.-S., E.H., I.G.-Á., and A.D. worked on conceptualization, methodology, investigation, analyzed the data, and outlined the manuscript. A.D., M.M., and M.Z. wrote the skeleton of the paper, and all authors contributed to the writing, review, and editing of the full version. All authors have read and agreed to the published version of the manuscript.

Funding: This work received no external funding.

Conflicts of Interest: The authors declare no conflict of interest.

References

1. Dahan, A.; Miller, J.M.; Hilfinger, J.M.; Yamashita, S.; Yu, L.X.; Lennernas, H.; Amidon, G.L. High-permeability criterion for BCS classification: Segmental/pH dependent permeability considerations. *Mol. Pharm.* **2010**, *7*, 1827–1834. [CrossRef] [PubMed]
2. Dahlgren, D.; Lennernas, H. Intestinal Permeability and Drug Absorption: Predictive Experimental, Computational and In Vivo Approaches. *Pharmaceutics* **2019**, *11*, 411. [CrossRef] [PubMed]
3. Fairstein, M.; Swissa, R.; Dahan, A. Regional-dependent intestinal permeability and BCS classification: Elucidation of pH-related complexity in rats using pseudoephedrine. *AAPS J.* **2013**, *15*, 589–597. [CrossRef] [PubMed]
4. Amidon, G.L.; Lennernas, H.; Shah, V.P.; Crison, J.R. A theoretical basis for a biopharmaceutic drug classification: The correlation of in vitro drug product dissolution and in vivo bioavailability. *Pharm. Res.* **1995**, *12*, 413–420. [CrossRef] [PubMed]
5. European Medicines Agency. *Guideline on the Investigation of Bioequivalence*; European Medicines Agency: Amsterdam, The Netherlands, 2010.
6. U.S. Department of Health and Human Services, Food and Drug Administration; Center for Drug Evaluation and Research. *Waiver of In-Vivo Bioavailability and Bioequivalence Studies for Immediate-Release Solid Oral Dosage Forms Based on a Biopharmaceutics Classification System. Guidance for Industry*; CDER: Silver Spring, MD, USA, 2017.
7. Garcia-Arieta, A.; Gordon, J. Bioequivalence requirements in the European Union: Critical discussion. *AAPS J.* **2012**, *14*, 738–748. [CrossRef] [PubMed]
8. Dahan, A.; Wolk, O.; Zur, M.; Amidon, G.L.; Abrahamsson, B.; Cristofoletti, R.; Groot, D.W.; Kopp, S.; Langguth, P.; Polli, J.E.; et al. Biowaiver Monographs for Immediate-Release Solid Oral Dosage Forms: Codeine Phosphate. *J. Pharm. Sci.* **2014**, *103*, 1592–1600. [CrossRef]
9. Ozawa, M.; Tsume, Y.; Zur, M.; Dahan, A.; Amidon, G.L. Intestinal permeability study of minoxidil: Assessment of minoxidil as a high permeability reference drug for biopharmaceutics classification. *Mol. Pharm.* **2015**, *12*, 204–211. [CrossRef]
10. Dahan, A.; Lennernäs, H.; Amidon, G.L. The Fraction Dose Absorbed, in Humans, and High Jejunal Human Permeability Relationship. *Mol. Pharm.* **2012**, *9*, 1847–1851. [CrossRef]
11. Lennernas, H. Regional intestinal drug permeation: Biopharmaceutics and drug development. *Eur. J. Pharm. Sci.* **2014**, *57*, 333–341. [CrossRef]
12. Zur, M.; Gasparini, M.; Wolk, O.; Amidon, G.L.; Dahan, A. The Low/High BCS Permeability Class Boundary: Physicochemical Comparison of Metoprolol and Labetalol. *Mol. Pharm.* **2014**, *11*, 1707–1714. [CrossRef]
13. Zur, M.; Hanson, A.S.; Dahan, A. The complexity of intestinal permeability: Assigning the correct BCS classification through careful data interpretation. *Eur. J. Pharm. Sci* **2014**, *61*, 11–17. [CrossRef] [PubMed]
14. Dahan, A.; Sabit, H.; Amidon, G.L. The H2 receptor antagonist nizatidine is a P-glycoprotein substrate: Characterization of its intestinal epithelial cell efflux transport. *AAPS J.* **2009**, *11*, 205–213. [CrossRef] [PubMed]
15. Lennernas, H. Human in vivo regional intestinal permeability: Importance for pharmaceutical drug development. *Mol. Pharm.* **2014**, *11*, 12–23. [CrossRef] [PubMed]
16. Ungell, A.L.; Nylander, S.; Bergstrand, S.; Sjoberg, A.; Lennernas, H. Membrane transport of drugs in different regions of the intestinal tract of the rat. *J. Pharm. Sci.* **1998**, *87*, 360–366. [CrossRef]

17. Corrigan, O.I. The biopharmaceutic drug classification and drugs administered in extended release (ER) formulations. *Adv. Exp. Med. Biol.* **1997**, *423*, 111–128. [CrossRef]
18. Tannergren, C.; Bergendal, A.; Lennernas, H.; Abrahamsson, B. Toward an increased understanding of the barriers to colonic drug absorption in humans: Implications for early controlled release candidate assessment. *Mol. Pharm.* **2009**, *6*, 60–73. [CrossRef]
19. Xu, J.; Lin, Y.; Boulas, P.; Peterson, M.L. Low colonic absorption drugs: Risks and opportunities in the development of oral extended release products. *Expert Opin. Drug Deliv.* **2018**, *15*, 197–211. [CrossRef]
20. Frishman, W.H. Carvedilol. *N. Engl. J. Med.* **1998**, *339*, 1759–1765. [CrossRef]
21. Kukin, M.L. β-Blockers in Chronic Heart Failure: Considerations for Selecting an Agent. *Mayo Clin. Proc.* **2002**, *77*, 1199–1206. [CrossRef]
22. Henderson, L.S.; Tenero, D.M.; Baidoo, C.A.; Campanile, A.M.; Harter, A.H.; Boyle, D.; Danoff, T.M. Pharmacokinetic and pharmacodynamic comparison of controlled-release carvedilol and immediate-release carvedilol at steady state in patients with hypertension. *Am. J. Cardiol.* **2006**, *98*, 17l–26l. [CrossRef]
23. Packer, M.; Lukas, M.A.; Tenero, D.M.; Baidoo, C.A.; Greenberg, B.H. Pharmacokinetic profile of controlled-release carvedilol in patients with left ventricular dysfunction associated with chronic heart failure or after myocardial infarction. *Am. J. Cardiol* **2006**, *98*, 39l–45l. [CrossRef] [PubMed]
24. Incecayir, T.; Tsume, Y.; Amidon, G.L. Comparison of the permeability of metoprolol and labetalol in rat, mouse, and Caco-2 cells: Use as a reference standard for BCS classification. *Mol. Pharm.* **2013**, *10*, 958–966. [CrossRef] [PubMed]
25. Brodde, O.E.; Kroemer, H.K. Drug-drug interactions of beta-adrenoceptor blockers. *Arzneim. Forsch.* **2003**, *53*, 814–822. [CrossRef]
26. Baris, N.; Kalkan, S.; Guneri, S.; Bozdemir, V.; Guven, H. Influence of carvedilol on serum digoxin levels in heart failure: Is there any gender difference? *Eur. J. Clin. Pharmacol.* **2006**, *62*, 535–538. [CrossRef] [PubMed]
27. Giessmann, T.; Modess, C.; Hecker, U.; Zschiesche, M.; Dazert, P.; Kunert-Keil, C.; Warzok, R.; Engel, G.; Weitschies, W.; Cascorbi, I.; et al. CYP2D6 genotype and induction of intestinal drug transporters by rifampin predict presystemic clearance of carvedilol in healthy subjects. *Clin. Pharmacol. Ther.* **2004**, *75*, 213–222. [CrossRef]
28. Hamed, R.; Awadallah, A.; Sunoqrot, S.; Tarawneh, O.; Nazzal, S.; AlBaraghthi, T.; Al Sayyad, J.; Abbas, A. pH-Dependent Solubility and Dissolution Behavior of Carvedilol-Case Example of a Weakly Basic BCS Class II Drug. *AAPS PharmSciTech* **2016**, *17*, 418–426. [CrossRef]
29. Varma, M.V.; Gardner, I.; Steyn, S.J.; Nkansah, P.; Rotter, C.J.; Whitney-Pickett, C.; Zhang, H.; Di, L.; Cram, M.; Fenner, K.S.; et al. pH-Dependent Solubility and Permeability Criteria for Provisional Biopharmaceutics Classification (BCS and BDDCS) in Early Drug Discovery. *Mol. Pharm.* **2012**, *9*, 1199–1212. [CrossRef]
30. Zur, M.; Cohen, N.; Agbaria, R.; Dahan, A. The biopharmaceutics of successful controlled release drug product: Segmental-dependent permeability of glipizide vs. metoprolol throughout the intestinal tract. *Int. J. Pharm.* **2015**, *489*, 304–310. [CrossRef]
31. Beig, A.; Miller, J.M.; Lindley, D.; Dahan, A. Striking the Optimal Solubility-Permeability Balance in Oral Formulation Development for Lipophilic Drugs: Maximizing Carbamazepine Blood Levels. *Mol. Pharm.* **2017**, *14*, 319–327. [CrossRef]
32. Fine-Shamir, N.; Beig, A.; Zur, M.; Lindley, D.; Miller, J.M.; Dahan, A. Toward Successful Cyclodextrin Based Solubility-Enabling Formulations for Oral Delivery of Lipophilic Drugs: Solubility–Permeability Trade-Off, Biorelevant Dissolution, and the Unstirred Water Layer. *Mol. Pharm.* **2017**, *14*, 2138–2146. [CrossRef]
33. Fine-Shamir, N.; Dahan, A. Methacrylate-Copolymer Eudragit EPO as a Solubility-Enabling Excipient for Anionic Drugs: Investigation of Drug Solubility, Intestinal Permeability, and Their Interplay. *Mol. Pharm.* **2019**, *16*, 2884–2891. [CrossRef] [PubMed]
34. Dahan, A.; West, B.T.; Amidon, G.L. Segmental-dependent membrane permeability along the intestine following oral drug administration: Evaluation of a triple single-pass intestinal perfusion (TSPIP) approach in the rat. *Eur. J. Pharm. Sci.* **2009**, *36*, 320–329. [CrossRef] [PubMed]
35. Lozoya-Agullo, I.; Zur, M.; Fine-Shamir, N.; Markovic, M.; Cohen, Y.; Porat, D.; Gonzalez-Alvarez, I.; Gonzalez-Alvarez, M.; Merino-Sanjuan, M.; Bermejo, M.; et al. Investigating drug absorption from the colon: Single-pass vs. Doluisio approaches to in-situ rat large-intestinal perfusion. *Int. J. Pharm.* **2017**, *527*, 135–141. [CrossRef] [PubMed]

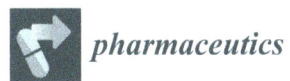

Article

Cubic Microcontainers Improve In Situ Colonic Mucoadhesion and Absorption of Amoxicillin in Rats

Juliane Fjelrad Christfort [1,*], Antonio José Guillot [2], Ana Melero [2,*], Lasse Højlund Eklund Thamdrup [1], Teresa M. Garrigues [2], Anja Boisen [1], Kinga Zór [1] and Line Hagner Nielsen [1]

1 Department of Health Technology, Technical University of Denmark, Ørsteds Plads, 2800 Kgs. Lyngby, Denmark; lhth@dtu.dk (L.H.E.T.); aboi@dtu.dk (A.B.); kinzo@dtu.dk (K.Z.); lihan@dtu.dk (L.H.N.)
2 Department de Farmàcia I Tecnología Farmacèutica, Avda. Vincent Andrés Estellés s/n, 46100 Burjassot (Valencia), Spain; antonio.guillot@uv.es (A.J.G.); teresa.garrigues@uv.es (T.M.G.)
* Correspondence: julchr@dtu.dk (J.F.C.); ana.melero@uv.es (A.M.)

Received: 24 March 2020; Accepted: 10 April 2020; Published: 14 April 2020

Abstract: An increased interest in colonic drug delivery has led to a higher focus on the design of delivery devices targeting this part of the gastrointestinal tract. Microcontainers have previously facilitated an increase in oral bioavailability of drugs. The surface texture and shape of microcontainers have proven to influence the mucoadhesion ex vivo. In the present work, these findings were further investigated using an in situ closed-loop perfusion technique in the rat colon, which allowed for simultaneous evaluation of mucoadhesion of the microcontainers as well as drug absorption. Cylindrical, triangular and cubic microcontainers, with the same exterior surface area, were evaluated based on in vitro release, in situ mucoadhesion and in situ absorption of amoxicillin. Additionally, the mucoadhesion of empty cylindrical microcontainers with and without pillars on the top surface was investigated. From the microscopy analysis of the colon sections after the in situ study, it was evident that a significantly higher percentage of cubic microcontainers than cylindrical microcontainers adhered to the intestinal mucus. Furthermore, the absorption rate constants and blood samples indicated that amoxicillin in cubic microcontainers was absorbed more readily than when cylindrical or triangular microcontainers were dosed. This could be due to a higher degree of mucoadhesion for these particular microcontainers.

Keywords: in situ perfusion; microdevices; shape; mucoadhesion; colon absorption

1. Introduction

Oral drug delivery remains the preferred administration route due to ease of use, flexibility and patient compliance [1]. Despite many advances in oral delivery systems [2–4], the design of 'the ideal delivery device' is still widely discussed and depends on the application.

In the past decades, an increased interest in colon drug delivery has led to significant research with a focus on designing delivery devices that target this part of the gastrointestinal (GI) tract [5]. In addition to local delivery, the colon has also been suggested as an interesting site for systemic drug delivery due to increased oral bioavailability for some drugs and longer transit time compared to the small intestine [6–8]. The prolonged transit time allows timing of the treatment to periods with maximal disease activity; for example, in diseases where symptoms are more pronounced in the morning (hypertension, asthma and arthritis) [7].

Mucoadhesion is an important factor in relation to targeted delivery to any part of the GI tract, since it can prolong the residence time and facilitate drug release in close proximity to the epithelium.

To understand mucoadhesion, six general theories have been proposed [9]. Amongst these are the wetting theory and the mechanical theory. The wetting theory is mainly applied to liquid or low-viscosity systems [9], while the mechanical theory can be applied to more rigid and adhesive materials. The mechanical theory explains mucoadhesion in terms of interlocking into irregularities on a rough surface [9,10]. Due to the complex nature of mucoadhesion, it is not likely that the phenomenon can be described by one of these theories alone [9]. Properties affecting mucoadhesion have been thoroughly investigated and it has been indicated that size and shape have a high impact on the mucoadhesive strength for micro- and nano-scale particles [11–13]. Advanced polymeric particles have paved the way for many new controlled drug delivery strategies [14]. However, as the field of drug delivery is moving towards more advanced microdevices, additional knowledge is needed to fully disclose and understand the influence of the multitude of parameters influencing mucoadhesion of drug delivery devices and the associated absorption of drugs.

Unidirectionally-releasing microdevices have been proposed for oral drug delivery to ensure a high local concentration of the active pharmaceutical ingredient (API) at the absorption site and to prolong the residence time [15,16]. The prolonged residence time is proposed to occur by decreased shear stress and increased retention [17]. For example, planar microdevices with a diameter of 200 μm were shown to enhance in vivo retention after oral dosing in mice [15]. These microdevices were found to adhere better than microspheres with the same surface area in the proximal and medial intestine. In the colon, however, the microspheres were retained approximately two times more than the microdevices [15]. The concept of planar microdevices was further developed with the inclusion of nanostraw structures on the surface, which was shown to enhance bioadhesion in a Caco-2 cell flow system when compared to similar microdevices without nanostraws [18]. Microcontainers, one type of unidirectionally-releasing microdevice, have previously been shown to improve oral bioavailability of drugs and provide inherent mucoadhesion [16,19]. Microcontainers are micrometer-sized devices (fabricated in polymers) with an inner cavity for storage of the API. Coating of the API-loaded cavity protects the content from the harsh environment of the stomach and provides unidirectional release at a relevant site in the GI tract [16]. Due to versatile fabrication processes, microcontainers have been fabricated in different materials, shapes and size ranges [20–22].

The influence of material composition, shape and size on the interaction with mucus has also been evaluated for microcontainers in an intestinal ex vivo perfusion model [22–24]. Here, triangular microcontainers adhered more readily in the mid-part of a porcine small intestinal section than cylindrical ones. Similarly, larger cone shaped microcontainers generally adhered better than cylindrical microcontainers with the same size [22,24]. When evaluating these microdevices fabricated in different materials in an ex vivo perfusion model, poly(lactic-co-glycolic acid) (PLGA) (50:50) microcontainers showed slightly higher mucoadhesion compared to polycaprolactone (PCL) and PLGA (75:25) microcontainers [23]. In a different study performed in the same model, there was a tendency that SU-8 microcontainers adhered better to the mucosa than PCL microcontainers with the same dimensions [22].

Techniques like the perfusion model described above, or atomic force microscopy (AFM), are commonly applied to study mucoadhesion ex vivo [25,26]. However, these techniques do not allow for simultaneous evaluation of the permeation across the intestinal barrier. In order to study API permeation, methods like in vitro studies with Caco-2 cells or ex vivo studies using an Ussing chamber setup are traditionally used [27,28].

A well-documented method to explore the performance of drug delivery systems in situ is the intestinal perfusion technique in rodents, introduced by Schanker in 1958 [29]. Several decades later, the technique is still widely applied in the field of intestinal absorption research due to its versatility [30–32]. Furthermore, the in situ technique provides the opportunity to investigate absorption and mucoadhesion simultaneously in a specific region of the intestine. These are important characteristics for evaluation of both local delivery and formulations aiming for prolonged release followed by absorption.

This in situ perfusion technique is applied in anesthetized rodents, where the relevant part of the intestine is isolated from nearby tissues, but not removed from the living organism. The perfusion can be performed as single-pass intestinal perfusion or with a closed-loop technique [32]. In both cases, the neural, endocrine, blood and lymphatic contributions are maintained during the experiment in order to simulate in vivo conditions. Both perfusion techniques have shown equally good correlations to literature values of the absorbed fraction of the oral dose (F_{abs}) in humans [32,33]. The closed-loop in situ perfusion technique based on Doluisio's method [34] has been widely applied for intestinal absorption of different drugs and in different regions of the intestine [35–37]. Earlier, the closed-loop intestinal perfusion technique has been applied to investigate the mechanisms governing absorption from drug suspensions [38] and drug-loaded microdevices [16] in the small intestine. The closed-loop perfusion technique has previously been validated to study colonic absorption [37], but has not yet been applied to study mucoadhesion and absorption simultaneously in this region of the GI tract.

Previously, we have seen that the shape and surface texture of microdevices influence mucoadhesion ex vivo [22,39]. More specifically, triangular microcontainers previously resulted in improved mucoadhesion in parts of a small intestinal section compared to cylindrical microcontainers [22]. However, these microcontainers were not normalized with respect to the surface area. Thus, it is unclear whether the shape or the difference in surface area was the reason for this observed effect. To elaborate on this, the present study aimed to evaluate differently shaped microcontainers, with the same exterior surface area, using a closed-loop in situ intestinal perfusion technique. This technique allowed us to simultaneously evaluate mucoadhesion of microcontainers and absorption of a model drug, amoxicillin, in the colon of rats. Cylindrical, triangular and cubic microcontainers were evaluated regarding in vitro release, in situ mucoadhesion and in situ absorption of amoxicillin. Additionally, the mucoadhesion of empty cylindrical microcontainers with pillars on the top surface were compared to a control without pillars.

2. Materials and Methods

2.1. Materials

Amoxicillin trihydrate was bought from TCI (Tokyo, Japan) and Eudragit® L100 was acquired from Evonik Industries (Essen, Germany). Dibutyl sebacate, isopropanol and potassium phosphate monobasic for the HPLC mobile phase were purchased from Sigma Aldrich (St. Louis, MO, USA). Methanol was bought from VWR International (Radnor, PA, USA).

The negative epoxy based photoresist SU-8 was used for production of microcontainers. Formulations with two different viscosities were used (i.e., SU-8 2035 and 2075) and the cross-linked structures were developed in Developer mr-Dev 600. Resist and developer were purchased from Micro Resist Technology GmbH (Berlin, Germany). Single-side polished ø100 mm Si substrates with a thickness of 525 µm were acquired from Topsil Globalwafers A/S (Frederikssund, Denmark).

For the phosphate buffered saline (PBS) used in the in situ perfusion studies, sodium chloride, potassium chloride, sodium phosphate dibasic and potassium phosphate monobasic were purchased from Scharlab (Barcelona, Spain). Animals were from Charles River Laboratories (Quebec, QC, Canada). Sylgaard 184 silicone elastomer kit was purchased from Dow Chemical (Midland, MI, USA). Ultrapure water used throughout the studies was obtained from a Q-POD® dispenser (Merck Millipore, Burlington, MA, USA).

2.2. Fabrication of SU-8 Microcontainers

Microcontainers with five different designs were used in these experiments. Amoxicillin-loaded microcontainers enteric coated with Eudragit® L100, were produced as 3D structures in three different shapes; cylindrical, equilateral triangular prism and quadrangular prism (Table 1). The central cylindrical compartment for drug loading was designed with a constant volume for all shapes. Furthermore, the three shapes were designed to have a constant outer surface area when neglecting the top surface (which was coated). By maintaining a constant interaction area, the studies aim to isolate the influence of geometry on the colonic mucoadhesion. In addition to the above mentioned microcontainers, cylindrical microcontainers with and without 35 µm pillars (in diameter) on the sidewalls were produced (Table 1).

Table 1. Design parameters of the microcontainers evaluated in the present study. Data represents mean ± SD and $n = 5$ unless otherwise specified.

Shape	Topology Image	Inner Diameter (µm)	Outer Diameter/Side Length [a] (µm)	Inner Height (µm)	Outer Height (µm)	Surface Area (Normalized to Cylinder)
Cylindrical		157.8 ± 2.2	304 ± 2.2	210.8 ± 3.1	247.8 ± 3.1	1.000 [b]
Cubic		157.6 ± 2.2	248.0 ± 2.2	211.0 ± 4.6	245.0 ± 4.6	0.985
Triangular		158.2 ± 2.2	342.0 ± 2.2	210.6 ± 4.2	245.4 ± 4.0	1.003
Cylindrical (reference) [c]		234.3 ± 2.2	324.7 ± 2.2	218.0 ± 3.0	252.0 ± 1.7	1.099
Cylindrical (reference) with pillars [d,e]		219.5 ± 2.2	323.7 ± 2.2	166.3 ± 1.5	202.8 ± 1.2	0.933

[a] the diameter for all cylindrical microcontainers and the side length for the cubic and triangular microcontainers.
[b] corresponding to 309243.3 µm^2. [c] $n = 3$. [d] $n = 6$. [e] pillar dimensions: 41 µm high with a diameter of 35 ± 2.2 µm.

All microcontainers were produced following an approach first introduced for drug delivery devices in [40], then adapted and modified in [41]. Starting out with clean Si substrates, a release layer consisting of 5 nm Ti and 20 nm Au was deposited (Temescal FC-2000, Ferrotec Corporation, Santa Clara, CA, USA) using electron-beam evaporation. The release layer ensures adequate adhesion during drug loading and lid coating, but allowed for harvesting the microcontainers without damaging the SU-8 structures. All microcontainers featured an approximately 35 µm thick bottom layer formed by spin coating SU-8 2035 (RCD8 manual spin coater, Süss MicroTec, Garching, Germany). This was followed by performing a soft bake at 50 °C for 2 h (ramping rate 2 °C/min, used for all baking steps), conducting UV exposure using doses in excess of 200 mJ/cm^2 and then carrying out a post exposure bake (PEB) at 50 °C for 6 h using the aforementioned ramping rate. The UV exposure was conducted using a maskless aligner (MLA100 Tabletop Maskless Aligner, Heidelberg Instruments, Heidelberg, Germany) or a conventional mask aligner (Karl Süss Mask Aligner MA6, Süss MicroTec, Garching, Germany) operated in soft contact mode. The sidewalls of the microcontainers were defined in SU-8 2075, which was spin coated and subject to a soft bake at 50 °C for 10 h. The UV exposure was conducted using a dose of 500 mJ/cm^2. For defining the cylindrical empty reference microcontainers with no pillars on the sidewalls, the mask aligner was operated in proximity exposure mode to avoid direct contact between the soda-lime glass mask and the SU-8. The remaining four microcontainer types were UV exposed using the maskless aligner. After UV exposure, a PEB of 10 h at 50 °C was carried out. To form the pillars on the sidewalls of one of the empty control microcontainer groups, a final layer of SU-8 2035 was spin coated, soft baked at 50 °C for 2 h, UV exposed using a dose of 200 mJ/cm^2 and finally subjected to a PEB at 50 °C for 6 h. The substrates, carrying the multitude of different drug delivery devices, were developed by immersion in two separate baths for 2 × 20 min and flushed with copious amounts of isopropanol before leaving the substrates to dry. Prior to drug loading and lid coating, the Si substrates were diced (Automatic Dicing Saw DAD 321, DISCO, Tokyo, Japan) into 12.8 × 12.8 mm² chips, each containing 625 microcontainers arranged in a 25 × 25 array.

The microcontainers were characterized using both conventional bright-field microscopy (Nikon Eclipse L200, Nikon Metrology, Tokyo, Japan) for extracting data on the horizontal dimensions and vertical scanning interferometry (PLu Neox 3D Optical Profiler, Sensofar Metrology, Barcelona, Spain) aimed at characterizing the vertical dimensions (i.e., inner and outer heights and pillar height). The results of the topology characterization are summarized in Table 1. For the horizontal measurements (i.e., diameters and side lengths), a value corresponding to the optical resolution multiplied by a factor of 3 was used. The optical resolution, R, of the used objective (20×, NA = 0.45) was evaluated as $R = (0.61\lambda)/NA$ where the illumination wavelength was $\lambda = 550$ nm. This resulted in the stated measurement uncertainty of ±2.2 µm. When considering the height measurements, we used the standard deviation based on an ensemble of measurements. Generally the horizontal dimensions are subject to small variations and the spread in the vertical dimensions are governed by the homogeneity of the spin coated SU-8 layers.

2.3. Loading of Amoxicillin into Microcontainers and Spray Coating with Eudragit® L100

For the in situ perfusion study, the microcontainer chips were loaded with amoxicillin as previously described [16,42]. Briefly, amoxicillin was manually distributed on the microcontainer chip and excess drug between the microcontainers was subsequently removed with an air gun. For the in vitro release studies, the microcontainers were loaded using a PDMS shadow mask to cover the chip area between the microcontainers, as previously described [43]. In both cases, the chip with microcontainers was weighed before and after loading to determine the loaded amount of amoxicillin. Visualization of the loading was carried out by scanning electron microscopy (SEM) using a Hitachi TM3030Plus tabletop microscope (Hitachi High-Technologies Europe, Krefeld, Germany).

A lid of Eudragit® L100 was deposited over the microcontainers as previously described [19], by spray coating an isopropanol solution with 1% *w/v* Eudragit® L100 and 5% *w/w* (in relation to the polymer) dibutyl sebacate. Briefly, the solution was sprayed over the amoxicillin-loaded microcontainers one chip at a time using an ultrasonic spray coater (Exactacoat system, Sono-Tek, Milton, NY, USA) with an Accumist nozzle operating at 120 kHz. Each chip was coated with 30 loops of two alternating spray paths having an offset of 2 mm, resulting in a total of 60 passages. Visualization of the coated microcontainers was carried out by SEM.

2.4. In Vitro Release Studies

The release of amoxicillin from the differently shaped microcontainers coated with Eudragit® L100 was measured using a µDISS Profiler™ (Pion Inc., Billerica, MA, USA), as previously described in the literature [16,19,42]. Initially, a calibration curve was prepared by addition of different volumes of amoxicillin in PBS stock solution to 10 mL PBS (pH 7.4) followed by measurements of UV absorbance in the range of 270–280 nm. For the release study, a microcontainer chip was placed on top of a cylindrical magnetic stirring bar with double-sided carbon tape, transferred to a sample vial and covered with 10 mL PBS at the same time as the experiment was started. Studies were performed at 37 °C with a stirring rate of 100 rpm, and the path length of the UV probes was 5 mm. UV measurements were carried out every 10 s until an amoxicillin release of 100% was observed after approximately 60 min.

2.5. Closed-Loop Colon Perfusion Study in Rats

Male Wistar rats were used in accordance with 2010/63/EU directive of 22 September 2010 regarding the protection of animals used for scientific experimentation. The Ethics Committee for Animal Experimentation of the University of Valencia approved the experimental protocols (code A1544541996825). Male Wistar rats weighing 240 ± 12 g were fasted for 3 h before the experiments with ad libitum access to water. The rats were anesthetized by intraperitoneal injection of pentobarbital sodium (40 mg/kg) prior to the surgical procedure.

The drug absorption rate constant of amoxicillin in the colon and the mucoadhesion of microcontainers were evaluated by the in situ closed-loop perfusion method based on Doluisio's technique [34]. Briefly, the animals were placed under a heating lamp and a midline abdominal incision was made to expose the intestine. The colon section was isolated by making two incisions; one after the caecum and the other just before the rectum. Two glass syringes connected to three-way stopcock valves were introduced in the incisions with the help of two cannulas, creating an isolated compartment as depicted in Figure 1. Procedures were performed with care to avoid disturbance of the intestinal blood supply and intestinal bleeding. In order to remove all intestinal content and wash the colon, the intestinal section was thoroughly flushed with PBS pre-heated to 37 °C. The colon was carefully placed back into the peritoneal cavity and the abdomen was covered with cotton wool pads to prevent peritoneal liquid evaporation and heat loss [16,32,35].

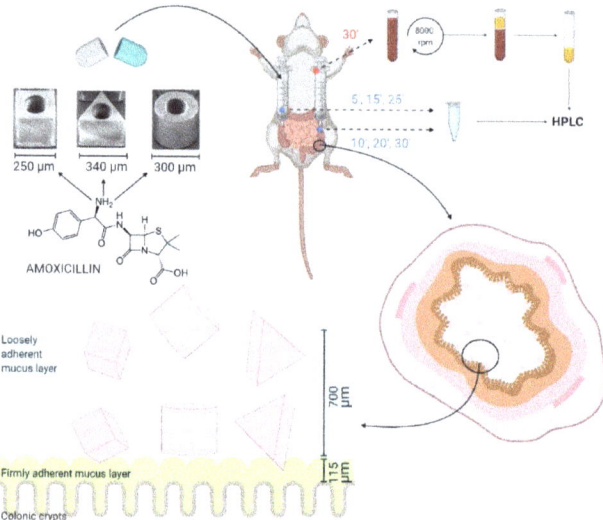

Figure 1. Schematic overview of the in situ colonic perfusion study. The different microcontainers were dosed through two cannulas connected to glass syringes creating a closed colon compartment. To investigate the absorption of amoxicillin, intestinal samples were collected from the two glass syringes every 5 min throughout the experiment and a blood sample was collected 30 min after the experiment. The plasma and intestinal samples were analyzed with high performance liquid chromatography (HPLC) to determine the concentration of amoxicillin. The mucoadhesion of the microcontainers was evaluated as the percentage adhering to the colonic section after the study.

A number of microcontainers, corresponding to 0.4 mg amoxicillin (120 cylindrical, 278 cubic or 136 triangular microcontainers) were dispersed in 5 mL pre-heated PBS and introduced through the cannulas into the isolated section. For the empty reference cylinders without and with pillars, 204 ± 25 and 223 ± 45 microcontainers, respectively, were dosed in the same manner. Samples of 150 µL were collected every 5 min up to a period of 30 min (Figure 1). Sample withdrawal was performed by pushing the luminal content from one syringe to the other, alternatively from the proximal syringe to the distal one and the other way around [44]. Intestinal samples were stored at −20 °C until further analysis.

Water flux absorption processed during the experiment could be significant, and hence it must be considered [45]. To do so, the volume of the intestinal content was measured in every animal after the whole procedure (V_t) and compared to the initial volume (V_0) of 5 mL. The drug concentration in the samples was corrected according to Equation (1):

$$C_t = C_e (V_t/V_0), \tag{1}$$

where C_t represents the concentration in the absence of water reabsorption at time t, and C_e is the experimental value. The corrected concentration, C_t, was then used to calculate the actual absorption rate coefficient in relation to the initial concentration (C_0) [45]. The absorption rate coefficients (k_a) of the compounds were determined by nonlinear regression analysis of the remaining concentrations in the intestinal lumen (C_t) versus time according to Equation (2):

$$C_t = C_0 \, e^{-k_a t} \tag{2}$$

After 30 min, a cardiac puncture was performed under anesthesia to collect the blood from the rat (Figure 1). The blood was collected in heparinized tubes and centrifuged at 10 °C and 6100× g for 8 min. The plasma was stored at −20 °C until further analysis. After the experiment, the isolated colon section was cut and placed onto a glass slide with the luminal side upwards to determine the number of microcontainers. A light microscope (Nikon Eclipse 50i, Nikon, Tokyo, Japan) with camera (Nikon digital camera, DXM1200C, Nikon, Tokyo, Japan) was used to visualize the microcontainers on the colon section.

2.6. High Performance Liquid Chromatography Analysis of Intestinal and Plasma Samples

The concentration of amoxicillin in the intestinal fluid and plasma was determined by high performance liquid chromatography (HPLC). HPLC analyses were performed on a Shimadzu HPLC system (Shimadzu, Kyoto, Japan). The system consisted of a CBM-20A system controller, SIL-20AC HT auto sampler, LC-20AD pump, DGU-20A5R degassing unit, CTO-20AC column oven, RID-20A refractive index detector, and SPD-30A photodiode array detector. The mobile phases consisted of A: phosphate buffer (6.8 g KH_2PO_4/L, pH 5) and B: acetonitrile, and the samples were run with an isocratic method with an A:B mobile phase ratio of 95:5 v/v. A Luna 5.0 µm C18 100 Å, 250 × 4.6 mm column (Phenomenex ApS, Værløse, Denmark) was used for the analyses and samples were run at 25 °C.

The intestinal samples were vortexed and centrifuged at 10,600× g for 10 min and the supernatant was transferred to HPLC vials with 300 µL flat bottom inserts (Frisenette, Knebel, Denmark). For the plasma samples, 60 µL plasma was mixed with 100 µL methanol and otherwise treated as described above for the intestinal samples. Calibration curves were prepared from stock solutions of amoxicillin in water. For the plasma sample analysis, accurate volumes of the stock solutions were mixed with plasma and methanol (same ratio as the samples) and treated the same way as the samples. A volume of 20 µL was injected and the flow rate was 0.8 mL/min with a run time of 10 min for each sample. The absorbance was measured at 230 nm.

2.7. Data Analysis

All data processing was performed in Microsoft Excel 2016 (Redmond, WA, USA), GraphPad Prism version 6.0 (GraphPad software, San Diego, CA, USA) and SPSS version 22.0 (IBM Corp, Armonk, NY, USA). The data is expressed as the mean ± standard deviation (SD) unless otherwise stated. Statistical differences were determined using one-way ANOVA followed by Games–Howell post-hoc analysis, where p-values below 5% were considered significant.

3. Results and Discussion

3.1. Microcontainer Characterization and Preparation

For the present study, which addresses the impact of microcontainer geometry on the colonic mucoadhesion and absorption during in situ experiments in rats, three 3D container designs were investigated: cylindrical, cubic and equilateral triangular (Table 1). The microcontainers all had a cylindrical center compartment for drug storage and the outer surface area (neglecting the top surface) was kept constant to ensure an identical interaction area between microcontainers with different shapes and the mucosal layer in the colon.

The microcontainers were loaded with 1.50 ± 0.27 mg, 0.89 ± 0.19 mg and 1.78 ± 0.18 mg amoxicillin per chip for the cylindrical, cubic and triangular microcontainers, respectively (Figure 2a–c). Despite having the same inner cavity volume for drug loading, the cubic microcontainers were loaded with significantly less amoxicillin than the two other shapes. This is ascribed to the manual loading process, where the additional corners can affect the loading efficiency. After drug loading, the microcontainers were coated with Eudragit® L100. Inspection with SEM showed uniform coatings covering the cavities of the drug-loaded microcontainers for all three shapes (Figure 2d–f).

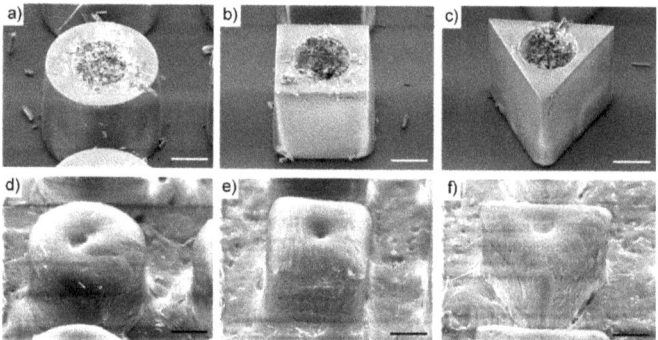

Figure 2. SEM images of a (**a**) cylindrical, (**b**) cubic and (**c**) triangular microcontainer loaded with amoxicillin and a (**d**) cylindrical, (**e**) cubic and (**f**) triangular microcontainer loaded with amoxicillin and coated with Eudragit® L100. All scale bars represent 100 µm.

Besides the three shapes described above, cylindrical reference microcontainers with pillars on the top surface of the sidewalls were also fabricated (but not loaded with drug) and the mucoadhesion of these were compared to the mucoadhesion of traditional empty cylinders of similar dimensions as the control (Table 1).

3.2. In Vitro Release Studies

To investigate the release rate, the in vitro release of amoxicillin from the microcontainers was evaluated on a µDISS Profiler™ in PBS at pH 7.4 (Figure 3).

For all three formulations, the loaded amount of amoxicillin was released after 60 min ($98 \pm 1\%$, $98 \pm 3\%$ and $94 \pm 3\%$ for the cylindrical, cubic and triangular microcontainers, respectively). The observed in vitro release of amoxicillin from the Eudragit® L100-coated microcontainers was expected since the coating dissolves at pH values above 6.0. After 30 min, a release of approximately 60% was observed for the cylindrical and triangular microcontainers, whereas there was a trend towards slower release of amoxicillin from the cubic ones ($44 \pm 10\%$ after 30 min).

After 45 min, at least 80% of the initial amoxicillin dose was released, which categorizes the formulation as an immediate release formulation according to the European Pharmacopoeia [46].

Comparable pH-dependent release profiles have previously been observed for drugs loaded in microcontainers and coated with Eudragit® L100 [16,47].

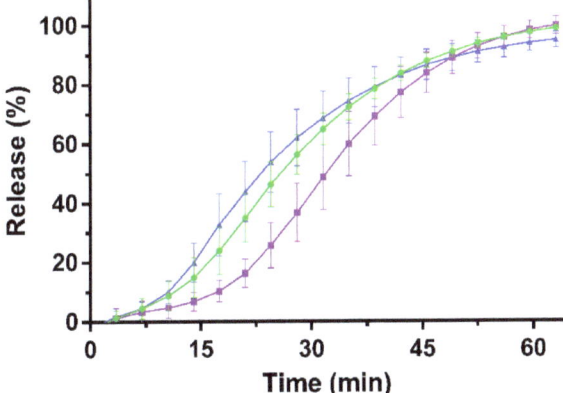

Figure 3. Amoxicillin in vitro release profiles as a function of time from —●— cylindrical, —■— cubic and —▲— triangular microcontainers in PBS (pH 7.4). All microcontainers were coated with Eudragit® L100. Data represent mean ± SD, $n = 4$.

3.3. In Situ Closed-Loop Colon Perfusion Study in Rats

The in situ closed-loop perfusion technique was applied to study the interaction between microcontainers and the colonic mucus layer, and whether this interaction affected the absorption of amoxicillin from the microcontainers compared to a control solution.

3.3.1. Mucoadhesion of Microcontainers

After 30 min of the perfusion study, the microcontainers were manually localized and counted by inspecting the colon sections under a light microscope (Figure 4). When qualitatively investigating the microcontainers retained in the colonic mucus, it was observed that the microcontainers were mainly found in clusters that were partly or completely covered by mucus (Figure 4). Similar clustering trends have previously been observed for other microdevices evaluated on a cell monolayer under flow [17].

The mucoadhesion of the microcontainers was quantified as the percentage of microcontainers adhering to the colonic mucus after 30 min compared to the total amount of microcontainers dosed (Figure 5). It was found that 12 ± 7% of the loaded cylindrical microcontainers were retained in the colonic mucus. In contrast, a significantly higher ($p = 0.019$) number of cubic microcontainers (33 ± 12%) were found to be retained in the colon sections after the same period of time (Figure 5). The percentage of the triangular microcontainers in the colonic mucus was 28 ± 26% and a higher inter-individual variation was observed for these rats compared to the rats in the other groups (Figure 5).

Based on the data presented in Figure 5, the only significant difference was between the cubic and cylindrical microcontainers loaded with amoxicillin. The absence of significant differences between the other groups can be explained through the rather large data distribution in the group dosed with triangular microcontainers, which varied between 3 and 81% (Figure 5). As expected, the shape with the least pronounced mucoadhesion was the cylindrical one, since this shape did not provide any corners or edges to allow for interaction with the mucus. The most mucoadhesive shape seemed to be the cube, although the differences were non-significant due to the large variations observed for triangular microcontainers. If the cubic and triangular microcontainers are analyzed based on geometry/topology, there are obvious differences between the two shapes. The cubic structures have 6 surfaces with approximately the same area and shape, 12 edges and 8 corners, whereas the triangles have 5 surfaces, 9 edges and 6 corners. We believe that the number of surfaces, corners and edges strongly influence the way the microcontainers are retained in the mucus. These shape differences would also result in different contact surfaces between the microcontainers and the mucus, and thus, differences in mucoadhesion according to the wetting theory [9]. The cylinders will for example have a much smaller contact surface with the mucus if they land on their curved side.

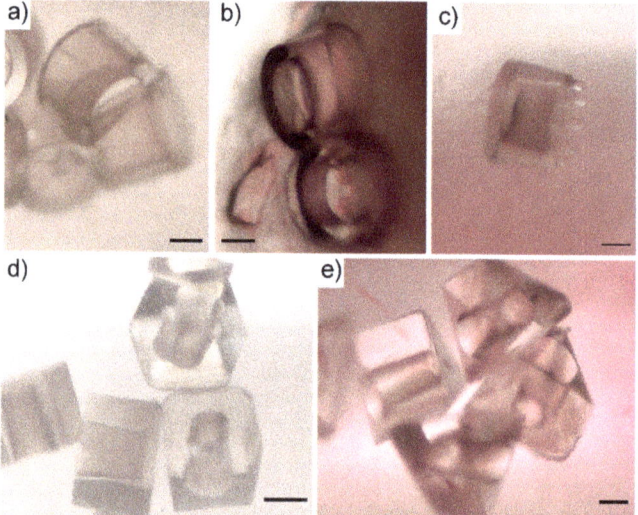

Figure 4. Microscopy images of microcontainers in colonic mucus following in situ perfusion studies. (**a,b**) cylindrical microcontainers, (**c**) pillared reference microcontainers, (**d**) cubic and (**e**) triangular microcontainers. All scale bars represent 100 μm.

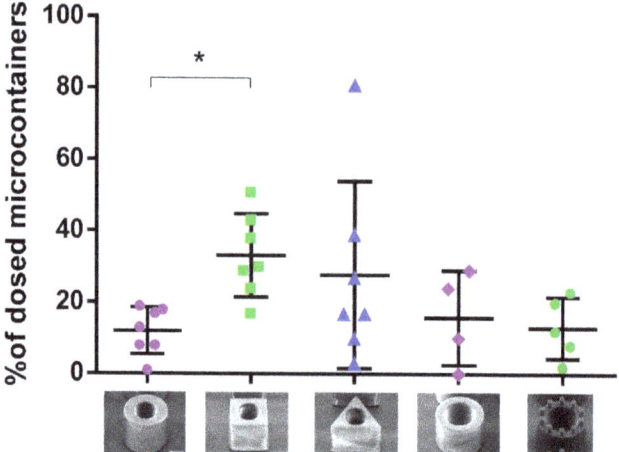

Figure 5. Mucoadhesion of the five microcontainer formulations expressed as percentage of dosed microcontainers still adhering to the mucus after the closed-loop intestinal perfusion study (mean ± SD, $n = 4$–7). * indicates a significant difference with a p-value below 5%.

A previous study investigated the mucoadhesion of cylindrical and triangular microcontainers in an ex vivo perfusion model and found triangular microcontainers to be significantly more mucoadhesive in the mid-part of the intestinal section [22]. This finding, in relation to the results in the present study about cubic microcontainers being more adhesive than cylindrical microcontainers, suggest that the presence of corners or edges can influence the mucoadhesion properties. However, the changing properties of the mucosa along the GI tract makes it difficult to directly extrapolate findings from one intestinal region to another.

We did not expect the material SU-8 to have any significant influence on mucoadhesion in itself. Even if SU-8 interacted with the mucus layer, the effect of this interaction would be similar for all the shapes since they have been normalized to have the same exterior surface area. Hence, we would not expect the differently shaped microcontainers to adhere differently as a result of interfacial interactions relating to material properties. Thus, we expect that the observed interaction with the intestinal mucosa is mostly due to mechanical detainment due to the differences in shape rather than chemical interactions.

In addition to the influence of the shape itself, the mucoadhesive effect of pillars applied to the top surface of cylinders was investigated (Figure 5). The amount of reference cylindrical microcontainers with pillars adhering to the colonic mucus was found to be 16 ± 13% after 30 min, which was very similar to the percentage of conventional reference and loaded cylinders (13 ± 9% and 12 ± 7%, respectively). In accordance with the mechanical theory of mucoadhesion described in the introduction, the pillars were introduced on the reference cylinders as bioinspired structures to increase adhesion by filling the imperfections of a rough surface. However, unexpectedly, no differences in mucoadhesion were observed by adding these small structures on top of the reference microcontainers. This could be attributed to the size or number of pillars, which might have been insufficient in order to interact with the mucus in a significant way. Finally, it was observed that handling of the reference microcontainers with pillars resulted in loss of some pillars when the microcontainers were evaluated with SEM before dosing, which could outweigh the potential adhesion effect of the pillars. To fully investigate the concept of surface structures further, additional studies are needed. Nevertheless, the microcontainers themselves seem to present adequate geometrical forms which can be detained in the mucus layer without help from smaller structures on the surface.

Surface modified microdevices have previously been found to increase adhesion in vitro and ex vivo [18]. However, these microdevices were not investigated in situ or in vivo and the surface structures on these devices were remarkably smaller (60–160 nm) than the pillars on the surface of the microcontainers in the present study (41 μm in height and 35 μm in diameter). In a different study, the impact of larger and more complex surface structures was investigated ex vivo and these were found to have a large impact on the adhesive properties of the microdevices [39].

When comparing the loaded and coated microcontainers to the empty reference microcontainers with and without pillars, it is important to consider the possible effect of the lid coating. Eudragit® polymers have previously been found to possess mucoadhesive properties when applied on nanocapsules [48]. Thus, the coating itself could influence the adhesion of the microcontainers even if Eudragit® L100 is expected to dissolve quickly at pH 7.4. However, all three types of cylindrical microcontainers appeared to result in similarly low mucoadhesion (Figure 5), which indicates that the shape is the most important factor for mucoadhesion in the present study.

In two euthanized rats dosed with cylindrical reference microcontainers, a remarkably smaller number of microcontainers were found to adhere after 30 min than for other rats dosed with reference cylinders. These findings indicate that the microcontainers interact differently with the colonic mucus in the presence of peristalsis, irrigation and water-resorption processes, which emphasizes the importance of evaluating mucoadhesion in situ as well as ex vivo.

3.3.2. Absorption of Amoxicillin

To address whether the mucus retention affected the absorption of amoxicillin from the microcontainers, blood and intestinal samples were collected. Based on the remaining concentrations in the intestinal lumen, the absorption rate constant (k_a) was calculated for amoxicillin in solution and amoxicillin dosed via cylindrical, cubic and triangular microcontainers (Figure 6). The values for k_a are relevant in order to evaluate how mucoadhesion affects the absorption of amoxicillin.

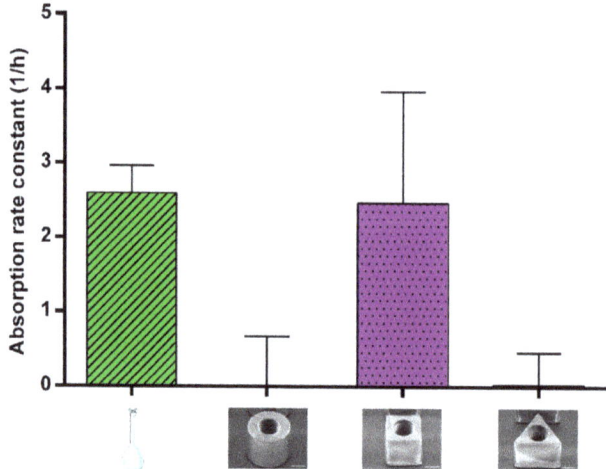

Figure 6. First-order absorption rate constants (k_a) calculated from the closed-loop intestinal perfusion studies for Eudragit® L100 coated microcontainers loaded with amoxicillin and for an amoxicillin control solution (mean ± SD, $n = 6$).

For amoxicillin in cubic microcontainers, k_a was calculated to be 2.5 ± 0.6 h^{-1}, which is not statistically different to the value obtained for the solution (2.6 ± 0.4 h^{-1}) (Figure 6). For cylinders and triangular prisms, k_a of amoxicillin was calculated to be 0.0 ± 0.7 h^{-1} and 0.0 ± 0.5 h^{-1}, respectively (Figure 6). In the case of the cubic microcontainers, absorption seems to be faster than the release, resulting in a positive k_a. This could be related to the slower in vitro release observed from this shape (Figure 3). On the contrary, the concentrations of amoxicillin measured in the lumen after dosing with cylindrical and triangular microcontainers appeared to be constant during the whole experiment. This could indicate that the absorption and release occurred with the same rate, and, thus, the absorbed amount of amoxicillin was continuously replaced by the released amount.

After 30 min, a blood sample was collected to compare k_a to the amount of amoxicillin absorbed from the colon during the experiment. In plasma, amoxicillin was mainly detected after dosing in solution and cubic microcontainers (0.26 ± 0.03 and 0.08 ± 0.02 µg/mL, respectively). On the contrary, amoxicillin could only be detected in plasma from one of the six rats dosed with triangular microcontainers (resulting in 0.02 ± 0.02 µg/mL for the group on average). Systemic uptake of amoxicillin was not detected in any of the blood samples from the rats dosed with cylindrical microcontainers. The absorption of amoxicillin has previously been shown to vary in different regions of the GI tract with limited absorption in the colon [49]. These region-dependent differences in absorption are believed to be caused by decreased levels of the uptake transport responsible for the absorption of amoxicillin [49,50].

In summary, the control solution and the cubic microcontainers were the formulations with the highest k_a, which also resulted in the highest concentration of amoxicillin in the plasma after 30 min. Amoxicillin dosed in the control solution had the obvious advantage that it was already in solution and available for absorption, whereas the amoxicillin powder inside the microcontainers needed more time to be released, solubilized and then absorbed. Based on the in vitro release profiles (Figure 3), only approximately 40% of the dose was expected to be released in the intestinal medium after 30 min, which could explain the observed difference in plasma concentrations. The different preconditions, but yet comparable performances, for the solution and the cubic microcontainers, suggested that the microcontainers must hold a different advantage, which might be related to the mucoadhesion. A high degree of mucoadhesion as observed for the cubic microcontainers would result in a high local concentration of amoxicillin facilitating the absorption.

Cylindrical microcontainers have previously been evaluated in an in situ closed loop perfusion model in the small intestine in order to investigate mucoadhesion and absorption of furosemide [16]. The microcontainers were found to adhere to the intestinal mucus and result in a higher absorption rate constant for furosemide when compared to a control solution [16]. The differences between this work and the present one can be attributed to the properties of the API and the intestinal section in which the absorption takes place.

4. Conclusions

In the present study, we investigated the influence of microdevice shape on colonic mucoadhesion and drug absorption by applying an in situ closed-loop intestinal perfusion technique. Cylindrical, triangular and cubic microcontainers were loaded with amoxicillin as a model drug and subsequently coated with Eudragit® L100. The amoxicillin release was evaluated in vitro and the absorption of amoxicillin and adhesion of microcontainers was evaluated in a closed-loop intestinal perfusion model in anesthetized rats.

In vitro, a complete amoxicillin release was observed after 60 min from the three types of microcontainers. From the microscopy analysis of the colon sections after the in situ perfusion study, it was evident that a significantly higher percentage of cubic microcontainers than cylindrical microcontainers (33 ± 12% and 12 ± 7%, respectively) was detained in the mucus. Additionally, the absorption rate constants and the blood samples indicated that amoxicillin in cubic microcontainers was absorbed more readily (2.5 ± 0.6 h^{-1} and 0.08 ± 0.02 µg/mL, respectively) than when cylindrical microcontainers (0.0 ± 0.7 h^{-1} and no absorption detected) or triangular microcontainers (0.0 ± 0.5 h^{-1} and 0.02 ± 0.02 µg/mL) were dosed. This could be due to a higher degree of mucoadhesion for these particular microcontainers.

With the present study, we have demonstrated that the in situ closed-loop intestinal perfusion model is a promising tool to evaluate overall performance of microdevices in a confined region of a rat intestine. Based on the presented results, the use of more complex microcontainer shapes including more edges and corners, such as star shapes, should be investigated in the future.

Author Contributions: Conceptualization, J.F.C., A.M., L.H.E.T., T.M.G., A.B., K.Z. and L.H.N.; methodology and supervision, J.F.C., A.M., A.B., K.Z. and L.H.N.; formal analysis, J.F.C., A.J.G., A.M., T.M.G., K.Z., L.H.N.; investigation and visualization, J.F.C., A.J.G., A.M., L.H.E.T.; resources, A.M. and A.B.; writing—original draft preparation, J.F.C., A.J.G. and L.H.E.T.; writing—review and editing, all authors; funding acquisition, T.M.G. and A.B. All authors have read and agreed to the published version of the manuscript.

Funding: This research was funded by the Novo Nordisk Foundation (NNF17OC0026910), MIMIO–Microstructures, microbiota and oral delivery and by the Danish National Research Foundation (DNRF122) and Villum Foundation (Grant No. 9301), Center for Intelligent Drug Delivery and Sensing Using Microcontainers and Nanomechanics (IDUN). Furthermore, the research was conducted with support from the University of Valencia precompetitive project UV-INV-PRECOMP12-80750 and GV/2013/086 project of the Valencian Government (Generalitat Valenciana).

Conflicts of Interest: The authors declare no conflict of interest.

References

1. Sastry, S.V.; Nyshadham, J.R.; Fix, J.A. Recent technological advances in oral drug delivery—A review. *Pharm. Sci. Technol. Today* **2000**, *3*, 138–145. [CrossRef]
2. Abramson, A.; Caffarel-Salvador, E.; Khang, M.; Dellal, D.; Silverstein, D.; Gao, Y.; Frederiksen, M.R.; Vegge, A.; Hubálek, F.; Water, J.J.; et al. An ingestible self-orienting system for oral delivery of macromolecules. *Science* **2019**, *363*, 611–615. [CrossRef] [PubMed]
3. Nemeth, C.L.; Lykins, W.R.; Tran, H.; ElSayed, M.E.H.; Desai, T.A. Bottom-Up Fabrication of Multilayer Enteric Devices for the Oral Delivery of Peptides. *Pharm. Res.* **2019**, *36*, 89. [CrossRef] [PubMed]

4. Nielsen, L.H.; Keller, S.S.; Boisen, A. Microfabricated devices for oral drug delivery. *Lab Chip* **2018**, *18*, 2348–2358. [CrossRef]
5. Lee, S.H.; Bajracharya, R.; Min, J.Y.; Han, J.-W.; Park, B.J.; Han, H.-K. Strategic Approaches for Colon Targeted Drug Delivery: An Overview of Recent Advancements. *Pharmaceutics* **2020**, *12*, 68. [CrossRef]
6. Basit, A.W.; Short, M.D.; McConnell, E.L. Microbiota-triggered colonic delivery: Robustness of the polysaccharide approach in the fed state in man. *J. Drug Target.* **2009**, *17*, 64–71. [CrossRef]
7. McConnell, E.L.; Liu, F.; Basit, A.W. Colonic treatments and targets: Issues and opportunities. *J. Drug Target.* **2009**, *17*, 335–363. [CrossRef]
8. Tubic-Grozdanis, M.; Hilfinger, J.M.; Amidon, G.L.; Kim, J.S.; Kijek, P.; Staubach, P.; Langguth, P. Pharmacokinetics of the CYP 3A substrate simvastatin following administration of delayed versus immediate release oral dosage forms. *Pharm. Res.* **2008**, *25*, 1591–1600. [CrossRef]
9. Smart, J.D. The basics and underlying mechanisms of mucoadhesion. *Adv. Drug Deliv. Rev.* **2005**, *57*, 1556–1568. [CrossRef]
10. Vinod, K.; Rohit, T.; Sandhya, S.; David, B.; Venkatram, R.B. A Critical Review on Mucoadhesive Drug Delivery Systems. *Hygeia J. Drugs Med.* **2012**, *4*, 7–28.
11. Champion, J.A.; Katare, Y.K.; Mitragotri, S. Particle shape: A new design parameter for micro- and nanoscale drug delivery carriers. *J. Control. Release* **2007**, *121*, 3–9. [CrossRef] [PubMed]
12. Shinde Patil, V.R.; Campbell, C.J.; Yun, Y.H.; Slack, S.M.; Goetz, D.J. Particle diameter influences adhesion under flow. *Biophys. J.* **2001**, *80*, 1733–1743. [CrossRef]
13. Pereira De Sousa, I.; Steiner, C.; Schmutzler, M.; Wilcox, M.D.; Veldhuis, G.J.; Pearson, J.P.; Huck, C.W.; Salvenmoser, W.; Bernkop-Schnürch, A. Mucus permeating carriers: Formulation and characterization of highly densely charged nanoparticles. *Eur. J. Pharm. Biopharm.* **2015**, *97*, 273–279. [CrossRef] [PubMed]
14. Varde, N.K.; Pack, D.W. Microspheres for controlled release drug delivery. *Expert Opin. Biol. Ther.* **2004**, *4*, 35–51. [CrossRef]
15. Chirra, H.D.; Shao, L.; Ciaccio, N.; Fox, C.B.; Wade, J.M.; Ma, A.; Desai, T.A. Planar Microdevices for Enhanced In Vivo Retention and Oral Bioavailability of Poorly Permeable Drugs. *Adv. Healthc. Mater.* **2014**, *3*, 1648–1654. [CrossRef]
16. Nielsen, L.H.; Melero, A.; Keller, S.S.; Jacobsen, J.; Garrigues, T.; Rades, T.; Müllertz, A.; Boisen, A. Polymeric microcontainers improve oral bioavailability of furosemide. *Int. J. Pharm.* **2016**, *504*, 98–109. [CrossRef]
17. Ainslie, K.M.; Lowe, R.D.; Beaudette, T.T.; Petty, L.; Bachelder, E.M.; Desai, T.A. Microfabricated devices for enhanced bioadhesive drug delivery: Attachment to and small-molecule release through a cell monolayer under flow. *Small* **2009**, *5*, 2857–2863. [CrossRef]
18. Fox, C.B.; Cao, Y.; Nemeth, C.L.; Chirra, H.D.; Chevalier, R.W.; Xu, A.M.; Melosh, N.A.; Desai, T.A. Fabrication of Sealed Nanostraw Microdevices for Oral Drug Delivery. *ACS Nano* **2016**, *10*, 5873–5881. [CrossRef]
19. Mazzoni, C.; Tentor, F.; Strindberg, S.A.; Nielsen, L.H.; Keller, S.S.; Alstrøm, T.S.; Gundlach, C.; Müllertz, A.; Marizza, P.; Boisen, A. From concept to in vivo testing: Microcontainers for oral drug delivery. *J. Control. Release* **2017**, *268*, 343–351. [CrossRef]
20. Petersen, R.S.; Mahshid, R.; Andersen, N.K.; Keller, S.S.; Hansen, H.N.; Boisen, A. Hot embossing and mechanical punching of biodegradable microcontainers for oral drug delivery. *Microelectron. Eng.* **2015**, *133*, 104–109. [CrossRef]
21. Abid, Z.; Strindberg, S.; Javed, M.M.; Mazzoni, C.; Vaut, L.; Nielsen, L.H.; Gundlach, C.; Petersen, R.S.; Müllertz, A.; Boisen, A.; et al. Biodegradable microcontainers—Towards real life applications of microfabricated systems for oral drug delivery. *Lab Chip* **2019**, *19*, 2905–2914. [CrossRef] [PubMed]
22. Mosgaard, M.D.; Strindberg, S.; Abid, Z.; Petersen, R.S.; Thamdrup, L.H.E.; Andersen, A.J.; Keller, S.S.; Müllertz, A.; Nielsen, L.H.; Boisen, A. Ex vivo intestinal perfusion model for investigating mucoadhesion of microcontainers. *Int. J. Pharm.* **2019**, *570*, 118658. [CrossRef] [PubMed]
23. Abid, Z.; Mosgaard, M.D.; Manfroni, G.; Petersen, R.S.; Nielsen, L.H.; Müllertz, A.; Boisen, A.; Keller, S.S. Investigation of Mucoadhesion and Degradation of PCL and PLGA Microcontainers for Oral Drug Delivery. *Polymers* **2019**, *11*, 1828. [CrossRef] [PubMed]
24. Vaut, L.; Scarano, E.; Tosello, G.; Boisen, A. Fully replicable and automated retention measurement setup for characterization of bio-adhesion. *HardwareX* **2019**, *6*, e00071. [CrossRef]
25. Sotres, J.; Jankovskaja, S.; Wannerberger, K.; Arnebrant, T. Ex-Vivo Force Spectroscopy of Intestinal Mucosa Reveals the Mechanical Properties of Mucus Blankets. *Sci. Rep.* **2017**, *7*, 1–14. [CrossRef]

26. Singh, I.; Rana, V. Techniques for the assessment of mucoadhesion in drug delivery systems: An overview. *J. Adhes. Sci. Technol.* **2012**, *26*, 2251–2267. [CrossRef]
27. Gamboa, J.M.; Leong, K.W. In vitro and in vivo models for the study of oral delivery of nanoparticles. *Adv. Drug Deliv. Rev.* **2013**, *65*, 800–810. [CrossRef] [PubMed]
28. Luo, Z.; Liu, Y.; Zhao, B.; Tang, M.; Dong, H.; Zhang, L.; Lv, B.; Wei, L. Ex vivo and in situ approaches used to study intestinal absorption. *J. Pharmacol. Toxicol. Methods* **2013**, *68*, 208–216. [CrossRef]
29. Schanker, L.S.; Tocco, D.J.; Brodie, B.B.; Hogben, C.A.M. Absorption of Drugs from the Rat Small Intestine. *J. Pharmacol. Exp. Ther.* **1958**, *123*, 81–88.
30. Stappaerts, J.; Brouwers, J.; Annaert, P.; Augustijns, P. In situ perfusion in rodents to explore intestinal drug absorption: Challenges and opportunities. *Int. J. Pharm.* **2015**, *478*, 665–681. [CrossRef]
31. Lennernäs, H. Regional intestinal drug permeation: Biopharmaceutics and drug development. *Eur. J. Pharm. Sci.* **2014**, *57*, 333–341. [CrossRef] [PubMed]
32. Lozoya-Agullo, I.; González-Álvarez, I.; Merino-Sanjuán, M.; Bermejo, M.; González-Álvarez, M. Preclinical models for colonic absorption, application to controlled release formulation development. *Eur. J. Pharm. Biopharm.* **2018**, *130*, 247–259. [CrossRef] [PubMed]
33. Lozoya-Agullo, I.; Zur, M.; Wolk, O.; Beig, A.; González-Álvarez, I.; González-Álvarez, M.; Merino-Sanjuán, M.; Bermejo, M.; Dahan, A. In-situ intestinal rat perfusions for human Fabs prediction and BCS permeability class determination: Investigation of the single-pass vs. the Doluisio experimental approaches. *Int. J. Pharm.* **2015**, *480*, 1–7. [CrossRef] [PubMed]
34. Doluisio, J.T.; Billups, N.F.; Dittert, L.W.; Sugita, E.T.; Swintosky, J.V. Drug Absorption I: An In Situ Rat Gut Technique Yielding Realistic Absorption Rates. *J. Pharm. Sci.* **1969**, *58*, 1196–1200. [CrossRef]
35. Lozoya-Agullo, I.; Gonzalez-Alvarez, I.; Zur, M.; Fine-Shamir, N.; Cohen, Y.; Markovic, M.; Garrigues, T.M.; Dahan, A.; Gonzalez-Alvarez, M.; Merino-Sanjuán, M.; et al. Closed-Loop Doluisio (Colon, Small Intestine) and Single-Pass Intestinal Perfusion (Colon, Jejunum) in Rat—Biophysical Model and Predictions Based on Caco-2. *Pharm. Res.* **2017**, *35*, 2. [CrossRef]
36. Ruiz-Picazo, A.; Lozoya-Agullo, I.; Ortiz-Azcarate, M.; Merino-Sanjuán, M.; González-Álvarez, M.; González-Álvarez, I.; Bermejo, M. Comparison of segmental-dependent permeability in human and in situ perfusion model in rat. *Eur. J. Pharm. Sci.* **2017**, *107*, 191–196. [CrossRef]
37. Lozoya-Agullo, I.; González-Álvarez, I.; González-Álvarez, M.; Merino-Sanjuán, M.; Bermejo, M. In Situ Perfusion Model in Rat Colon for Drug Absorption Studies: Comparison with Small Intestine and Caco-2 Cell Model. *J. Pharm. Sci.* **2015**, *104*, 3136–3145. [CrossRef]
38. Xu, Y.; Wang, Y.; Li, X.M.; Huang, Q.; Chen, W.; Liu, R.; Chen, B.; Wei, P. Study on the release of fenofibrate nanosuspension in vitro and its correlation with in situ intestinal and in vivo absorption kinetics in rats. *Drug Dev. Ind. Pharm.* **2014**, *40*, 972–979. [CrossRef]
39. Vaut, L.; Juszczyk, J.; Kamguyan, K.; Jensen, K.; Tosello, G.; Boisen, A. 3D Printing of Reservoir Devices for Oral Drug Delivery and Enhanced Mucoadhesion. *ACS Biomater. Sci. Eng.* **2020**, *6*, 2478–2486. [CrossRef]
40. Tao, S.L.; Popat, K.; Desai, T.A. Off-wafer fabrication and surface modification of asymmetric 3D SU-8 microparticles. *Nat. Protoc.* **2007**, *1*, 3153–3158. [CrossRef]
41. Nielsen, L.H.; Keller, S.S.; Gordon, K.C.; Boisen, A.; Rades, T.; Müllertz, A. Spatial confinement can lead to increased stability of amorphous indomethacin. *Eur. J. Pharm. Biopharm.* **2012**, *81*, 418–425. [CrossRef] [PubMed]
42. Nielsen, L.H.; Rades, T.; Boyd, B.; Boisen, A. Microcontainers as an oral delivery system for spray dried cubosomes containing ovalbumin. *Eur. J. Pharm. Biopharm.* **2017**, *118*, 13–20. [CrossRef] [PubMed]
43. Kamguyan, K.; Thamdrup, L.H.E.; Vaut, L.; Nielsen, L.H.; Zor, K.; Boisen, A. A Flexible and Precise Masking Technique for Microfabricated Devices Based on Physicochemical Properties of Polydimethylsiloxane. *Under Rev. J. Appl. Polym. Sci.* **2020**.
44. Tuğcu-Demiröz, F.; Gonzalez-Alvarez, I.; Gonzalez-Alvarez, M.; Bermejo, M. Validation of phenol red versus gravimetric method for water reabsorption correction and study of gender differences in Doluisio's absorption technique. *Eur. J. Pharm. Sci.* **2014**, *62*, 105–110. [CrossRef] [PubMed]
45. Martín-Villodre, A.; Plá-Delfina, J.M.; Moreno, J.; Pérez-Buendía, D.; Miralles, J.; Collado, E.F.; Sánchez-Moyano, E.; Pozo, A. del Studies on the reliability of a bihyperbolic functional absorption model. II. Phenylalkylamines. *J. Pharmacokinet. Biopharm.* **1987**, *15*, 633–643.

46. Dissolution test for solid dosage forms. In *European Pharmacopeia*, 8th ed.; Council of Europe: Strasbourg, France, 2013; Volume 1, pp. 288–295.
47. Nielsen, L.H.; Nagstrup, J.; Gordon, S.; Keller, S.S.; Østergaard, J.; Rades, T.; Müllertz, A.; Boisen, A. pH-triggered drug release from biodegradable microwells for oral drug delivery. *Biomed. Microdevices* **2015**, *17*, 55. [CrossRef]
48. Chaves, P.D.S.; Frank, L.A.; Frank, A.G.; Pohlmann, A.R.; Guterres, S.S.; Beck, R.C.R. Mucoadhesive Properties of Eudragit®RS100, Eudragit®S100, and Poly(ε-caprolactone) Nanocapsules: Influence of the Vehicle and the Mucosal Surface. *AAPS PharmSciTech* **2018**, *19*, 1637–1646. [CrossRef]
49. Barr, W.H.; Zola, E.M.; Candler, E.L.; Hwang, S.-M.; Tendolkar, A.V.; Shamburek, R.; Parker, B.; Hilty, M.D. Differential absorption of amoxicillin from the human small and large intestine. *Clin. Pharmacol. Ther.* **1994**, *56*, 279–285. [CrossRef]
50. Tannergren, C.; Bergendal, A.; Lennernäs, H.; Abrahamsson, B. Toward an increased understanding of the barriers to colonic drug absorption in humans: Implications for early controlled release candidate assessment. *Mol. Pharm.* **2009**, *6*, 60–73. [CrossRef]

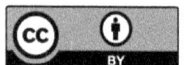

© 2020 by the authors. Licensee MDPI, Basel, Switzerland. This article is an open access article distributed under the terms and conditions of the Creative Commons Attribution (CC BY) license (http://creativecommons.org/licenses/by/4.0/).

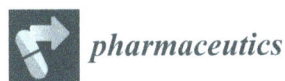

Review

The Segregated Intestinal Flow Model (SFM) for Drug Absorption and Drug Metabolism: Implications on Intestinal and Liver Metabolism and Drug–Drug Interactions

K. Sandy Pang *, H. Benson Peng and Keumhan Noh

Leslie Dan Faculty of Pharmacy, University of Toronto, Toronto, ON M5S 3M2, Canada; hao.peng@mail.utoronto.ca (H.B.P.); keumhan.noh@utoronto.ca (K.N.)
* Correspondence: ks.pang@utoronto.ca; Tel.: +1-416-978-6164

Received: 12 March 2020; Accepted: 27 March 2020; Published: 1 April 2020

Abstract: The properties of the segregated flow model (SFM), which considers split intestinal flow patterns perfusing an active enterocyte region that houses enzymes and transporters (<20% of the total intestinal blood flow) and an inactive serosal region (>80%), were compared to those of the traditional model (TM), wherein 100% of the flow perfuses the non-segregated intestine tissue. The appropriateness of the SFM model is important in terms of drug absorption and intestinal and liver drug metabolism. Model behaviors were examined with respect to intestinally (M1) versus hepatically (M2) formed metabolites and the availabilities in the intestine (F_I) and liver (F_H) and the route of drug administration. The %contribution of the intestine to total first-pass metabolism bears a reciprocal relation to that for the liver, since the intestine, a gateway tissue, regulates the flow of substrate to the liver. The SFM predicts the highest and lowest M1 formed with oral (po) and intravenous (iv) dosing, respectively, whereas the extent of M1 formation is similar for the drug administered po or iv according to the TM, and these values sit intermediate those of the SFM. The SFM is significant, as this drug metabolism model explains route-dependent intestinal metabolism, describing a higher extent of intestinal metabolism with po versus the much reduced or absence of intestinal metabolism with iv dosing. A similar pattern exists for drug–drug interactions (DDIs). The inhibitor or inducer exerts its greatest effect on victim drugs when both inhibitor/inducer and drug are given po. With po dosing, more drug or inhibitor/inducer is brought into the intestine for DDIs. The bypass of flow and drug to the enterocyte region of the intestine after intravenous administration adds complications to in vitro–in vivo extrapolations (IVIVE).

Keywords: segregated flow intestinal model (SFM); traditional model (TM); route-dependent intestinal metabolism; first-pass effect; drug-drug interactions; DDI; in vitro in vivo extrapolations; IVIVE

1. The Intestine–Liver Unit

The extent of the absorption of orally administered drugs is controlled by the intestine and liver, which are anatomically linked as a serial unit that is sequentially perfused by the circulation (Figure 1). The intestine is the gateway tissue to the liver and is important for drug absorption and first-pass removal. The superior mesenteric artery (SMA) supplies blood to the small intestine and its venous drainage, together with venous returns from the spleen, pancreas, gallbladder and gastrointestinal tract (GIT) including the stomach, constitute the hepatic portal vein flow (Q_{PV}), which is approximately 75% of the total liver blood flow, Q_H. Together with the hepatic artery (Q_{HA}), the remaining 25% of Q_H, the dual flows collectively perfuse the liver.

The intestine is endowed with absorptive transmembrane transporters in simple columnar, epithelial cells known as enterocytes that line the inner surfaces of the small intestine. These cells contain numerous protrusions known as the villi and microvilli that increase the surface area multiple-fold to absorb drug molecules or nutrients from the gut lumen. Intestinal absorption models have been classically linked to drug properties and the dosage form (pKa, logP, and solubility), as well as the physiology of the gastrointestinal tract (pH, gastrointestinal transit time, gastric emptying time, surface area, and microbiota) that control the fraction of dose absorbed (F_a) [1–11]. In addition to passive diffusion, absorptive transporters known as the apical solute carrier transporters (SLC), as exemplified by the PEPT1 (oligopeptide transporter 1), OATP1A2, OATP2B1 (the organic anion transporting polypeptide 1A1 and 2B1), MCT1 (the monocarboxylic acid transporter 1), ASBT (apical sodium dependent bile acid transporter) that reclaims bile acids, and OCT (organic cation transporter), facilitate the entry of weak acids and weak bases [12–18]. Counterbalancing drug entry are the efflux transporters—the P-gp (P-glycoprotein), BCRP (breast cancer resistance protein) and MRP2 (multidrug resistance-associated protein 2) that mediate drug or metabolite secretion back to the intestinal lumen [19,20], and this backward flux tends to reduce the net absorption of solutes. The OSTα and OSTβ (organic solute transporter α and β, half-transporters) transport bile acids out of the enterocytes [21]. It is well recognized that P-gp is capable of secreting highly lipophilic drugs [22,23]. Since lipophilic drugs with high solubility and permeability (Biopharmaceutical Classification System or BCS, Class I) are readily reabsorbed, the excretory function of P-gp is readily nullified [24]. The significance of P-gp, being more abundant distally in the ileum is, therefore, reduced for drugs that are readily reabsorbed [20,23,25,26]. However, for highly soluble but poorly permeable Class III BCS drugs, P-gp is more effective in reducing intestinal drug absorption [7]. It is also notable that drug permeability can be influenced by the pH of the intestinal lumen that becomes more and more basic and in turn, influence the extent of drug absorbed [3,8]. Segment-dependent decline in membrane permeability, reduced surface area from the duodenum to ileum [27] and pH changes along the intestine [8,28] are noted. These variables will modulate the extent of passive drug absorption.

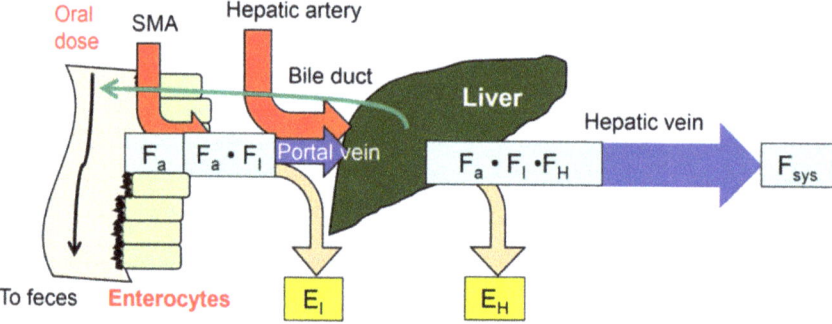

Figure 1. The intestine as a gateway tissue to the liver. Because of intestinal removal [extraction ratio, E_I or $(1 - F_I)$], the drug entering the liver is reduced, and the liver may further remove the drug with a liver extraction ratio (E_H) to effect first-pass metabolism. The fraction absorbed, F_a and F_I or $(1 - E_I)$, and F_H or $(1 - E_H)$ influence the systemic bioavailability, F_{sys}. This figure was reproduced with permission from Noh and Pang [18], Wiley, 2019.

After crossing the intestinal membrane, the drug is met with metabolizing enzymes such as the cytochromes P450 3A (CYP3A) and UDP-glucuronosyltransferases, UGTs [29–32]. The most abundant CYP isoform is CYP3A4, which exceeds other isoforms such as 2C9, 2C19 > 2J2 > 2D6 that are present in lower quantities [31,33–35]. UGT 1A (1A1, 1A6, 1A5, 1A8, and 1A10) and 2B (2B7, 2B15, and 2B17) subfamilies are present to mediate the glucuronidation of morphine, raloxifene, mycophenolate, bisphenol A and gemfibrozil [36–40]. The intestinal metabolic activities for CYP3A4 and some of the UGTs are comparable to, or higher than, those in the liver [31,41,42]. Cytosolic glutathione S-transferases [43,44] are found abundantly, whereas epoxide hydrolases [43] and sulfotransferases (SULT) [45] are present at much lower quantities in the intestine.

The availability of the intestine (F_I) after intestinal metabolism or secretion is defined as $(1 - E_I)$ [where E_I is the intestinal extraction ratio], and hepatic availability, F_H, is given by $(1 - E_H)$ [where E_H is the hepatic extraction ratio]. The overall systemic availability, F_{sys}, is given by $F_aF_IF_H$. Following oral (po) drug dosing, the fraction of the dose absorbed (F_a) is attributed to dosage forms and/or solubility properties, intestinal removal via metabolism or secretion (defined by the intestinal extraction ratio, E_I), and liver removal (defined as the hepatic extraction ratio, E_H), respectively. The product of the availabilities, $F_aF_IF_H$, constitute the net fraction, the systemic availability, F_{sys}. For this reason, the intestine and liver are both capable of removing a significant proportion of the orally administered dose, a phenomenon known as the first-pass effect [46]. The extent of intestinal versus liver removal of drugs is therefore intimately related [47–50].

2. Reason or Need for Intestinal Flow Models

Although the development of clearance concepts for the intestine has lagged behind that for the liver [51–53], there have been some activities trending towards the fabrication of a useful and meaningful intestine clearance model to predict the extent of removal and examine how the intestine influences the rate of liver removal according to the route of drug administration. The correct intestinal model will exert serious implications in terms of drug–drug interactions (DDIs) with inducers or inhibitors, or in terms of in vitro–in vivo extrapolation (IVIVE).

3. Route-Dependent Intestinal Metabolism

Midazolam is a prototypic probe substrate of CYP3A4 metabolism that is often utilized for the screening of CYP3A4 and CYP3A5 activities in inhibition or induction studies [42,54–58]. Midazolam is metabolized by both the intestine and liver [42,59]. For the completely absorbed drug ($F_a \sim 1$), there was a dramatically lower intestinal extraction ratio ($E_I = 0.08$), measured across the arterial and hepatic portal venous blood for midazolam after its intravenous administration among anhepatic patients whose livers were removed during transplantation surgery [59]. In comparison, the mean fraction metabolized across the intestinal mucosa when given intraduodenally was much higher ($E_I = 0.43$). This first, direct evidence uniquely shows route-dependent metabolism of the small intestine. Clinically, the erythromycin breath test relates well to the midazolam unbound liver clearance and not correlated to the intestinal clearance [60]. For radiolabeled (-)morphine that forms morphine 3-glucuronide (M3G) in both the intestine and liver, M3G was absent and undetectable in the vascularly perfused rat intestine preparation when morphine from the reservoir recirculated the rat intestine, a scenario akin to the systemic administration of morphine. This contrasts the copious presence of the radiolabeled M3G metabolite in both the intestinal lumen and reservoir after the intraduodenal administration of morphine into the gut lumen [61]. Additional animal and human studies attest to the same trend of a higher extent of intestinal metabolism after oral (po) than after intravenous (iv) drug administration (Table 1). These examples serve as direct evidence that display route-dependent metabolism of the small intestine. There will be a corresponding route-dependent change in the proportion of liver metabolites formed as well, since the unmetabolized drug leaving the intestine now enters the liver for further processing.

Table 1. Examples of route-dependent intestinal metabolism.

Compound	System	Enzyme/Metabolite	Examples	References
Enalapril	Perfused rat intestine–liver preparation	Esterase/enalaprilat	Enalaprilat formed from enalapril after po administration but not systemic administration	[62]
Acetaminophen	Perfused rat small intestine preparation	Ugt1a6/acetaminophen glucuronide	Metabolite observed after intraduodenal but not systemic dosing	[63]
(-)-6-aminocarbovir (6AC)	Perfused rat small intestine preparation	Adenosine deaminase activates (-)-carbovir to 6AC	6AC was highly extracted by intestine after luminal dosing (0.54) compared to reservoir dosing (0.08)	[64]
Morphine	Perfused rat small intestine preparation	Ugt2b1/ morphine 3-glucuronide (M3G)	M3G appeared after intraduodenal but not systemic dosing	[61]
L-754,394, (furanopyridine derivative)	Rats and dogs in vivo and rat liver perfusion	Cyp3a/ epoxide intermediate	Inhibition of L-754,394 and its metabolites by Cyp3a is much greater for po than iv administration of drug	[65]
Cyclosporine	Human in vivo	CYP3A4/AM1 and AM9	Metabolites: AM1 and AM9 are lower after iv compared to po	[66]
Verapamil	Human in vivo	CYP3A4 and 3A5/ norverapamil	Metabolite, norverapamil formation after po > iv	[67]
Hydralazine	Human in vivo	Acetyltransferase/ 3-methyl-striazolo-3,4, α-phthalazine (MTP)	More MTP formation observed after oral dosing than iv dosing	[68]
Cyclobenzaprine	Human in vivo	UGT/ cyclobenzaprine glucuronide (CBG)	Formation of CBG was greater for the oral than for parenteral case	[69]
Midazolam (MDZ)	Human in vivo	CYP3A4/ 1'-OH and 4-OH MDZ	E_I after intraduodenal administration >> E_I for iv administration	[59,70]
Methyldopa	Human in vivo	SULT/ methyldopa sulfate (MS)	Greater formation of MS after po than iv dosing of M	[71]
Quinidine	Human in vivo	CYP3A/ 3-hydroxyquinidine	More 3-hydroxyquinidine formed via oral compared to iv route	[72]

4. Intestinal Flow Models: Segregated Flow (SFM), Q_{Gut}, and Traditional (TM) Models

Compartmental models are ill equipped to examine the extent of drug metabolism among metabolizing tissues or organs that are arranged serially. Hence, physiologically based pharmacokinetic (PBPK) modeling of the intestine and liver works a lot better. The approach has been used to appraise the extent of intestine vs. liver removal of drugs [48,49,73–78]. Here, the view is that the intestine is perfused 100% by superior mesenteric arterial flow (Q_{SMA}), which drains into the portal venous blood (Q_{PV}) for the traditional intestinal model (TM), and, upon combining with Q_{HA}, these flows in turn perfuse the liver. However, the TM would not explain route-dependent intestinal metabolism on midazolam [59] and morphine [61], which propelled us to develop useful intestinal flow models that can describe this phenomenon. The segregated flow model (SFM) describes a split flow pattern, as proposed by Klippert and Noordhoek [79], with a lower flow rate perfusing the active, enterocyte region (f_Q or fraction of the total intestinal flow, <20%) that houses the enzymes and absorptive/efflux transporters, and the remainder flow (>80%) perfusing the non-active, serosal region has since surfaced [80]. With oral administration, the entire dose amount needs to cross into the enterocyte region—the volume of which is conveniently viewed as ($f_Q \cdot V_{int}$), where V_{int} (or V_I) is the volume of the total intestine—whereas, for intravenous dosing, <20% of the drug in the circulation reaches the enterocyte region, and this will effectively reduce the rate of drug removal by the intestine. The segregated flow behavior of the intestine is found to explain route-dependent intestinal removal observed for many drugs.

A similar flow model, the Q_{Gut} model [81–83], was coined as a minimal model based on the well-stirred model equation for the liver, namely, $F_I = \frac{Q_{Gut}}{Q_{Gut}+fu_B CL_{int}^I}$ [49], after the equation of Yang et al. [83] was corrected upon substitution of fu_B for the unbound fraction to intestinal tissue, fu_I. Since the villous flow (Q_{villi}) is 6% of the cardiac output as 19 L/h, the ratio of the Q_{villi}/Q_{PV} or f_Q value for the Q_{Gut} model is as high as 0.484 for a lipophilic drug such as midazolam [81–83]. Notably, f_Q is different among these flow models: the SFM ($f_Q < 0.2$), Q_{Gut} model ($f_Q = 0.484$) and TM ($f_Q = 1$). The f_Q value is expected to affect the extent of intestine and liver removal (E_I and E_H) in the intestine–liver unit with respect to the route of drug administration.

5. Equations for Prediction of Route-Dependent Intestinal Removal

There are major differences in drug distribution and therefore intestinal drug clearance when the drug is entering from gut lumen into the villous tip or from the circulation (drug given intravenously) (Figure 2). For the TM, whereby the total intestinal flow perfuses the entire intestine ($f_Q = 1$), there is no difference in the distribution and clearance of drug between oral and intravenous administration when the enterocyte and serosal regions are meshed together (Figure 2A). After po administration, the drug is absorbed into the enterocyte (yellow arrow) and is well distributed in the enterocyte (right graph); the distribution of drug into the enterocyte is also similar after intravenous administration, and the drug is again well-distributed into the enterocyte ($f_Q = 1$). For the SFM (Figure 2B), the extent of distribution after po dosing for a rapidly absorbed drug is similar to that as for TM. Since the enterocyte region is perfused with a lower flow rate ($f_Q \cdot Q_{PV}$) according to the SFM, its drug extraction ratio for $E_{I,po,SFM}$ is therefore slightly higher than that for the TM, $E_{I,po,TM}$, as the drug is associated with a longer transit time in the tissue [18]. However for iv dosing, there is a reduced distribution of drug reaching the enterocyte due to the reduced intestinal flow ($f_Q < 0.2$), and there will be a smaller intestinal clearance pursuant to intravenous dosing (Figure 2B). Thus $E_{I,po,SFM} > E_{I,iv,SFM}$ or $F_{I,iv,SFM} > F_{I,po,SFM}$ (Figure 2B) when the drug is shunted away from the enterocyte region, especially for highly permeable drugs entering the intestinal tissue from the circulation than from the gut lumen [18,80].

The explicit solutions for both the TM and SFM (and Q_{Gut} model) are provided by Sun and Pang [84], who placed the intestine and liver into simple or semi-physiologically based pharmacokinetic (PBPK) models upon viewing both metabolic as well as transport (basolateral influx and efflux) pathways in the intestine and liver (Figure 3). The only difference between the TM and SFM (or Q_{Gut} model) is the presence of an additional intestinal compartment, since the intestine is now denoted as two subcompartments, the enterocyte and serosa, for the SFM and Q_{Gut} model. For simplistic assignment of the volume and flow, $f_Q \times$ volume or flow are used to designate the enterocyte volume and flow, respectively, and $(1 - f_Q) \times$ volume or flow are used to denote the serosal volume and flow, respectively. A common solution ([Equation (1)] now surfaces to represent the systemic bioavailability with oral administration [84]. This common equation may be used to describe bioavailability, F_{sys}, when $f_Q = 1$, 0.484 and <0.2, respectively, for the TM, Q_{Gut} model, and the SFM.

$$\frac{AUC_{po}/Dose_{po}}{AUC_{iv}/Dose_{iv}} = F_{sys} = F_a\, F_I F_H$$

$$F_a \left[\frac{f_Q Q_{PV} CL_{d2}^I}{f_Q Q_{PV} CL_{d2}^I + (f_Q Q_{PV} + fu_B CL_{d1}^I)[CL_{int,met1}^I + CL_{int,met2}^I + CL_{int,sec}^I(1-F_a)]} \right] \left[\frac{Q_H(CL_{d2}^H + CL_{int,H}^H)}{Q_H(CL_{d2}^H + CL_{int,H}^H) + fu_B CL_{d1}^H CL_{int,H}^H} \right] \quad (1)$$

where CL_{d1}^I is the influx transport clearance and CL_{d2}^I is the efflux transport clearance. $CL_{int,met}^I$ is the intestinal intrinsic metabolic clearance (for pathways 1 or 2) and $CL_{int,sec}^I$ is the secretory intestinal intrinsic clearance. In the liver, the sum of $CL_{int,sec}^H$ and $CL_{int,met}^H$ is CL_{int}^H; fu_B is the unbound fraction in blood, and Q_{PV} and Q_H are the portal venous flow and total liver blood flow, respectively. The superscripts I and H denote the intestine and liver, respectively. Notably, the unbound fractions of drug in intestine and liver tissue (fu_I and fu_H) are canceled out in the manipulation.

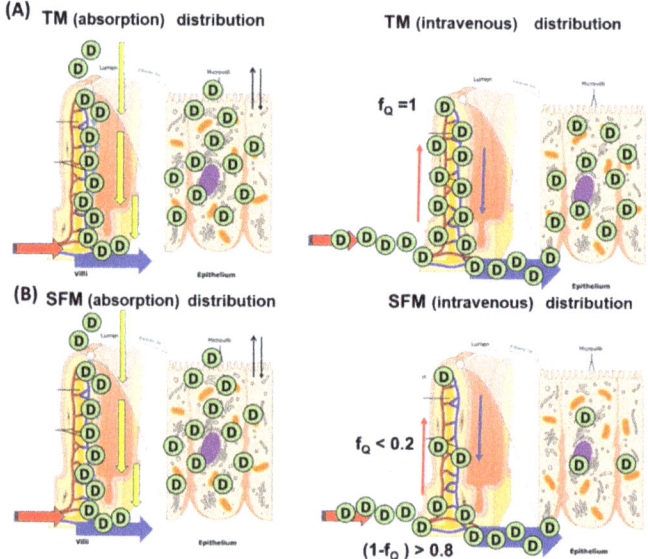

Figure 2. Schematic of drug molecules (D) traversing the intestinal membrane and entering the enterocyte for the tradtional model (TM) (**A**) and segregated flow model (SFM) (**B**). After po admininstration, the drug is absorbed into the enterocyte (yellow arrow) and distributed abundantly in the epithelisum (adjacent) for both the TM and SFM. After intravenous administration, the drug is distributed to the same extent in the epithelium according to the TM ($f_Q = 1$) while the SFM ($f_Q < 0.2$) predicts a much lower distribution of drug in enterocytes. This figure was reproduced with permission from Noh and Pang [18], Wiley, 2019.

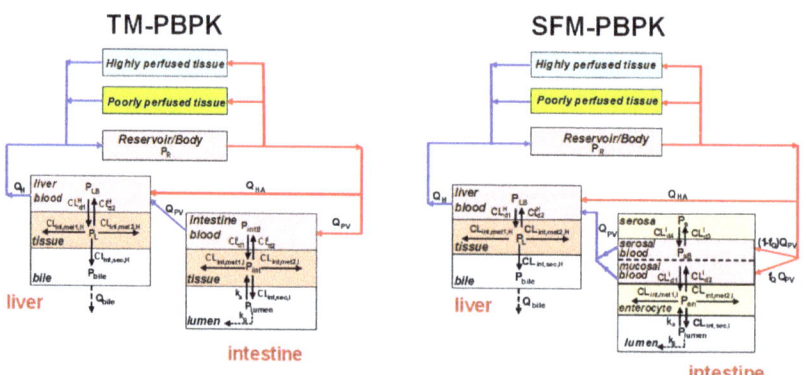

Figure 3. Physiologically based pharmacokinetic (PBPK) models depicting the intestine as a single tissue or compartment for the TM (left) or as the two subcompartments, the enterocyte and serosal subcompartments for the SFM (right), perfused by segregated flows. This figure was reproduced with permission from Sun and Pang [84], Springer, 2010.

For a drug in the circulation entering the intestine, the rate of drug removal by the enterocyte is $f_Q \cdot Q_{PV}(1 - F_I) \cdot C_A$, but there is no removal by the serosal region (Figure 4). The split flow pattern for the SFM or Q_{Gut} model results in a flow-averaged outflow, portal venous concentration, $\overline{C}_{PV}$ [49].

$$\overline{C}_{PV} = \frac{f_Q Q_{PV} F_I C_A + (1 - f_Q) Q_{PV} C_A}{Q_{PV}} = C_A [f_Q F_I + (1 - f_Q)] \qquad (2)$$

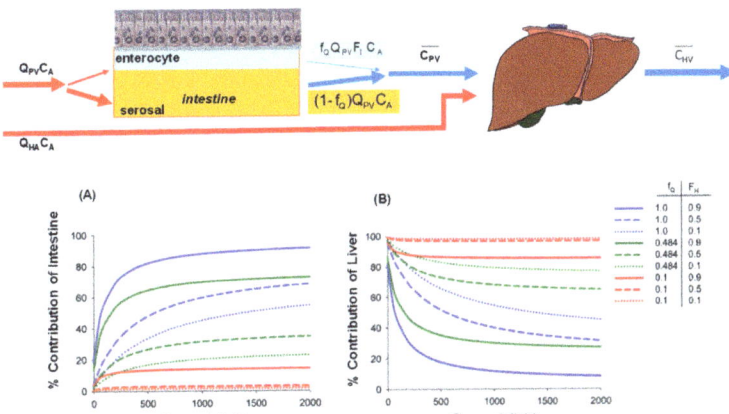

Figure 4. Drug removal by the intestine–liver unit: the intestine controls the substrate flux to the liver. The contributions of intestinal (**A**) and liver (**B**) removal are given by Equations (3) and (4). The drug in the circulation enters two subcompartments of the intestine—the enterocyte and serosal compartments. Removal by the enterocyte but not seroal compartment results in a flow-averaged portal venous concentration,$\overline{C}_{PV}$. If intestinal removal is high, the contribution by the liver is opposite and will be low. This figure was modified with permission from Pang and Chow [49], ASPET, 2012.

This flow-averaged portal venous concentration is then combined with the arterial concentration (C_A) to perfuse the liver. Along the same line of reasoning, the rates of removal of drug by the intestine and liver or the fractional contributions are given by,

$$\frac{v_I}{v_I+v_H} = \frac{f_Q Q_{PV}(1-F_I)}{f_Q Q_{PV}(1-F_I) + E_H \langle Q_{PV}[f_Q F_I + (1-f_Q)] + Q_{HA} \rangle} \quad (3)$$

and

$$\frac{v_H}{v_I+v_H} = \frac{E_H \langle Q_{PV}[f_Q F_I + (1-f_Q)] + Q_{HA} \rangle}{f_Q Q_{PV}(1-F_I) + E_H \langle Q_{PV}[f_Q F_I + (1-f_Q)] + Q_{HA} \rangle} \quad (4)$$

The contributions of the intestine (v_I) and liver (v_H) in first-pass removal are hence described by Equations (3) and (4). With f_Q values = 1 (left) (TM), = 0.1 (SFM), or = 0.484 (Q_{Gut} model) and with the assumption that Q_{PV} is approximated by Q_{SMA}, simulations show that, for a drug entering the intestine from the circulation, the TM predicts the highest intestinal contribution by the intestine–liver unit, whereas the SFM predicts the least; the Q_{Gut} model predicts values somewhere in the middle (Figure 4A). The importance of the intestine increases when the liver possesses a low enzymatic removal capacity (high F_H). Under the same scenario, results for the %contribution by the liver are the exact opposites, since there is a reciprocal relation to the intestine (Figure 4B). For the SFM, which suggests a lower contribution of metabolism by the intestine for drugs entering from the circulation, the contribution by the liver to first-pass removal is higher than those predicted for the TM and Q_{Gut} model, since there is a greater substrate flux entering the liver that will result in a greater %contribution by the liver, especially for high E_H drugs.

6. Is the SFM the Better Intestinal Flow Model Compared to the TM?

Theoretical development of the SFM readily explains the observed higher E_I for midazolam and morphine given orally versus intravenously (also Table 1), as do many other drug examples or substrates. When different sets of in vivo or intestinal perfusion data were fitted to the TM versus the

SFM, fits to the SFM were all superior over those for the TM. The fitted values of f_Q were all <0.2, and the SFM was shown to better the TM statistically among all examples (Table 2). The villous flow pattern to the enterocyte region [85], being a low fraction (<0.2), has also been suggested by Granger et al. [86]. A better discrimination between the TM and SFM occurs when metabolite data are present, as provided by the example of morphine, which forms morphine-3-glucuronide (M3G) by the intestine and liver in the rat in vivo. The discriminatory power for the morphine study was further provided by the biliary versus urinary excretion ratio of the metabolite, M3G, which is unable to cross the liver membrane due to its polarity [87]. The M3G presence in bile suggests that the origin of the metabolite is from the liver. The urinary morphine 3-glucuronide originates from both intestinal and liver metabolism, and the observed ratio of M3G in urine/bile associated with intraduodenal morphine dosing was 2.55-fold that with intravenous morphine administration, as predicted for the SFM [76]. The observations for morphine and morphine 3-glucuronide correlated much better with the predictions from the SFM than from TM.

Table 2. Fitted values of f_Q in rodents in vivo and in perfusion preparations.

Drug	Fraction of Intestinal Flow to Enterocytes (f_Q)	Experimental Condition	References
Benzoic acid	0.07	Rat liver perfusion	[88]
Codeine	0.16	Rat in vivo	[77]
Digoxin	0.20	Rat intestinal perfusion	[26]
Digoxin	0.16	Mouse in vivo	[89]
Morphine	0.10	Rat in vivo	[76]
Morphine	0.024	Rat intestinal perfusion	[80]
1,25-Dihydroxyvitamin D_3	0.11	Mouse in vivo	[87]

By contrast, there is practically no difference in the fitted results between the SFM and TM for codeine, the inactive precursor that is N-demethylated to form morphine [77]. At first glance, the similarity of both the SFM and TM fits is unique, suggesting that the drug is not subject to intestinal metabolism. For codeine, rat Cyp2d1 (human CYP2D6) is of very low abundance in the intestine, and intestinal metabolism of codeine is very low. For that reason, the agreement of the TM and SFM fits to the codeine data infer a lack of intestine metabolism for codeine. We also recently observed the same pattern for the pan-inhibitor, ketoconazole, after oral and intravenous administration to the rat (unpublished information, Keumhan Noh, Lilly Xu, and K. Sandy Pang).

6.1. Implications on Formation of Intestinal and Liver Metabolites

Noh and Pang [18] examined the formation of the metabolites: M1 from intestine and M2 from liver, as well as extraction ratios of the intestine with the route of drug administration. For TM, the simulations verified that $F_{I,po,TM} = F_{I,iv,TM}$ for highly permeable drugs, but $F_{I,po,SFM} < F_{I,iv,SFM}$ for SFM and $F_{I,po,SFM} < F_{I,po,TM} = F_{I,iv,TM} < F_{I,iv,SFM}$. The SFM predicts the highest formation of the M1 metabolite with oral dosing but the lowest formation of M1 with intravenous administration; the converse should occur for M2 formation from liver. From M1/M2, the ratio would further unveil that there is more M2 formation arising via the iv route because of direct delivery of drug via the hepatic artery to the liver. Additionally, M1 is less formed according to the SFM for drugs administered iv than po. For this reason, the ratio M1/M2 would always be smaller after intravenous administration according to the SFM as well as TM (Figure 5).

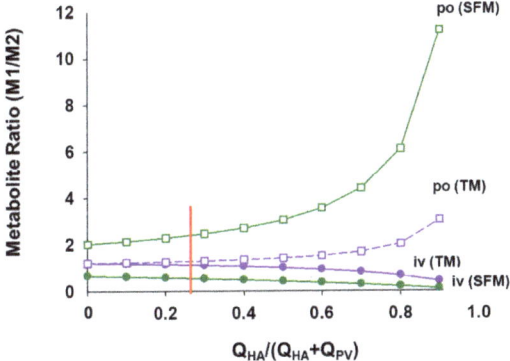

Figure 5. Formation of M1 and M2, specific metabolites formed by the intestine and liver, respecitvely, as simulated by Noh and Pang [18]. The hepatic arterial flow (Q_{HA}), normally 25% of total liver blood flow (shown where red line is), delivers the drug directly into the liver, and this contributes M2 formation. Additionally, M2 formation is highest according to the SFM for iv drug administration wherein M1 formation is low due to the low f_Q. For the TM, the extent of M2 formation is identical for a drug given orally and intravenously, when there is no Q_{HA} flow; the extent increases with increasing Q_{HA}. This figure was reproduced with permission from Noh and Pang [18], Wiley, 2019.

6.2. Implications of the SFM on Drug–Drug Interactions (DDIs)

Another reason for properly selecting the intestine flow model is on the prediction of DDI with an inducer or inhibitor. Because >80% intestinal flow bypasses the enterocytes according to the SFM, the route of administration of the inhibitor/inducer, if oral, should be much more effective than the intravenous route, with the underlying reason that the inhibitor/inducer concentrations would be higher in the enterocyte region. Hence, the extent of DDIs is dependent on how the victim drug or inhibitor/inducer is administered and which intestinal flow model, TM or SFM, prevails (Table 3). For midazolam given intravenously (2 mg) or orally (6 mg) to humans, its AUC_{iv} increased 5-fold, whereas AUC_{po} increased 16-fold upon pretreatment with 3 po doses of 200 mg ketoconazole orally at 12 h prior to midazolam dosing, and twice at every 12 h thereafter [57]. For digoxin (1 mg), the inducer rifampin (600 mg daily po for 15 days) produced a dramatic lowering of AUC_{po} but not AUC_{iv} of digoxin due to a 3.5-fold induction of intestinal P-gp protein [20]. In monkeys, ketoconazole inhibited the metabolism of simvastatin, a typical Cyp3a substrate, when given orally and increased the AUC_{po} 5 to 10x, without changing AUC_{iv} for simvastatin given intravenously [90]. For midazolam, oral treatment (50 mg/kg/day for 4 days) of dexamethasone increased the V_{max} values for 1'-hydroxylation and 4-hydroxylation of midazolam in rat intestinal microsomes much more than that with iv dexamethasone [91]. For digoxin given to Wistar rats, purple grape juice (inhibitor of transporter or enzymes) increased the AUC_{po} (73%) but not AUC_{iv} for digoxin [92]. There exist many other examples attesting to this interesting DDI pattern for orally but not intravenously administered victim drugs in the presence of inhibitors or inducers, also given orally (Table 3). These examples confirm the observation that inhibitors or inducers of intestinal enzymes act best after oral administration, since the concentration attained will be highest within the intestine, and the same goes for the victim drug. The inhibition expected for the SFM should be the greatest, and hence this would also create opposite changes in liver metabolism, since inhibition of the intestine leads to a greater flux of substrate towards liver metabolism.

Table 3. Greater inhibitory or inductive effects after oral administration than iv administration for drug–drug interactions (DDIs) of the intestine.

Compound	Inducer/Inhibitor (Dosing Route)	Enzyme /Transporter	Outcome	Reference
	Induction Studies			
Alfentanil	Rifampicin (po)	CYP	Decrease in $AUC_{po}/AUC_{iv} = 8.2$	[93]
Cyclosporin	Rifampicin (po)	CYP	Decrease in $AUC_{po}/AUC_{iv} = 2.6$	[94]
Digoxin	Rifampicin (po)	P-gp	Decrease in $AUC_{po}/AUC_{iv} = 1.3$	[20]
Indinavir	Dexamethasone (po)	CYP and P-gp	Decrease in $AUC_{po}/AUC_{iv} = 2.3$	[24]
Methadone	Rifampicin (po)	CYP	Decrease in $AUC_{po}/AUC_{iv} = 1.4$	[95]
Midazolam	Rifampicin (po)	CYP	Decrease in $AUC_{po}/AUC_{iv} = 4.4$	[96]
Nifedipine	Rifampicin (po)	CYP	Decrease in $AUC_{po}/AUC_{iv} = 8.5$	[97]
Talinolol	Rifampicin (po)	P-gp	Decrease in $AUC_{po}/AUC_{iv} = 1.7$	[98]
Tacrolimus	Rifampicin (po)	CYP	Decrease in $AUC_{po}/AUC_{iv} = 2.0$	[99]
Temsirolimus	Rifampicin (po)	CYP	Decrease in $AUC_{po}/AUC_{iv} = 1.3$	[100]
	Inhibition Studies			
Alfentanil	Grapefruit juice (po) Troleandomycin (po)	CYP	Increase in $AUC_{po}/AUC_{iv} = 1.5\text{–}2.6$	[93]
Atorvastatin	Itraconazole (iv)	CYP and P-gp	$AUC_{iv\ +INH}/AUC_{iv,control} = 1.3$ $AUC_{po\ +INH}/AUC_{po\ control} = 2.2$	[101]
Cyclosporine	Carvedilol (po) Grapefruit juice (po) Ketoconazole (po)	CYP	Increase of $AUC_{po}/AUC_{iv} = 1.5\text{–}2.8$	[66,102,103]
Felodipine	Grapefruit juice (po)	CYP	Increase of $AUC_{po}/AUC_{iv} = 1.9$	[104]
Losartan	Ticlopidine (po)	CYP	Increase of $AUC_{po}/AUC_{iv} = 1.2$	[105]
Midazolam	Clarithromycin (po) Diltiazem (po) Erythromycin (po) Fluconazole (po) Grapefruit juice (po) Itraconazole (po) Ketoconazole (po) Saquinavir (po) Voriconazole (po)	CYP	Increase of $AUC_{PO}/AUC_{IV} = 1.4\text{–}3.2$	[57,91,93,106–111]
Nifedipine	Grapefruit juice (po) licochalcone A (po)	CYP	Increase in $AUC_{po}/AUC_{iv} = 1.2\text{–}1.4$	[112,113]
Saquanvir	Grapefruit juice (po)	CYP	Increase in $AUC_{po}/AUC_{iv} = 1.7$	[114]
Simvastatin	Ketoconazole (po)	CYP	Increase in $AUC_{po}/AUC_{iv} = 5.0$	[90]
Tacrolimus	Ketoconazole (po)	CYP	Increase in $AUC_{po}/AUC_{iv} = 1.4$	[115]

Noh and Pang [18] recently explored the properties of the SFM and TM models with respect to inhibitors via simulations. Within the assigned, limited parameter space set forth for the drug example, the reduction in M1 formation is highest when both inhibitor (intestine inhibition constant, $K_i = 2\ \mu M$) and drug are both given orally, and least or almost unaltered at all when the drug is given intravenously (Figure 6A). Inhibition of metabolism is revealed by the higher drug AUC in the presence of the inhibitor. Often, changes in metabolite patterns are able to reveal inhibition of enzymes within the tissue. For TM, the same extent of M1 formation occurs for both intravenous and oral drug administration, and inhibition of M1 formation is the same after iv or po drug administration. For SFM, a greater extent of inhibition exists for the drug given orally and least when given intravenously. Liver metabolism is in turn affected upon inhibition of the intestinal metabolism, and an inverse relation to that for the intestine is found.

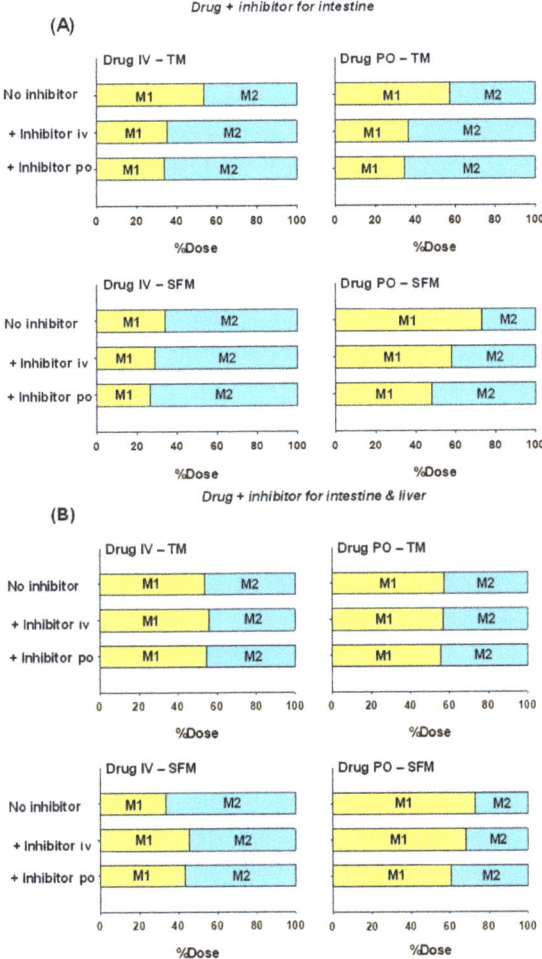

Figure 6. Simulation of intestinally (M1) and hepatically (M2) formed metabolites. For simulation, M1 and M2 were assumed to be inhibited within the intestine only (**A**), and both the intestine and liver (**B**) for a drug example ([18]; data in Table 6 of the reference). The simulation showed that the SFM predicted the highest and lowest M1 formation after oral and intravenous drug admintration, respectively, and the TM predicts a similar extent. The inhibition on intestinal metabolism is the greatest when both the inhibitor and drug are given orally, as predicted by the SFM (**A**). When both intestine and liver metabolism is inhibited, the pattern of change is not readily predictable (**B**). A greater liver inhibition exists after iv drug administration, and the extent of inhibition within the liver can exceed that in the intestine (**B**). This figure was reproduced with permission from data in Table 6 of Noh and Pang [18], Wiley, 2019.

The patterns of intestinal and liver metabolites formed upon inhibition of both the intestine and liver are less revealing as to which tissue is being inhibited, since the proportions of M1 to M2 formed do not always change in the same direction. When inhibition occurring for both the intestine and liver (same K_i = 2 µM for M1 and M2 formation), the fluctuations for M1 and M2 are small for the TM and SFM for oral drug administration when inhibition of the intestine is highest. Although inhibition is noted for the victim drug, the extent of M1 formation may even increase due to inhibition of liver metabolism to a greater extent for the drug given intravenously due to the higher input with Q_{HA}, with inhibition of the liver being more severe than for the intestine (Figure 6B). It is surmised that the extent of change here depends very much on the parameter space and susceptibility of the intestine versus the liver to the inhibitor and route of administration. But a higher AUC of the drug is strong evidence for the presence of the inhibitor on intestinal and liver metabolism.

6.3. Changes in Intestinal and Liver Metabolism with Respect to Flow to Intestine and Liver

Different flow rates to the enterocyte region in the intestine–liver unit would affect intestinal and liver drug processing differentially. An increase in Q_{PV} decreases the $E_{I,po}$ (increased $F_{I,po}$), allowing for more substrate flow to the liver for both the TM and SFM. With the greater substrate flux but faster transit in the liver, the rate of liver metabolism may remain the same although the increase in liver blood flow increases the CL_H [47,50]. The converse is also true, with a lower Q_{PV} or $Q_{SMA,}$ an increase in E_I and a lower flux to the liver will result.

6.4. Implications of the SFM on IVIVE

The IVIVE of transporter function is difficult to deduce when different transit times in GIT, gastric emptying rates, varying pH, and microenvironment exist [116]. The permeability, apical absorptive transporters, and split flow pattern of the intestine to the enterocyte and serosal regions, and efflux transporters complicate the IVIVE picture in the prediction of F_a and F_I. In terms of IVIVE, Kadono et al. [117] employed permeability measurements in artificial membranes to obtain F_a from the apparent permeability (P_{app}) with the parallel artificial membrane permeability assay (PAMPA) and obtain F_a and F_I from a scaling factor against a standard such as midazolam using the Yang equation [83]. In addition, IVIVE may be poor for the SFM due to the split flow behavior of the intestinal models, when there is incomplete accessibility of the substrate in circulation to reach enterocytes to fully recruit the intestinal metabolic activity, and this translates to poor IVIVE for the liver. Moreover, methods for identification of intestinal enzymatic activities vary. There are differences in the intestinal functional activity with the mucosal scraping and buffer isolation methods [70,118]. Paine et al. [70] found CYP3A content in each intestinal segment as 30.6, 22.6 and 16.6 pmol/mg mucosal microsomal protein, with similar K_m towards midazolam but varying V_{max} values. von Richter et al. [119] showed that the CYP3A4 in isolated enterocytes (76 pmol/mg homogenate protein corresponded to 210 pmol/mg microsomal protein) and was 3.2-fold higher than that in corresponding liver samples, whereas the P-gp content was 7.2-fold higher in enterocyte homogenate than in liver. The CYP3A4 content from the isolated cell method is higher than that from mucosal scraping. Moreover, intestinal metabolism may occur within cells that are shed into the gut lumen that possess copious metabolic activities in the lumen [118]. Nishimuta et al. [120] employed human intestinal and human microsomes to predict the CYP3A intrinsic metabolic clearance for human intestinal microsomes (HIM) versus human liver microsomes (HLM) ($CL_{int,HIM}$ and $CL_{int,HLM}$, corrected by the ratio of $CL_{int,HIM}$ to $CL_{int,HLM}$), and alamethicin-activated HIM for the clearance of UGT substrates. The CYP3A intestinal intrinsic clearance ($CL_{int,I,CYP3A}$) was highly correlated to hepatic intrinsic clearance ($CL_{int,L,CYP3A}$), being 2.2-fold higher in liver, although the correlation was poorer for UGTs. Ito and Houston [34] scaled up the $CL_{int,H}$ with an empirical scaling factor (SF) of 6.2 g protein/kg weight to compensate for the extent of underprediction for IVIVE in rats. Allometric scaling shows that in vitro microsomal data consistently underestimate $CL_{int,met,I}$ and $CL_{int,met,H}$. Hence, scaling and IVIVE remain somewhat empirical approaches.

7. Other Intestinal Models

Our laboratory has extended the SFM to the segmental, segregated flow model (SSFM) to accommodate transporter and enzyme heterogeneity [121]. However, we have oversimplified the segments as a 1/3 of the total volume, flow and permeability characteristics (Figure 7), even knowing that the surface area, permeability, and lengths of the segments of the digestive tract differed [27]. We found higher abundance P450 activity in the proximal region but higher localization of P-gp in the distal region; this pattern produced the lowest availability in drug absorption (Figure 8). This same trend was confirmed by Watanabe et al. [122] years later in a simulation study. The transporter distributions and functions along the intestinal segments reveal similar transporter and drug metabolizing enzyme distribution patterns along the small intestine for rodents and humans (Table 4). Therefore, the rat may be used to predict drug transport across the small intestine in humans. The same extrapolation, however, is not recommended for drug metabolizing enzymes due to the known species differences observed among animal species [123]. The TM- or SFM-PBPK models have been developed to encompass heterogeneity of transporters and enzymes for improved prediction of PK, including polymorphism and sex differences in enzymes, and tease out contributions of intestine and liver in first-pass metabolism (Table 4). Other factors on the physiology of the GIT may also be considered. It is known that the duodenum is the shortest segment and is approximately 1/5 and 1/7 the lengths of the jejunum and ileum, respectively [28]. As shown by the transport of substrates in segments using chamber or single-pass segmental perfusion, drug permeability, revealed with use of a deconvolution-permeability model, is higher in the jejunum [124,125]. Moreover, the pH and transit times in the duodenum, jejunum and ileum differed [28]. Dressman et al. [3] described, in the continuous absorption model, that the GIT is a continuous tube with varying spatial properties on permeability and solubility and pH, surface area, lengths, diameters, gastric emptying [4], highlighting the importance of gastric emptying time, small intestinal transit time, and effective surface area for absorption [5]. There are other models that accommodate variation in villi surface area, in drug permeability along the intestinal segment. Wu [126] applied the SSFM to examine enterohepatic circulation of glucuronides and found that the processes is affected by segmental distribution of enzymes. With accountability of segmental CYP and P-gp activities, reasonable absorption, efflux, and metabolism are observed for midazolam and compound S [25].

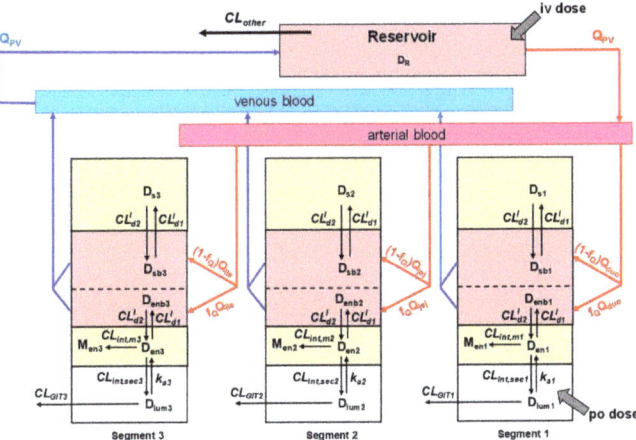

Figure 7. An expanded intestinal flow model—the segmental segregated flow PBPK model depicting the intestine as three different segmental regions with segregated flows to the enterocyte and serosal subcompartments. This figure was reproduced with permission from [121], ASPET, 2003.

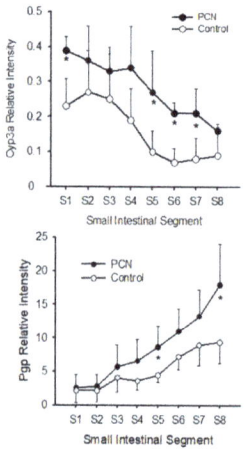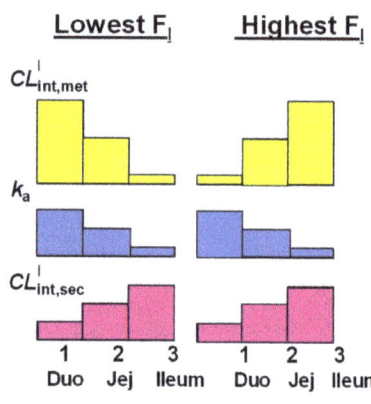

Figure 8. Heterogeneous distribution of Cyp3a and P-gp in the rat intestine, and changes accompanying the inducer, pregnenolone 16α-carbonitrile (PCN) on intestinal bioavailablity. Both P-gp and Cyp3a relative protein expressions were determined by Western blotting (see referecne 26). The scale on the y-axes of the left panel represents an arbitray scale. Segments 1, 2, 7, and 8 are the duodenal, proximal jejunal, distal jejunal and ileal segments, respectively. The symbols, duo and jej of the left panel denote the duodenum and jejunum, respectively. This figure was reproduced with permission from [26], ASPET, 2006.

Commercially available softwares on drug absorption include Simcyp® (advanced dissolution absorption metabolism (ADAM) model is implemented in Simcyp®), GastroPlus and GI-Sim [127], and GUT framework [128], which tackle the subject of drug absorption. Although the same input parameters may be used, the software show different F_a prediction characteristics depending on the rate-limiting steps of oral drug absorption [127]. The advanced compartmental absorption transit model or ACAT model [9], first conceived by Yu and Amidon [2] as the compartment absorption model [1], has evolved to include permeability (in silico properties derived from chemical structure), logP, pKa, particle size and dose. Dissolution that is based on the Nernst–Brunner modification of the Noyes–Whitney equation is implemented. The influx and efflux transporters [129], pH and pKa, and heterogeneous enzyme distribution are recognized as important processes of the software [2,10,11]. Other considerations include the microbiota and composition. It appears that most of these models deal with dosage form and drug properties and may not have considered the segregated flow behavior of the intestine. A suggestion is for these software developers to consider first finalizing their software based on the absorption of a drug solution while incorporating flow and enzyme/transporter heterogeneity, then combining this to another model with the drug and intestine properties (logP, pKa, particle size, pH, surface area) to consider drug absorption.

Table 4. Heterogeneous distribution of enzymes and transporters in animal and human intestine.

Transporter/Enzyme	Segmental Distribution	References
Animals		
Apical sodium-dependent bile acid transporter (Asbt)	highest at ileum duodenum < jejunum < ileum	[130,131]
Nucleoside transporters (Cnt)	highest in jejunum	[132]
Monocarboxylic acid transporter (Mct1)	duodenum < jejunum > ileum	[88]
Organic cation transporter 1 (Oct1)	duodenum < jejunum < ileum	[133]

Table 4. *Cont.*

Transporter/Enzyme	Segmental Distribution	References
Organic cation transporter 3 (Oct3)	duodenum < jejunum < ileum	[133]
Organic anion transporting polypeptide 3 (Oatp3)	highest in jejunum	[133]
Oligopeptide transporter 1 (PepT1)	duodenum > jejunum > ileum	[133]
Multidrug resistance-associated protein 2 (Mrp2)	duodenum > jejunum > ileum	[133]
Multidrug resistance-associated protein 3 (Mrp 3)	duodenum < jejunum < ileum	[133]
Multidrug resistance-associated protein 4 (Mrp 4)	duodenum > ileum > jejunum	[88]
P-glycoprotein (P-gp)	duodenum < jejunum < ileum	[26]
Organic solute transporter α-β (Ostα,β)	duodenum > jejunum > ileum	[21]
Cytochrome P450 3A (Cyp3a)	duodenum ~ jejunum > ileum	[134,135]
Estrone sulfatase	duodenum > jejunum > ileum	[136]
Glutathione S-Transferase (Gst)	duodenum > jejunum > ileum	[137]
UDP-Glucuronosyltransferase (Ugt)	duodenum ~ jejunum > ileum	[138]
Humans		
ASBT	duodenum < ileum	[139]
OATP2B1	duodenum < ileum	[140]
PEPT1	slightly increasing jejunum > ileum > duodenum duodenum ~ ileum	[19,139]
MCT1	slightly decreasing duodenum > ileum	[19]
CNT11 CNT2	even duo > ileum	[138]
OCT1	even	[19]
OCTN1	duodenum < ileum	[138]
OCTN2	even	[19,139]
MRP3	even	[19]
P-gp	ileum > jejunum > proximal	[19,25,28,140]
BCRP	even jejunum > ileum > duodenum	[19,55,141]
MRP2 mRNA MRP1 protein MRP2 protein	slightly decreasing proximal > distal even	[19,142]
MRP1 to 5 MRP2 to MRP6 MRP4	duodenum < jejunum and ileum	[141,143,144]
CYP3A4	proximal > distal	[25,28]
UGT1A1 UGT1A3 UGT1A4 UGT1A5 UGT1A6 UGT1A7 UGT1A8 UGT1A9 UGT1A10 UGT2B4 UGT2B7 UGT2B10 UGT2B15	duodenum ~ jejunum and ileum duodenum ~ jejunum and ileum duodenum ~ jejunum and ileum duodenum ~ jejunum and ileum duodenum > jejunum and ileum duodenum ~ jejunum and ileum duodenum ~ jejunum and ileum duodenum ~ jejunum and ileum duodenum and jejunum > ileum duodenum and jejunum < ileum duodenum and jejunum < ileum duodenum and jejunum < ileum duodenum < jejunum and ileum	[145]
SULT1A1, 1A3, 1B1, 1E1 SULT2A1	jejunum < ileum jejunum > ileum	[146]
GST GST	jejunum > ileum jejunum ~ ileum	[147]

8. Conclusions

This review has highlighted that metabolite formation and DDIs of the intestine are not well predicted by the traditional intestinal flow model (TM) with respect to the routes of administration of drug and inhibitor. Instead, we recognize the importance of the segregated flow model (SFM) as the premier model to examine intestinal drug metabolism. The evidence in the literature is compelling in support of the SFM based on route-dependent intestinal metabolism. The higher propensity of inhibition with oral and not intravenous dosing is indisputable. Implementation of the SFM is just an additional intestinal compartment away, and this PBPK segregated intestinal flow model (SFM) should be expanded to encompass heterogeneity of transporters and enzymes (SSFM) for improved prediction of PK, including polymorphism and sex differences in enzymes to tease out contributions of intestine and liver in first-pass metabolism. This type of metabolism model could now be coupled with an absorption model to fully investigate the different aspects of F_a, F_I and F_H. We encourage the use of the more "bottom–up" approach in PBPK modeling to provide mechanistic insight into intestinal metabolism/transport [148] by incorporating the SFM into the model. Another improvement could be made is when the Q_{SMA} is not assumed to equal Q_{PV}. The difference in flow (Q_{PV}-Q_{SMA}) is due to the venous returns from the coeliac and splenic arteries, and stomach and mesenteries. These venous returns would join that from the small intestine (Q_{SMA}) and the hepatic arterial flow to perfuse the liver [149,150].

Funding: This research received no external funding.

Acknowledgments: We thank Qi Joy Yang for discussion.

Conflicts of Interest: The authors declare no conflict of interest.

References

1. Yu, L.X.; Lipka, E.; Crison, J.R.; Amidon, G.L. Transport approaches to the biopharmaceutical design of oral drug delivery systems: Prediction of intestinal absorption. *Adv. Drug Deliv. Rev.* **1996**, *19*, 359–376. [CrossRef]
2. Yu, L.X.; Amidon, G.L. A compartmental absorption and transit model for estimating oral drug absorption. *Int. J. Pharm.* **1999**, *186*, 119–125. [CrossRef]
3. Dressman, J.B.; Thelen, K.; Jantratid, E. Towards quantitative prediction of oral drug absorption. *Clin. Pharmacokinet.* **2008**, *47*, 655–667. [CrossRef] [PubMed]
4. Willmann, S.; Schmitt, W.; Keldenich, J.; Dressman, J.B. A physiologic model for simulating gastrointestinal flow and drug absorption in rats. *Pharm. Res.* **2003**, *20*, 1766–1771. [CrossRef]
5. Willmann, S.; Edginton, A.N.; Dressman, J.B. Development and validation of a physiology-based model for the prediction of oral absorption in monkeys. *Pharm. Res.* **2007**, *24*, 1275–1282. [CrossRef]
6. Dahan, A.; West, B.T.; Amidon, G.L. Segmental-dependent membrane permeability along the intestine following oral drug administration: Evaluation of a triple single-pass intestinal perfusion (TSPIP) approach in the rat. *Eur. J. Pharm. Sci.* **2009**, *36*, 320–329. [CrossRef]
7. Dahan, A.; Amidon, G.L. Segmental dependent transport of low permeability compounds along the small intestine due to P-glycoprotein: The role of efflux transport in the oral absorption of bcs class iii drugs. *Mol. Pharm.* **2009**, *6*, 19–28. [CrossRef]
8. Dahan, A.; Miller, J.M.; Hilfinger, J.M.; Yamashita, S.; Yu, L.X.; Lennernäs, H.; Amidon, G.L. High-permeability criterion for BCS classification: Segmental/pH dependent permeability considerations. *Mol. Pharm.* **2010**, *7*, 1827–1834. [CrossRef]
9. Agoram, B.; Woltosz, W.S.; Bolger, M.B. Predicting the impact of physiological and biochemical processes on oral drug bioavailability. *Adv. Drug Deliv. Rev.* **2001**, *50* (Suppl. 1), S41–S67. [CrossRef]
10. Daga, P.R.; Bolger, M.B.; Haworth, I.S.; Clark, R.D.; Martin, E.J. Physiologically based pharmacokinetic modeling in lead optimization. 1. Evaluation and adaptation of GastroPlus to predict bioavailability of medchem series. *Mol. Pharm.* **2018**, *15*, 821–830. [CrossRef]
11. Hens, B.; Bolger, M.B. Application of a dynamic fluid and pH model to simulate intraluminal and systemic concentrations of a weak base in GastroPlus^{TM}. *J. Pharm. Sci.* **2019**, *108*, 305–315. [CrossRef]
12. Tsuji, A.; Tamai, I. Carrier-mediated intestinal transport of drugs. *Pharm. Res.* **1996**, *13*, 963–977. [CrossRef] [PubMed]
13. Adibi, S.A. The oligopeptide transporter (PEPT-1) in human intestine: Biology and function. *Gastroenterology* **1997**, *113*, 332–340. [CrossRef]

14. Zhang, L.; Brett, C.M.; Giacomini, K.M. Role of organic cation transporters in drug absorption and elimination. *Ann. Rev. Pharmacol. Toxicol.* **1998**, *38*, 431–460. [CrossRef]
15. Brandsch, M.; Knutter, I.; Leibach, F.H. The intestinal H+/peptide symporter PEPT1: Structure-affinity relationships. *Eur. J. Pharm. Sci.* **2004**, *21*, 53–60. [CrossRef]
16. Terada, T.; Inui, K. Peptide transporters: Structure, function, regulation and application for drug delivery. *Curr. Drug Metab.* **2004**, *5*, 85–94. [CrossRef] [PubMed]
17. Muller, J.; Keiser, M.; Drozdzik, M.; Oswald, S. Expression, regulation and function of intestinal drug transporters: An update. *Biol. Chem.* **2017**, *398*, 175–192. [CrossRef] [PubMed]
18. Noh, K.; Pang, K.S. Theoretical consideration of the properties of intestinal flow models on route-dependent drug removal: Segregated flow (SFM) vs. traditional (TM). *Biopharm. Drug Dispos.* **2019**, *40*, 195–213. [CrossRef] [PubMed]
19. Englund, G.; Rorsman, F.; Ronnblom, A.; Karlbom, U.; Lazorova, L.; Grasjo, J.; Kindmark, A.; Artursson, P. Regional levels of drug transporters along the human intestinal tract: Co-expression of ABC and SLC transporters and comparison with Caco-2 cells. *Eur. J. Pharm. Sci.* **2006**, *29*, 269–277. [CrossRef]
20. Greiner, B.; Eichelbaum, M.; Fritz, P.; Kreichgauer, H.P.; Von Richter, O.; Zundler, J.; Kroemer, H.K. The role of intestinal P-glycoprotein in the interaction of digoxin and rifampin. *J. Clin. Investig.* **1999**, *104*, 147–153. [CrossRef]
21. Dawson, P.A.; Hubbert, M.; Haywood, J.; Craddock, A.L.; Zerangue, N.; Christian, W.V.; Ballatori, N. The heteromeric organic solute transporter alpha-beta, Ostα-Ostβ, is an ileal basolateral bile acid transporter. *J. Biol. Chem.* **2005**, *280*, 6960–6968. [CrossRef] [PubMed]
22. Abbott, N.J.; Khan, E.U.; Rollinson, C.M.; Reichel, A.; Janigro, D.; Dombrowski, S.M.; Dobbie, M.S.; Begley, D.J. Drug resistance in epilepsy: The role of the blood-brain barrier. *Novartis Found. Symp.* **2002**, *243*, 38–47. [PubMed]
23. Fromm, M.F.; Kim, R.B.; Stein, C.M.; Wilkinson, G.R.; Roden, D.M. Inhibition of p-glycoprotein-mediated drug transport: A unifying mechanism to explain the interaction between digoxin and quinidine. *Circulation* **1999**, *99*, 552–557. [CrossRef] [PubMed]
24. Lin, J.H.; Chiba, M.; Chen, I.W.; Nishime, J.A.; DeLuna, F.A.; Yamazaki, M.; Lin, Y.J. Effect of dexamethasone on the intestinal first-pass metabolism of indinavir in rats: Evidence of cytochrome P-450 A and P-glycoprotein induction. *Drug Metab. Dispos.* **1999**, *27*, 1187–1193.
25. Bruyère, A.; Decleves, X.; Bouzom, F.; Ball, K.; Marques, C.; Treton, X.; Pocard, M.; Valleur, P.; Bouhnik, Y.; Panis, Y.; et al. Effect of variations in the amounts of P-glycoprotein (ABCB1), BCRP (ABCG2) and CYP3A4 along the human small intestine on PBPK models for predicting intestinal first pass. *Mol. Pharm.* **2010**, *7*, 1596–1607. [CrossRef]
26. Liu, S.; Tam, D.; Chen, X.; Pang, K.S. P-glycoprotein and an unstirred water layer barring digoxin absorption in the vascularly perfused rat small intestine preparation: Induction studies with pregnenolone-16alpha-carbonitrile. *Drug Metab. Dispos.* **2006**, *34*, 1468–1479. [CrossRef]
27. Helander, H.F.; Fandriks, L. Surface area of the digestive tract—Revisited. *Scand. J. Gastroenterol.* **2014**, *49*, 681–689. [CrossRef]
28. Badhan, R.; Penny, J.; Galetin, A.; Houston, J.B. Methodology for development of a physiological model incorporating CYP3A and P-glycoprotein for the prediction of intestinal drug absorption. *J. Pharm. Sci.* **2009**, *98*, 2180–2197. [CrossRef]
29. Fisher, M.B.; Paine, M.F.; Strelevitz, T.J.; Wrighton, S.A. The role of hepatic and extrahepatic UDP-glucuronosyltransferases in human drug metabolism. *Drug Metab. Rev.* **2001**, *33*, 273–297. [CrossRef]
30. Mizuma, T. Intestinal glucuronidation metabolism may have a greater impact on oral bioavailability than hepatic glucuronidation metabolism in humans: A study with raloxifene, substrate for UGT1A1, 1A8, 1A9, and 1A10. *Int. J. Pharm.* **2009**, *378*, 140–141. [CrossRef]
31. Paine, M.F.; Hart, H.L.; Ludington, S.S.; Haining, R.L.; Rettie, A.E.; Zeldin, D.C. The human intestinal cytochrome P-450 "pie". *Drug Metab. Dispos.* **2006**, *34*, 880–886. [CrossRef] [PubMed]
32. Radominska-Pandya, A.; Little, J.M.; Pandya, J.T.; Tephly, T.R.; King, C.D.; Barone, G.W.; Raufman, J.P. UDP-glucuronosyltransferases in human intestinal mucosa. *Biochim. Biophys. Acta* **1998**, *1394*, 199–208. [CrossRef]
33. Barter, Z.E.; Bayliss, M.K.; Beaune, P.H.; Boobis, A.R.; Carlile, D.J.; Edwards, R.J.; Houston, J.B.; Lake, B.G.; Lipscomb, J.C.; Pelkonen, O.R.; et al. Scaling factors for the extrapolation of in vivo metabolic drug clearance

from in vitro data: Reaching a consensus on values of human microsomal protein and hepatocellularity per gram of liver. *Curr. Drug Metab.* **2007**, *8*, 33–45. [CrossRef]

34. Ito, K.; Houston, J.B. Prediction of human drug clearance from in vitro and preclinical data using physiologically based and empirical approaches. *Pharm. Res.* **2005**, *22*, 103–112. [CrossRef]

35. Shin, H.C.; Kim, H.R.; Cho, H.J.; Yi, H.; Cho, S.M.; Lee, D.G.; Abd El-Aty, A.M.; Kim, J.S.; Sun, D.; Amidon, G.L. Comparative gene expression of intestinal metabolizing enzymes. *Biopharm. Drug Dispos.* **2009**, *30*, 411–421. [CrossRef] [PubMed]

36. Bullingham, R.E.; Nicholls, A.J.; Kamm, B.R. Clinical pharmacokinetics of mycophenolate mofetil. *Clin. Pharmacokinet.* **1998**, *34*, 429–455. [CrossRef]

37. Inoue, H.; Yuki, G.; Yokota, H.; Kato, S. Bisphenol a glucuronidation and absorption in rat intestine. *Drug Metab. Dispos.* **2003**, *31*, 140–144. [CrossRef]

38. Iwamoto, K.; Klaassen, C.D. First-pass effect of nalorphine in rats. *J. Pharmcol. Exp. Ther.* **1977**, *203*, 365–376.

39. Kosaka, K.; Sakai, N.; Endo, Y.; Fukuhara, Y.; Tsuda-Tsukimoto, M.; Ohtsuka, T.; Kino, I.; Tanimoto, T.; Takeba, N.; Takahashi, M.; et al. Impact of intestinal glucuronidation on the pharmacokinetics of raloxifene. *Drug Metab. Dispos.* **2011**, *39*, 1495–1502. [CrossRef]

40. Tukey, R.H.; Strassburg, C.P. Genetic multiplicity of the human UDP-glucuronosyltransferases and regulation in the gastrointestinal tract. *Mol. Pharmacol.* **2001**, *59*, 405–414. [CrossRef]

41. Kemp, D.C.; Fan, P.W.; Stevens, J.C. Characterization of raloxifene glucuronidation in vitro: Contribution of intestinal metabolism to presystemic clearance. *Drug Metab. Dispos.* **2002**, *30*, 694–700. [CrossRef] [PubMed]

42. Thummel, K.E.; O'Shea, D.; Paine, M.F.; Shen, D.D.; Kunze, K.L.; Perkins, J.D.; Wilkinson, G.R. Oral first-pass elimination of midazolam involves both gastrointestinal and hepatic CYP3A-mediated metabolism. *Clin. Pharmacol. Ther.* **1996**, *59*, 491–502. [CrossRef]

43. De Waziers, I.; Cugnenc, P.H.; Yang, C.S.; Leroux, J.P.; Beaune, P.H. Cytochrome P 450 isoenzymes, epoxide hydrolase and glutathione transferases in rat and human hepatic and extrahepatic tissues. *J. Pharmacol. Exp. Ther.* **1990**, *253*, 387–394. [PubMed]

44. Ozer, N.; Erdemli, O.; Sayek, I.; Ozer, I. Resolution and kinetic characterization of glutathione S-transferases from human jejunal mucosa. *Biochem. Med. Metab. Biol.* **1990**, *44*, 142–150. [CrossRef]

45. Maiti, S.; Chen, G. Ethanol up-regulates phenol sulfotransferase (Sult1a1) and hydroxysteroid sulfotransferase (Sult2a1) in rat liver and intestine. *Arch. Physiol. Biochem.* **2015**, *121*, 68–74. [CrossRef]

46. Gibaldi, M.; Boyes, R.N.; Feldman, S. Influence of first-pass effect on availability of drugs on oral administration. *J. Pharm. Sci.* **1971**, *60*, 1338–1340. [CrossRef]

47. Chen, J.; Pang, K.S. Effect of flow on first-pass metabolism of drugs: Single pass studies on 4-methylumbelliferone conjugation in the serially perfused rat intestine and liver preparations. *J. Pharmcol. Exp. Ther.* **1997**, *280*, 24–31.

48. Hirayama, H.; Pang, K.S. First-pass metabolism of gentisamide: Influence of intestinal metabolism on hepatic formation of conjugates. Studies in the once-through vascularly perfused rat intestine-liver preparation. *Drug Metab. Dispos.* **1990**, *18*, 580–587.

49. Pang, K.S.; Chow, E.C.Y. Commentary: Theoretical predictions of flow effects on intestinal and systemic availability in physiologically based pharmacokinetic intestine models: The traditional model, segregated flow model, and Q_{Gut} model. *Drug Metab. Dispos.* **2012**, *40*, 1869–1877. [CrossRef]

50. Pang, K.S.; Mulder, G.J. The effect of hepatic blood flow on formation of metabolites. *Drug Metab. Dispos.* **1990**, *18*, 270–275.

51. Pang, K.S.; Han, Y.R.; Noh, K.; Lee, P.I.; Rowland, M. Hepatic clearance concepts and misconceptions: Why the well-stirred model is still used even though it is not physiologic reality? *Biochem. Pharmacol.* **2019**, *169*, 113596. [CrossRef]

52. Pang, K.S.; Rowland, M. Hepatic clearance of drugs. I. Theoretical considerations of a "well-stirred" model and a "parallel tube" model. Influence of hepatic blood flow, plasma and blood cell binding, and the hepatocellular enzymatic activity on hepatic drug clearance. *J. Pharmacokinet. Biopharm.* **1977**, *5*, 625–653. [CrossRef]

53. Roberts, M.S.; Rowland, M. A dispersion model of hepatic elimination: 1. *Formulation of the model and bolus considerations J. Pharmacokinet. Biopharm.* **1986**, *14*, 227–260. [CrossRef] [PubMed]

54. Chapron, B.; Risler, L.; Phillips, B.; Collins, C.; Thummel, K.; Shen, D. Reversible, time-dependent inhibition of CYP3A-mediated metabolism of midazolam and tacrolimus by telaprevir in human liver microsomes. *J. Pharm. Pharm. Sci.* **2015**, *18*, 101–111. [CrossRef] [PubMed]
55. Guo, H.; Liu, C.; Li, J.; Zhang, M.; Hu, M.; Xu, P.; Liu, L.; Liu, X. A mechanistic physiologically based pharmacokinetic-enzyme turnover model involving both intestine and liver to predict CYP3A induction-mediated drug-drug interactions. *J. Pharm. Sci.* **2013**, *102*, 2819–2836. [CrossRef] [PubMed]
56. Shirasaka, Y.; Chang, S.Y.; Grubb, M.F.; Peng, C.C.; Thummel, K.E.; Isoherranen, N.; Rodrigues, A.D. Effect of CYP3A5 expression on the inhibition of CYP3A-catalyzed drug metabolism: Impact on modeling cyp3a-mediated drug-drug interactions. *Drug Metab. Dispos.* **2013**, *41*, 1566–1574. [CrossRef]
57. Tsunoda, S.M.; Velez, R.L.; Von Moltke, L.L.; Greenblatt, D.J. Differentiation of intestinal and hepatic cytochrome P450 3A activity with use of midazolam as an in vivo probe: Effect of ketoconazole. *Clin. Pharmacol. Ther.* **1999**, *66*, 461–471. [CrossRef]
58. Wang, J.S.; Wen, X.; Backman, J.T.; Taavitsainen, P.; Neuvonen, P.J.; Kivisto, K.T. Midazolam alpha-hydroxylation by human liver microsomes in vitro: Inhibition by calcium channel blockers, itraconazole and ketoconazole. *Pharmacol. Toxicol.* **1999**, *85*, 157–161. [CrossRef]
59. Paine, M.F.; Shen, D.D.; Kunze, K.L.; Perkins, J.D.; Marsh, C.L.; McVicar, J.P.; Barr, D.M.; Gillies, B.S.; Thummel, K.E. First-pass metabolism of midazolam by the human intestine. *Clin. Pharmacol. Ther.* **1996**, *60*, 14–24. [CrossRef]
60. Lown, K.S.; Thummel, K.E.; Benedict, P.E.; Shen, D.D.; Turgeon, D.K.; Berent, S.; Watkins, P.B. The erythromycin breath test predicts the clearance of midazolam. *Clin. Pharmacol. Ther.* **1995**, *57*, 16–24. [CrossRef]
61. Doherty, M.M.; Pang, K.S. Route-dependent metabolism of morphine in the vascularly perfused rat small intestine preparation. *Pharm. Res.* **2000**, *17*, 291–298. [CrossRef] [PubMed]
62. Pang, K.S.; Cherry, W.F.; Ulm, E.H. Disposition of enalapril in the perfused rat intestine-liver preparation: Absorption, metabolism and first-pass effect. *J. Pharmacol. Exp. Ther.* **1985**, *233*, 788–795. [PubMed]
63. Pang, K.S.; Yuen, V.; Fayz, S.; Te Koppele, J.M.; Mulder, G.J. Absorption and metabolism of acetaminophen by the in situ perfused rat small intestine preparation. *Drug Metab. Dispos.* **1986**, *14*, 102–111.
64. Wen, Y.; Remmel, R.P.; Zimmerman, C.L. First-pass disposition of (-)-6-aminocarbovir in rats. I. Prodrug activation may be limited by access to enzyme. *Drug Metab. Dispos.* **1999**, *27*, 113–121.
65. Sahali-Sahly, Y.; Balani, S.K.; Lin, J.H.; Baillie, T.A. In vitro studies on the metabolic activation of the furanopyridine l-754,394, a highly potent and selective mechanism-based inhibitor of cytochrome P450 3A4. *Chem. Res. Toxicol.* **1996**, *9*, 1007–1012. [CrossRef] [PubMed]
66. Ducharme, M.P.; Warbasse, L.H.; Edwards, D.J. Disposition of intravenous and oral cyclosporine after administration with grapefruit juice. *Clin. Pharmacol. Ther.* **1995**, *57*, 485–491. [CrossRef]
67. Darbar, D.; Fromm, M.F.; Dell'Orto, S.; Kim, R.B.; Kroemer, H.K.; Eichelbaum, M.; Roden, D.M. Modulation by dietary salt of verapamil disposition in humans. *Circulation* **1998**, *98*, 2702–2708. [CrossRef]
68. Talseth, T. Studies on hydralazine. III. Bioavailability of hydralazine in man. *Eur. J. Clin. Pharmacol.* **1976**, *10*, 395–401. [CrossRef] [PubMed]
69. Till, A.E.; Constanzer, M.L.; Demetriades, J.; Irvin, J.D.; Lee, R.B.; Ferguson, R.K. Evidence for route dependent biotransformation of cyclobenzaprine hydrochloride. *Biopharm. Drug Dispos.* **1982**, *3*, 19–28. [CrossRef]
70. Paine, M.F.; Khalighi, M.; Fisher, J.M.; Shen, D.D.; Kunze, K.L.; Marsh, C.L.; Perkins, J.D.; Thummel, K.E. Characterization of interintestinal and intraintestinal variations in human CYP3A-dependent metabolism. *J. Pharmacol. Exp. Ther.* **1997**, *283*, 1552–1562.
71. Kwan, K.C.; Foltz, E.L.; Breault, G.O.; Baer, J.E.; Totaro, J.A. Pharmacokinetics of methyldopa in man. *J. Pharmacol. Exp. Ther.* **1976**, *198*, 264–277. [PubMed]
72. Darbar, D.; Dell'Orto, S.; Morike, K.; Wilkinson, G.R.; Roden, D.M. Dietary salt increases first-pass elimination of oral quinidine. *Clin. Pharmacol. Ther.* **1997**, *61*, 292–300. [CrossRef]
73. Mano, Y.; Sugiyama, Y.; Ito, K. Use of a physiologically based pharmacokinetic model for quantitative prediction of drug-drug interactions via CYP3A4 and estimation of the intestinal availability of CYP3A4 substrates. *J. Pharm. Sci.* **2015**, *104*, 3183–3193. [CrossRef] [PubMed]
74. Marzolini, C.; Rajoli, R.; Battegay, M.; Elzi, L.; Back, D.; Siccardi, M. Physiologically based pharmacokinetic modeling to predict drug-drug interactions with efavirenz involving simultaneous inducing and inhibitory effects on cytochromes. *Clin. Pharmacokinet.* **2017**, *56*, 409–420. [CrossRef]

75. Quinney, S.K.; Galinsky, R.E.; Jiyamapa-Serna, V.A.; Chen, Y.; Hamman, M.A.; Hall, S.D.; Kimura, R.E. Hydroxyitraconazole, formed during intestinal first-pass metabolism of itraconazole, controls the time course of hepatic CYP3A inhibition and the bioavailability of itraconazole in rats. *Drug Metab. Dispos.* **2008**, *36*, 1097–1101. [CrossRef]
76. Yang, Q.J.; Fan, J.; Chen, S.; Liu, L.; Sun, H.; Pang, K.S. Metabolite kinetics: The segregated flow model for intestinal and whole body physiologically based pharmacokinetic modeling to describe intestinal and hepatic glucuronidation of morphine in rats in vivo. *Drug Metab. Dispos.* **2016**, *44*, 1123–1138. [CrossRef]
77. Noh, K.; Chen, S.; Yang, Q.J.; Pang, K.S. Physiologically based pharmacokinetic modeling revealed minimal codeine intestinal metabolism in first-pass removal in rats. *Biopharm. Drug Dispos.* **2017**, *38*, 50–74. [CrossRef]
78. Zhang, X.; Quinney, S.K.; Gorski, J.C.; Jones, D.R.; Hall, S.D. Semiphysiologically based pharmacokinetic models for the inhibition of midazolam clearance by diltiazem and its major metabolite. *Drug Metab. Dispos.* **2009**, *37*, 1587–1597. [CrossRef]
79. Klippert, P.J.M.; Noordhoek, J. Influence of administration route and blood sampling site on the area under the curve. Assessment of gut wall, liver, and lung metabolism from a physiological model. *Drug Metab. Dispos.* **1983**, *11*, 62–66.
80. Cong, D.; Doherty, M.; Pang, K.S. A new physiologically based, segregated-flow model to explain route-dependent intestinal metabolism. *Drug Metab. Dispos.* **2000**, *28*, 224–235.
81. Gertz, M.; Harrison, A.; Houston, J.B.; Galetin, A. Prediction of human intestinal first-pass metabolism of 25 CYP3A substrates from in vitro clearance and permeability data. *Drug Metab. Dispos.* **2010**, *38*, 1147–1158. [CrossRef] [PubMed]
82. Gertz, M.; Houston, J.B.; Galetin, A. Physiologically based pharmacokinetic modeling of intestinal first-pass metabolism of CYP3A substrates with high intestinal extraction. *Drug Metab. Dispos.* **2011**, *39*, 1633–1642. [CrossRef] [PubMed]
83. Yang, J.; Jamei, M.; Yeo, K.R.; Tucker, G.T.; Rostami-Hodjegan, A. Prediction of intestinal first-pass drug metabolism. *Curr. Drug Metab.* **2007**, *8*, 676–684. [CrossRef] [PubMed]
84. Sun, H.; Pang, K.S. Physiological modeling to understand the impact of enzymes and transporters on drug and metabolite data and bioavailability estimates. *Pharm. Res.* **2010**, *27*, 1237–1254. [CrossRef]
85. Svanvik, J. Mucosal blood circulation and its influence on passive absorption in the small intestine. An experimental study in the cat. *Acta Physiol. Scand. Suppl.* **1973**, *385*, 1–44.
86. Granger, D.N.; Richardson, P.D.; Kvietys, P.R.; Mortillaro, N.A. Intestinal blood flow. *Gastroenterology* **1980**, *78*, 837–863. [CrossRef]
87. Yang, Q.J.; Bukuroshi, P.; Quach, H.P.; Chow, E.C.Y.; Pang, K.S. Highlighting vitamin D receptor-targeted activities of 1α,25-dihydroxyvitamin D_3 in mice via physiologically based pharmacokinetic-pharmacodynamic modeling. *Drug Metab. Dispos.* **2018**, *46*, 75–87. [CrossRef]
88. Cong, D.; Fong, A.K.; Lee, R.; Pang, K.S. Absorption of benzoic acid in segmental regions of the vascularly perfused rat small intestine preparation. *Drug Metab. Dispos.* **2001**, *29*, 1539–1547.
89. Chow, E.C.; Durk, M.R.; Cummins, C.L.; Pang, K.S. 1α,25-Dihydroxyvitamin D_3 upregulates P-glycoprotein activities via the vitamin D receptor and not farnesoid X receptor in both *fxr(-/-)* and *fxr(+/+)* mice, and increased renal and brain efflux of digoxin in mice in vivo. *J. Pharmacol. Exp. Ther.* **2011**, *337*, 846–859. [CrossRef]
90. Ogasawara, A.; Utoh, M.; Nii, K.; Ueda, A.; Yoshikawa, T.; Kume, T.; Fukuzaki, K. Effect of oral ketoconazole on oral and intravenous pharmacokinetics of simvastatin and its acid in cynomolgus monkeys. *Drug Metab. Dispos.* **2009**, *37*, 122–128. [CrossRef]
91. Eeckhoudt, S.L.; Horsmans, Y.; Verbeeck, R.K. Differential induction of midazolam metabolism in the small intestine and liver by oral and intravenous dexamethasone pretreatment in rat. *Xenobiotica* **2002**, *32*, 975–984. [CrossRef]
92. Song, X.; Ju, Y.; Zhao, H.; Qiu, W. Effect of purple grape juice on the pharmacokinetics of digoxin: Results of a food-drug interaction study. *Int. J. Clin. Pharmacol. Ther.* **2019**, *57*, 101–109. [CrossRef] [PubMed]
93. Westphal, K.; Weinbrenner, A.; Zschiesche, M.; Franke, G.; Knoke, M.; Oertel, R.; Fritz, P.; Von Richter, O.; Warzok, R.; Hachenberg, T.; et al. Induction of P-glycoprotein by rifampin increases intestinal secretion of talinolol in human beings: A new type of drug/drug interaction. *Clin. Pharmacol. Ther.* **2000**, *68*, 345–355. [CrossRef] [PubMed]

94. Hebert, M.F.; Fisher, R.M.; Marsh, C.L.; Dressler, D.; Bekersky, I. Effects of rifampin on tacrolimus pharmacokinetics in healthy volunteers. *J. Clin. Pharmacol.* **1999**, *39*, 91–96. [CrossRef] [PubMed]
95. Boni, J.; Leister, C.; Burns, J.; Cincotta, M.; Hug, B.; Moore, L. Pharmacokinetic profile of temsirolimus with concomitant administration of cytochrome P450-inducing medications. *J. Clin. Pharmacol.* **2007**, *47*, 1430–1439. [CrossRef] [PubMed]
96. Dong, J.; Yu, X.; Wang, L.; Sun, Y.B.; Chen, X.J.; Wang, G.J. Effects of cyclosporin a and itraconazole on the pharmacokinetics of atorvastatin in rats. *Acta Pharmacol. Sin.* **2008**, *29*, 1247–1252. [CrossRef]
97. Amioka, K.; Kuzuya, T.; Kushihara, H.; Ejiri, M.; Nitta, A.; Nabeshima, T. Carvedilol increases ciclosporin bioavailability by inhibiting P-glycoprotein-mediated transport. *J. Pharm. Pharmacol.* **2007**, *59*, 1383–1387. [CrossRef]
98. Gomez, D.Y.; Wacher, V.J.; Tomlanovich, S.J.; Hebert, M.F.; Benet, L.Z. The effects of ketoconazole on the intestinal metabolism and bioavailability of cyclosporine. *Clin. Pharmacol. Ther.* **1995**, *58*, 15–19. [CrossRef]
99. Lundahl, J.; Regardh, C.G.; Edgar, B.; Johnsson, G. Effects of grapefruit juice ingestion—Pharmacokinetics and haemodynamics of intravenously and orally administered felodipine in healthy men. *Eur. J. Clin. Pharmacol.* **1997**, *52*, 139–145. [CrossRef]
100. Yang, S.H.; Cho, Y.A.; Choi, J.S. Effects of ticlopidine on pharmacokinetics of losartan and its main metabolite exp-3174 in rats. *Acta Pharmacol. Sin.* **2011**, *32*, 967–972. [CrossRef]
101. Gorski, J.C.; Jones, D.R.; Haehner-Daniels, B.D.; Hamman, M.A.; O'Mara, E.M., Jr.; Hall, S.D. The contribution of intestinal and hepatic CYP3A to the interaction between midazolam and clarithromycin. *Clin. Pharmacol. Ther.* **1998**, *64*, 133–143. [CrossRef]
102. Kupferschmidt, H.H.; Ha, H.R.; Ziegler, W.H.; Meier, P.J.; Krahenbuhl, S. Interaction between grapefruit juice and midazolam in humans. *Clin. Pharmacol. Ther.* **1995**, *58*, 20–28. [CrossRef]
103. Olkkola, K.T.; Ahonen, J.; Neuvonen, P.J. The effects of the systemic antimycotics, itraconazole and fluconazole, on the pharmacokinetics and pharmacodynamics of intravenous and oral midazolam. *Anesth. Anal.* **1996**, *82*, 511–516.
104. Olkkola, K.T.; Aranko, K.; Luurila, H.; Hiller, A.; Saarnivaara, L.; Himberg, J.J.; Neuvonen, P.J. A potentially hazardous interaction between erythromycin and midazolam. *Clin. Pharmacol. Ther.* **1993**, *53*, 298–305. [CrossRef] [PubMed]
105. Palkama, V.J.; Ahonen, J.; Neuvonen, P.J.; Olkkola, K.T. Effect of saquinavir on the pharmacokinetics and pharmacodynamics of oral and intravenous midazolam. *Clin. Pharmacol. Ther.* **1999**, *66*, 33–39. [CrossRef]
106. Saari, T.I.; Laine, K.; Leino, K.; Valtonen, M.; Neuvonen, P.J.; Olkkola, K.T. Effect of voriconazole on the pharmacokinetics and pharmacodynamics of intravenous and oral midazolam. *Clin. Pharmacol. Ther.* **2006**, *79*, 362–370. [CrossRef]
107. Choi, J.S.; Choi, J.S.; Choi, D.H. Effects of licochalcone a on the bioavailability and pharmacokinetics of nifedipine in rats: Possible role of intestinal CYP3A4 and P-gp inhibition by licochalcone a. *Biopharm. Drug Dispos.* **2014**, *35*, 382–390. [CrossRef]
108. Rashid, T.J.; Martin, U.; Clarke, H.; Waller, D.G.; Renwick, A.G.; George, C.F. Factors affecting the absolute bioavailability of nifedipine. *Br. J. Clin. Pharmacol.* **1995**, *40*, 51–58. [CrossRef]
109. Kupferschmidt, H.H.; Fattinger, K.E.; Ha, H.R.; Follath, F.; Krahenbuhl, S. Grapefruit juice enhances the bioavailability of the hiv protease inhibitor saquinavir in man. *Br. J. Clin. Pharmacol.* **1998**, *45*, 355–359. [CrossRef]
110. Floren, L.C.; Bekersky, I.; Benet, L.Z.; Mekki, Q.; Dressler, D.; Lee, J.W.; Roberts, J.P.; Hebert, M.F. Tacrolimus oral bioavailability doubles with coadministration of ketoconazole. *Clin. Pharmacol. Ther.* **1997**, *62*, 41–49. [CrossRef]
111. Harwood, M.D.; Neuhoff, S.; Carlson, G.L.; Warhurst, G.; Rostami-Hodjegan, A. Absolute abundance and function of intestinal drug transporters: A prerequisite for fully mechanistic in vitro-in vivo extrapolation of oral drug absorption. *Biopharm. Drug Dispos.* **2013**, *34*, 2–28. [CrossRef]
112. Kadono, K.; Akabane, T.; Tabata, K.; Gato, K.; Terashita, S.; Teramura, T. Quantitative prediction of intestinal metabolism in humans from a simplified intestinal availability model and empirical scaling factor. *Drug Metab. Dispos.* **2010**, *38*, 1230–1237. [CrossRef] [PubMed]

113. Glaeser, H.; Drescher, S.; Van der Kuip, H.; Behrens, C.; Geick, A.; Burk, O.; Dent, J.; Somogyi, A.; Von Richter, O.; Griese, E.U.; et al. Shed human enterocytes as a tool for the study of expression and function of intestinal drug-metabolizing enzymes and transporters. *Clin. Pharmacol. Ther.* **2002**, *71*, 131–140. [CrossRef] [PubMed]
114. Von Richter, O.; Burk, O.; Fromm, M.F.; Thon, K.P.; Eichelbaum, M.; Kivisto, K.T. Cytochrome P450 3A4 and P-glycoprotein expression in human small intestinal enterocytes and hepatocytes: A comparative analysis in paired tissue specimens. *Clin. Pharmacol. Ther.* **2004**, *75*, 172–183. [CrossRef] [PubMed]
115. Nishimuta, H.; Sato, K.; Yabuki, M.; Komuro, S. Prediction of the intestinal first-pass metabolism of CYP3A and UGT substrates in humans from in vitro data. *Drug Metab. Pharmacokinet.* **2011**, *26*, 592–601. [CrossRef]
116. Tam, D.; Tirona, R.G.; Pang, K.S. Segmental intestinal transporters and metabolic enzymes on intestinal drug absorption. *Drug Metab. Dispos.* **2003**, *31*, 373–383. [CrossRef]
117. Watanabe, T.; Maeda, K.; Nakai, C.; Sugiyama, Y. Investigation of the effect of the uneven distribution of CYP3A4 and P-glycoprotein in the intestine on the barrier function against xenobiotics: A simulation study. *J. Pharm. Sci.* **2013**, *102*, 3196–3204. [CrossRef]
118. Cao, X.; Gibbs, S.T.; Fang, L.; Miller, H.A.; Landowski, C.P.; Shin, H.C.; Lennernäs, H.; Zhong, Y.; Amidon, G.L.; Yu, L.X.; et al. Why is it challenging to predict intestinal drug absorption and oral bioavailability in human using rat model. *Pharm. Res.* **2006**, *23*, 1675–1686. [CrossRef]
119. Chen, X.; Chen, F.; Liu, S.; Glaeser, H.; Dawson, P.A.; Hofmann, A.F.; Kim, R.B.; Shneider, B.L.; Pang, K.S. Transactivation of rat apical sodium-dependent bile acid transporter and increased bile acid transport by $1\alpha,25$-dihydroxyvitamin D_3 via the vitamin d receptor. *Mol. Pharmacol.* **2006**, *69*, 1913–1923. [CrossRef]
120. Mottino, A.D.; Hoffman, T.; Dawson, P.A.; Luquita, M.G.; Monti, J.A.; Sanchez Pozzi, E.J.; Catania, V.A.; Cao, J.; Vore, M. Increased expression of ileal apical sodium-dependent bile acid transporter in postpartum rats. *Am. J. Physiol. Gastrointest. Liver Physiol.* **2002**, *282*, G41–G50. [CrossRef]
121. Ngo, L.Y.; Patil, S.D.; Unadkat, J.D. Ontogenic and longitudinal activity of Na(+)-nucleoside transporters in the human intestine. *Am. J. Physiol. Gastrointest. Liver Physiol.* **2001**, *280*, G475–G481. [CrossRef] [PubMed]
122. Chow, E.C.; Sun, H.; Khan, A.A.; Groothuis, G.M.; Pang, K.S. Effects of $1\alpha,25$-dihydroxyvitamin D_3 on transporters and enzymes of the rat intestine and kidney in vivo. *Biopharm. Drug Dispos.* **2010**, *31*, 91–108. [PubMed]
123. Liu, B.; Crewe, H.K.; Ozdemir, M.; Rowland Yeo, K.; Tucker, G.; Rostami-Hodjegan, A. The absorption kinetics of ketoconazole plays a major role in explaining the reported variability in the level of interaction with midazolam: Interplay between formulation and inhibition of gut wall and liver metabolism. *Biopharm. Drug Dispos.* **2017**, *38*, 260–270. [CrossRef] [PubMed]
124. Bolger, M.B.; Lukacova, V.; Woltosz, W.S. Simulations of the nonlinear dose dependence for substrates of influx and efflux transporters in the human intestine. *AAPS J.* **2009**, *11*, 353–363. [CrossRef] [PubMed]
125. Jones, H.M.; Chen, Y.; Gibson, C.; Heimbach, T.; Parrott, N.; Peters, S.A.; Snoeys, J.; Upreti, V.V.; Zheng, M.; Hall, S.D. Physiologically based pharmacokinetic modeling in drug discovery and development: A pharmaceutical industry perspective. *Clin. Pharmacol. Ther.* **2015**, *97*, 247–262. [CrossRef]
126. Jamei, M.; Bajot, F.; Neuhoff, S.; Barter, Z.; Yang, Z.; Rostami-Hodjegan, A.; Rowland-Yeo, K. A mechanistic framework for in vitro–in vivo extrapolation of liver membrane transporters: Ppion of drug–drug interaction between rosuvastatin and cyclosporine. *Clin. Pharmacokinet.* **2014**, *53*, 73–87. [CrossRef] [PubMed]
127. Bi, Y.; Deng, J.; Murry, D.J.; An, G. A whole-body physiologically based pharmacokinetic model of gefitinib in mice and scale-up to humans. *AAPS J.* **2015**, *18*. [CrossRef]
128. Kharasch, E.D.; Walker, A.; Hoffer, C.; Sheffels, P. Intravenous and oral alfentanil as in vivo probes for hepatic and first-pass cytochrome P450 3A activity: Noninvasive assessment by use of pupillary miosis. *Clin. Pharmacol. Ther.* **2004**, *76*, 452–466. [CrossRef] [PubMed]
129. Hebert, M.F.; Roberts, J.P.; Prueksaritanont, T.; Benet, L.Z. Bioavailability of cyclosporine with concomitant rifampin administration is markedly less than predicted by hepatic enzyme induction. *Clin. Pharmacol. Ther.* **1992**, *52*, 453–457. [CrossRef]
130. Mitschke, D.; Reichel, A.; Fricker, G.; Moenning, U. Characterization of cytochrome p450 protein expression along the entire length of the intestine of male and female rats. *Drug Metab. Dispos.* **2008**, *36*, 1039–1045. [CrossRef]
131. Huijghebaert, S.M.; Sim, S.M.; Back, D.J.; Eyssen, H.J. Distribution of estrone sulfatase activity in the intestine of germfree and conventional rats. *J. Steroid Biochem.* **1984**, *20*, 1175–1179. [CrossRef]

132. Pinkus, L.M.; Ketley, J.N.; Jakoby, W.B. The glutathione S-transferases as a possible detoxification system of rat intestinal epithelium. *Biochem. Pharmacol.* **1977**, *26*, 2359–2363. [CrossRef]
133. Koster, A.S.; Frankhuijzen-Sierevogel, A.C.; Noordhoek, J. Glucuronidation of morphine and six beta 2-sympathomimetics in isolated rat intestinal epithelial cells. *Drug Metab. Dispos.* **1985**, *13*, 232–238. [PubMed]
134. Meier, Y.; Eloranta, J.J.; Darimont, J.; Ismair, M.G.; Hiller, C.; Fried, M.; Kullak-Ublick, G.A.; Vavricka, S.R. Regional distribution of solute carrier mRNA expression along the human intestinal tract. *Drug Metab. Dispos.* **2007**, *35*, 590–594. [CrossRef]
135. Mouly, S.; Paine, M.F. P-glycoprotein increases from proximal to distal regions of human small intestine. *Pharm. Res.* **2003**, *20*, 1595–1599. [CrossRef]
136. Haslam, I.S.; Wright, J.A.; O'Reilly, D.A.; Sherlock, D.J.; Coleman, T.; Simmons, N.L. Intestinal ciprofloxacin efflux: The role of breast cancer resistance protein (ABCG2). *Drug Metab. Dispos.* **2011**, *39*, 2321–2328. [CrossRef]
137. Berggren, S.; Gall, C.; Wollnitz, N.; Ekelund, M.; Karlbom, U.; Hoogstraate, J.; Schrenk, D.; Lennernäs, H. Gene and protein expression of P-glycoprotein, MRP1, MRP2, and CYP3A4 in the small and large human intestine. *Mol. Pharm.* **2007**, *4*, 252–257. [CrossRef]
138. Prime-Chapman, H.M.; Fearn, R.A.; Cooper, A.E.; Moore, V.; Hirst, B.H. Differential multidrug resistance-associated protein 1 through 6 isoform expression and function in human intestinal epithelial Caco-2 cells. *J. Pharmacol. Exp. Ther.* **2004**, *311*, 476–484. [CrossRef]
139. Zimmermann, C.; Gutmann, H.; Hruz, P.; Gutzwiller, J.P.; Beglinger, C.; Drewe, J. Mapping of multidrug resistance gene 1 and multidrug resistance-associated protein isoform 1 to 5 mRNA expression along the human intestinal tract. *Drug Metab. Dispos.* **2005**, *33*, 219–224. [CrossRef]
140. Strassburg, C.P.; Kneip, S.; Topp, J.; Obermayer-Straub, P.; Barut, A.; Tukey, R.H.; Manns, M.P. Polymorphic gene regulation and interindividual variation of UDP-glucuronosyltransferase activity in human small intestine. *J. Biol. Chem.* **2000**, *275*, 36164–36171. [CrossRef] [PubMed]
141. Teubner, W.; Meinl, W.; Florian, S.; Kretzschmar, M.; Glatt, H. Identification and localization of soluble sulfotransferases in the human gastrointestinal tract. *Biochem. J.* **2007**, *404*, 207–215. [CrossRef] [PubMed]
142. Khuruna, S.; Corbally, M.T.; Manning, F.; Armenise, T.; Kierce, B.; Kitty, C. Glutathione S-transferase: A potential new marker of intestinal ischemia. *J. Pediatr. Surg.* **2002**, *37*, 1543–1548. [CrossRef] [PubMed]
143. Dahlgren, D.; Lennernäs, H. Intestinal permeability and drug absorption: Predictive experimental, computational and in vivo approaches. *Pharmaceutics* **2019**, *11*, 411. [CrossRef] [PubMed]
144. Dahlgren, D.; Roos, C.; Lundqvist, A.; Abrahamsson, B.; Tannergren, C.; Hellstrom, P.M.; Sjögren, E.; Lennernäs, H. Regional intestinal permeability of three model drugs in human. *Mol. Pharm.* **2016**, *13*, 3013–3021. [CrossRef] [PubMed]
145. Wu, B. Use of physiologically based pharmacokinetic models to evaluate the impact of intestinal glucuronide hydrolysis on the pharmacokinetics of aglycone. *J. Pharm. Sci.* **2012**, *101*, 1281–1301. [CrossRef] [PubMed]
146. Sjögren, E.; Thorn, H.; Tannergren, C. In silico modeling of gastrointestinal drug absorption: Predictive performance of three physiologically based absorption models. *Mol. Pharm.* **2016**, *13*, 1763–1778. [CrossRef]
147. Matsumura, N.; Hayashi, S.; Akiyama, Y.; Ono, A.; Funaki, S.; Tamura, N.; Kimoto, T.; Jiko, M.; Haruna, Y.; Sarashina, A.; et al. Prediction characteristics of oral absorption simulation software evaluated using structurally diverse low-solubility drugs. *J. Pharm. Sci.* **2019**, *109*, 1403–1416. [CrossRef]
148. Kharasch, E.D.; Hoffer, C.; Whittington, D.; Sheffels, P. Role of hepatic and intestinal cytochrome P450 3A and 2B6 in the metabolism, disposition, and miotic effects of methadone. *Clin. Pharmacol. Ther.* **2004**, *76*, 250–269. [CrossRef]
149. Gorski, J.C.; Vannaprasaht, S.; Hamman, M.A.; Ambrosius, W.T.; Bruce, M.A.; Haehner-Daniels, B.; Hall, S.D. The effect of age, sex, and rifampin administration on intestinal and hepatic cytochrome P450 3A activity. *Clin. Pharmacol. Ther.* **2003**, *74*, 275–287. [CrossRef]
150. Holtbecker, N.; Fromm, M.F.; Kroemer, H.K.; Ohnhaus, E.E.; Heidemann, H. The nifedipine-rifampin interaction. Evidence for induction of gut wall metabolism. *Drug Metab. Dispos.* **1996**, *24*, 1121–1123.

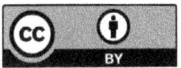

© 2020 by the authors. Licensee MDPI, Basel, Switzerland. This article is an open access article distributed under the terms and conditions of the Creative Commons Attribution (CC BY) license (http://creativecommons.org/licenses/by/4.0/).

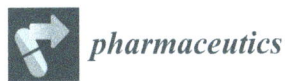

Review

Enteroendocrine Hormone Secretion and Metabolic Control: Importance of the Region of the Gut Stimulation

Cong Xie [1], Karen L. Jones [1,2], Christopher K. Rayner [1,3] and Tongzhi Wu [1,2,4,*]

1. Adelaide Medical School and Centre of Research Excellence (CRE) in Translating Nutritional Science to Good Health, The University of Adelaide, Adelaide 5005, Australia; c.xie@adelaide.edu.au (C.X.); karen.jones@adelaide.edu.au (K.L.J.); chris.rayner@adelaide.edu.au (C.K.R.)
2. Endocrine and Metabolic Unit, Royal Adelaide Hospital, Adelaide 5005, Australia
3. Department of Gastroenterology and Hepatology, Royal Adelaide Hospital, Adelaide 5005, Australia
4. Institute of Diabetes, School of Medicine, Southeast University, Nanjing 210009, China
* Correspondence: tongzhi.wu@adelaide.edu.au

Received: 31 July 2020; Accepted: 19 August 2020; Published: 21 August 2020

Abstract: It is now widely appreciated that gastrointestinal function is central to the regulation of metabolic homeostasis. Following meal ingestion, the delivery of nutrients from the stomach into the small intestine (i.e., gastric emptying) is tightly controlled to optimise their subsequent digestion and absorption. The complex interaction of intraluminal nutrients (and other bioactive compounds, such as bile acids) with the small and large intestine induces the release of an array of gastrointestinal hormones from specialised enteroendocrine cells (EECs) distributed in various regions of the gut, which in turn to regulate gastric emptying, appetite and postprandial glucose metabolism. Stimulation of gastrointestinal hormone secretion, therefore, represents a promising strategy for the management of metabolic disorders, particularly obesity and type 2 diabetes mellitus (T2DM). That EECs are distributed distinctively between the proximal and distal gut suggests that the region of the gut exposed to intraluminal stimuli is of major relevance to the secretion profile of gastrointestinal hormones and associated metabolic responses. This review discusses the process of intestinal digestion and absorption and their impacts on the release of gastrointestinal hormones and the regulation of postprandial metabolism, with an emphasis on the differences between the proximal and distal gut, and implications for the management of obesity and T2DM.

Keywords: nutrient digestion; nutrient absorption; gastrointestinal hormone; postprandial glycaemia; energy intake; region of the gut; obesity; type 2 diabetes

1. Introduction

As the key interface between ingested nutrients and the body, the gastrointestinal tract is now recognised to play a central role in regulating postprandial metabolism. During the fasting state, ghrelin is released from the gastric Gr-cells to drive food intake [1]. After meal ingestion, the stomach accommodates the nutrients, grinds digestible solids into small particles, and releases the resultant chyme into the small intestine in a regulated fashion to optimise intestinal digestion and absorption. It is now widely appreciated that distinctive enteroendocrine cells (EECs) scattered along the gastrointestinal tract, comprising up to 1% of the gut epithelium, constitute the largest endocrine organ in the body, accounting for the release of an array of peptides that orchestrate appetite, energy intake and the blood glucose responses to meals [2]. Of particular importance are cholecystokinin (CCK) and glucose-dependent insulinotropic polypeptide (GIP) released from the upper small intestine, and glucagon-like peptide-1 (GLP-1) and peptide YY (PYY) secreted mainly from the distal gut. These integrated hormonal responses convey important regulatory signals governing subsequent gastric emptying, insulin and glucagon secretion from the pancreas, energy intake, and postprandial glycaemic control. Stimulation of gastrointestinal postprandial hormone secretion, therefore, represents an attractive strategy for the management of metabolic disorders, such as obesity and type 2 diabetes mellitus (T2DM) [2]. Given that the distribution of the respective types of EECs varies substantially along the gastrointestinal tract, the region of the gut exposed to intraluminal stimuli is likely to be of major relevance to the secretion profile of gastrointestinal hormones and associated metabolic responses. This review discusses nutrient digestion and absorption along the gastrointestinal tract and how these processes influence the secretion of GIP, CCK, GLP-1 and PYY, and highlights the importance of which region of the gut is stimulated to the secretory profiles of these gastrointestinal hormones, the regulation of postprandial metabolism, and the implications for the management of obesity and T2DM. Other hormones, such as ghrelin and leptin, are also important metabolic regulators, but are not specifically discussed as they are outside the scope of this review.

2. Nutrient Transport, Digestion, and Absorption

Following meal ingestion, the stomach stores the ingested content and grinds digestible solids into small particles prior to delivering them into the small intestine. The latter occurs at a relatively constant caloric rate (in the range of 1–4 kcal/min in healthy individuals), driven by antral and duodenal contractions against tonic and phasic pyloric pressures [3], to optimise the subsequent digestion and absorption of nutrients in the small intestine. Due to the inactivation of salivary amylase in the gastric environment, there is limited digestion of carbohydrate in the stomach, whereas fat and protein are digested into lipid emulsions [4] and oligopeptides [5], respectively. Upon entering the duodenum, nutrients stimulate the release of a range of digestive enzymes from the exocrine pancreas and bile acids from the gallbladder, influenced by both the load and composition of the meal. Starch is broken down by pancreatic α-amylase and disaccharidases into glucose and other monosaccharides (e.g., fructose and galactose) [6]. Dietary fat (90–95% in the form of triglycerides) is digested by pancreatic lipase, a process relying largely on emulsification by bile acids, to form monoacylglycerol, glycerol and free fatty acids [4]. Digestion of protein involves both pancreatic enzymes, including chymotrypsin and trypsin, and aminopeptidases secreted by the small intestine mucosa, and yields individual amino acids, dipeptides and tripeptides [5].

The digestive products are transported by peristalsis and absorbed by passive diffusion and/or active transport via distinctive transporters at specific regions of the gut. For example, absorption of glucose involves both active transport from the lumen into the enterocytes via sodium-glucose cotransporter 1 (SGLT-1) and facilitated diffusion across the basolateral side of enterocytes through the glucose transporter 2 (GLUT2), taking place predominantly in the upper small intestine [7–10]. Unlike glucose, fructose is absorbed mainly through GLUT5 [11], which is well expressed in both the human jejunum and ileum [12]. Dietary fat typically binds to bile acids to form mixed micelles, which are absorbed by fatty acid transport proteins (FATPs) (e.g., FATP4 and FAT/CD36) and Niemann-Pick C1 like-1 (NPC1L1) [13,14]. Although a small fraction of bile acids are absorbed passively in the jejunum, the majority of them (~90%) are actively absorbed in the ileum through the apical sodium-dependent bile acid transporter (ASBT) [15]. The uptake of amino acids depends on a variety of "amino acid transport systems" that preferentially transport amino acids of similar biophysical properties [16,17], whereas dipeptides and tripeptides are absorbed via the proton-dependent intestinal peptide transporter 1 (PEPT1) [18]. The large intestine hosts a diversity of gut bacteria, which are involved in the fermentation of products that escape digestion/absorption in the small intestine, such as dietary fibre, resistant starches and proteins, leading to the production of short-chain fatty acids (SCFAs) which can be absorbed through facilitated diffusion [19–21].

3. Secretion and Actions of Gastrointestinal Hormones

While intestinal EECs maintain a low secretory profile during fasting, the interaction between intraluminal contents and EECs during the digestive process represents the main driver of the secretion of gastrointestinal hormones. The latter, including GLP-1, GIP, CCK and PYY released from distinctive EECs in various regions of the gastrointestinal tract (Figure 1), are now recognised as key regulators of energy intake and postprandial glucose metabolism (Figure 2).

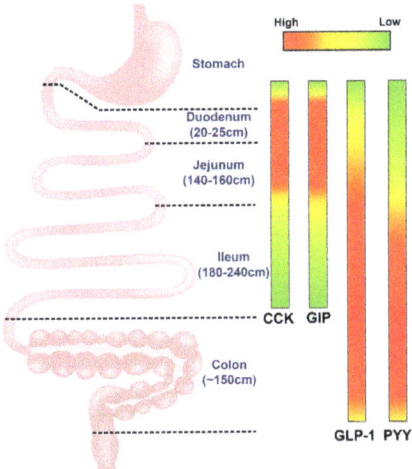

Figure 1. The density of enteroendocrine cells (EECs) secreting cholecystokinin (CCK), glucose-dependent insulinotropic polypeptide (GIP), glucagon-like peptide 1 (GLP-1) and peptide YY (PYY) in the duodenum, jejunum, ileum and colon.

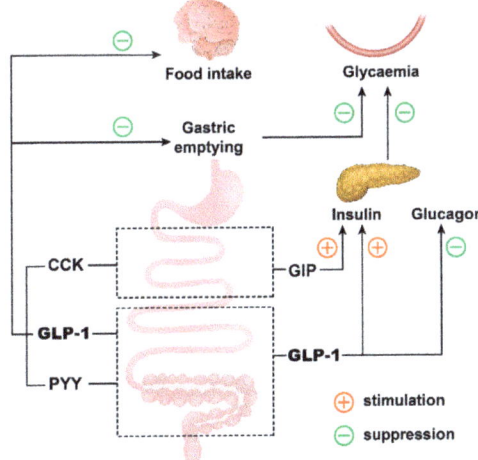

Figure 2. The roles of gastrointestinal hormones, including cholecystokinin (CCK), glucose-dependent insulinotropic polypeptide (GIP), glucagon-like peptide 1 (GLP-1) and peptide YY (PYY), released in response to meal ingestion, in the regulation of gastric emptying, postprandial glycemia and energy intake.

EECs are equipped with a variety of chemo-sensors linking the sensing of intraluminal stimuli to the secretion of gastrointestinal hormones. For example, carbohydrates can be detected by both their sweet taste through sweet taste receptors (STRs) [22–24], and via the glucose transporters, SGLT-1 and GLUT2 [25,26], although stimulation of STRs by artificial sweeteners alone does not seem to be sufficient to induce GLP-1 or GIP secretion in humans [23,27]. EEC sensing of intraluminal fat is dependent on the degree of its digestion [28–30] and involves a number of G protein-coupled receptors (GPRs), such as GPR40, GPR119 and GPR120 [31–33], and intestinal fat transporters FATP4 and FAT/CD36 [34,35]. Amino acids are detected by the calcium-sensing receptors (CasR) [25,36] and amino acid transporters [37,38]. Non-nutritive compounds are also effectively sensed by EECs. In particular, bile acids are known to induce GLP-1 and PYY secretion via inhibition of nuclear farnesoid X receptor (FXR) [39] and/or stimulation of Takeda G-protein coupled receptor 5 (TGR-5) [40,41]. Of note, TGR5 is expressed on the basolateral membrane of EECs [42], such that intestinal bile acid absorption is necessary to achieve TGR5 activation [41,42]. There is recent evidence that a group of specialized GPRs responsible for the sensing of bitter taste (i.e., bitter taste receptors; BTRs) are also abundantly expressed on EECs. Activation of BTRs on EECs by a variety of natural or chemosynthetic bitter taste compounds, therefore, has the potential to trigger the secretion of gastrointestinal hormones [43].

3.1. Glucagon-Like Peptide-1 (GLP-1)

GLP-1 is secreted from the enteroendocrine L-cells located mainly in the ileum and colon in response to each of the macronutrients, although fat, relative to glucose and protein, is generally more potent at stimulating GLP-1 secretion when administered into the duodenum in humans [44,45]. However, in patients who have undergone Roux-en-Y gastric bypass, oral ingestion of glucose was shown to be more effective than fat or protein to stimulate GLP-1 secretion [46]. The discrepancy observed in the latter is likely to be attributable to the influence of gastric emptying and digestion of fat or protein. Other bioactive compounds released into the lumen following meal ingestion, such as bile acids, are also responsible for postprandial GLP-1 secretion [41,47]. After its secretion, GLP-1 is rapidly inactivated by the enzyme dipeptidyl peptidase IV (DPP-4) with a half-life of 1–2 min, such that only 10–15% intact GLP-1 reaches the peripheral circulation [48,49]. While obesity is associated with attenuated GLP-1 secretion, accumulating evidence suggests that the latter is otherwise unaltered in patients with T2DM [50,51]. Importantly, the action of GLP-1 is also relatively well preserved in T2DM [51].

GLP-1 binds to its receptor, expressed in a variety of metabolic tissues, to regulate glucose, lipid and energy metabolism. Within the pancreas, GLP-1 stimulates insulin secretion from the pancreatic β-cells and suppresses glucagon secretion from the α-cells in a glucose-dependent manner [52]. For this reason, GLP-1-based glucose-lowering therapies, in general, entail a low risk of hypoglycaemia. Although there is preclinical evidence that GLP-1 receptor signalling is involved in β-cell survival and regeneration [53], such effects have not been established in humans. Within the liver, GLP-1-signalling is linked to the control of endogenous glucose production, an effect that can be independent of changes in insulin or glucagon [54]. Moreover, GLP-1 slows gastric emptying in both healthy individuals and those with T2DM [55–58]. That the reduction in postprandial glycaemia induced by exogenous GLP-1 is associated with less, rather than more, postprandial insulin secretion suggests that the slowing of gastric emptying outweighs its insulinotropic effect in controlling postprandial glycaemia [59]. In contrast to the GLP-1 receptor agonists, the DPP-4 inhibitors—which prolong the half-life of endogenous GLP-1—have little, if any, effect on gastric emptying [60,61].

Effects of GLP-1 signalling on lipid metabolism have been noted in both preclinical and clinical studies. GLP-1 has been shown to inhibit the production of lipid proteins (e.g., apolipoprotein B-48 (apob-48)) that are involved in the synthesis and transport of chylomicrons in the enterocytes, thereby improving lipid metabolism in rodents [62,63]. Similarly, the GLP-1 receptor agonist, exenatide, and the DPP-4 inhibitor, sitagliptin, have been shown to reduce plasma apob-48 concentrations in humans [64,65], while in obesity, treatment with GLP-1 receptor agonists improves dyslipidaemia [66].

GLP-1 also has the capacity to regulate energy intake and expenditure. Both exogenous GLP-1 and the GLP-1 receptor agonists suppress energy intake [50,67], and this effect has been shown to be mediated primarily via vagal afferents [68,69] and the activation of GLP-1 receptors in the central nervous system [70,71]. GLP-1 receptor agonists are therefore often associated with weight loss in both obesity and T2DM [48,72]. The role of GLP-1 in the regulation of energy expenditure is controversial. In mice, GLP-1 receptor agonists have been reported to induce browning of white adipose tissue and increase β-oxidation of fatty acids [73–75], and administration of both GLP-1 receptor agonists and DPP-4 inhibitors increases energy expenditure and reduces body weight [75–78]. However, a recent meta-analysis suggests that GLP-1 receptor agonists have little, if any, effect on energy expenditure in humans [79]. Although inhibition of DPP-4 by vildagliptin was found to augment the energy expenditure response to an intraduodenal fat infusion in healthy humans [80], this effect was not evident in patients with T2DM [81]. That antagonism of GLP-1 signalling by exendin (9–39) increased energy expenditure in the latter group during treatment with vildagliptin suggests that endogenous GLP-1 signalling may rather be associated with suppression of energy expenditure [81].

3.2. Glucose-Dependent Insulinotropic Polypeptide (GIP)

GIP is released from the enteroendocrine K-cells, distributed predominantly in the upper small intestine [51]. GIP is also co-expressed with GLP-1 in a subset of "K/L-cells" in the duodenum and proximal jejunum [82,83]. Similar to GLP-1, GIP is released in response to macronutrients—with fat being a more potent stimulus than glucose or protein [44]—and rapidly inactivated by DPP-4 after secretion [51,84]. However, the secretion of GIP does not seem to be affected by T2DM or obesity [50].

In health, GIP stimulates insulin secretion in a glucose-dependent manner by binding to the GIP receptor expressed on the pancreatic β-cells [85], which contributes equally with GLP-1 to the augmented insulin response that is observed during enteral glucose administration when compared to an "isoglycaemic" intravenous glucose infusion, i.e., the so-called the "incretin effect". However, the insulinotropic effect of GIP is markedly diminished in patients with T2DM [49,86]. Unlike GLP-1, GIP stimulates glucagon secretion from the pancreatic α-cells, particularly in the face of hypoglycaemia [87], and has little effect on appetite [88] or gastrointestinal motility [89]. Moreover, GIP exhibits numerous extra-glycaemic actions; blockade of GIP signalling in mice preferentially increases fat oxidation [90–92], reduces fat accumulation in adipocytes [90,92,93] and skeletal muscle [91,92], decreases triglyceride deposition in the liver [90,93], and prevents the development of obesity [90,91,94] in the context of overfeeding. In line with these findings, the antagonism of the GIP receptor is associated with reduced blood flow and triglyceride deposition in adipose tissue in healthy subjects [95]. Although compounds that display dual GIP and GLP-1 receptor agonism appear to be more effective for weight loss and glycaemic control than the GLP-1 receptor agonists, liraglutide and dulaglutide, in patients with T2DM [96,97], the relative contribution of GIP signalling to this superiority remains to be characterized in humans. Counterintuitively, acute administration of exogenous GIP failed to show any effect on energy intake or expenditure, but rather, augmented postprandial glycaemia in patients with T2DM receiving long-acting GLP-1 receptor agonists [98]. The mechanism underlying this phenomenon is unclear, but may be related to the stimulation of glucagon by intravenous GIP administration [86,98].

3.3. Cholecystokinin (CCK)

CCK is secreted from the enteroendocrine I-cells located in the duodenum and upper jejunum [1]. In mice, there is also evidence that a subset of EECs co-express CCK, GIP, GLP-1 and PYY in the proximal small intestine [83,99]. However, this is unlikely to be the case in humans, since exposure to glucose in the proximal 60 cm segment of the small intestine, while inducing substantial GIP and CCK secretion, does not affect GLP-1 secretion [100]. CCK is secreted within 10–15 min in response to oral ingestion of macronutrients (fat > protein > carbohydrate) [1]. This is critical for subsequent digestion since CCK stimulates the release of digestive enzymes and bile from the pancreas and the gallbladder, respectively.

Exogenous CCK is reported to attenuate the postprandial glycaemic excursion in humans. This effect is secondary to the slowing of gastric emptying, rather than a direct effect on glucose metabolism; intravenous administration of CCK at physiological doses diminishes the glycaemic response to an oral, but not an intraduodenal, glucose load in healthy males [101]. Similarly, in patients with well-controlled T2DM, the administration of CCK at a physiological dose (0.4 pmol/kg/min) was shown to slow gastric emptying and reduce postprandial blood glucose excursions [102]. However, for those with longstanding T2DM, both the secretion and action of CCK appear to be impaired, due probably to the development of autonomic neuropathy [3,103]. In addition to its effects on upper gastrointestinal motor function, CCK has an established role in the regulation of appetite through both vagal and endocrine pathways. In rats, the effect of exogenous CCK to suppress food intake was abolished by small-molecule CCK antagonists or after vagotomy [104]. Similarly, intravenous infusion of CCK at both physiological (0.6–0.8 pmol/kg/min) and supraphysiological doses (1.8 and 2.6 pmol/kg/min) suppresses hunger and energy intake in healthy subjects [105–107], effects abolished in the presence of a CCK antagonist [108]. In a population-based study, genetic polymorphisms of the CCK receptor, e.g., increased CCK_H3 haplotype frequency, may be responsible for over-eating in obesity [109]. However, acute administration of exogenous CCK showed a comparable effect on suppressing appetite in non-diabetic obese and lean subjects [110].

3.4. Peptide YY (PYY)

PYY is a 36-amino-acid peptide co-released with GLP-1 from L-cells [111]. Like other gastrointestinal hormones, postprandial secretion of PYY is dependent on the composition and load of macronutrients [112–115]. In contrast to GLP-1 and GIP, enzymatic conversion of PYY1-36 to PYY3-36 by DPP-4 is necessary for the systemic effects of PYY, namely suppression of appetite and slowing of gastric emptying [1].

PYY participates in the regulation of appetite and energy intake. PYY-null mice exhibit increased daily food intake and weight gain when compared with wild type mice, and this phenotype is reversed with PYY3-36 administration [115]. PYY binds to Neuropeptide Y receptor Y2 (NPY2R), which is highly expressed in the hypothalamic arcuate nucleus [116]. That the effect of PYY on energy intake is abolished in NPY2R knockout mice and by the selective NPY2R antagonist BIIE0246, suggests a key role of NPY2R signalling in mediating the effect of PYY to suppress energy intake [117,118]. In healthy humans, postprandial PYY levels are positively correlated with changes in satiety scores [119,120], and intravenous PYY(3-36) infusion (up to 0.8 pmol/kg/min) reduces food intake in a dose-dependent manner [121,122]. Recently, the long-acting PYY3-36 analogue, mAb-cycPYY, was shown to reduce food intake and body weight over 7 days in rhesus macaques, effects further augmented when combined with the GLP-1 receptor agonist, liraglutide [123].

PYY may be also involved in the regulation of postprandial glycaemia, given its effect to slow gastric emptying in both rodents and humans [124–127]. Furthermore, PYY may influence insulin secretin; PYY1-36, but not PYY3-36, was found to inhibit insulin secretion from the pancreatic β-cells ex vivo [128–130], and isolated islets from PYY-knockout mice showed higher glucose-induced insulin levels [131]. PYY-knockout mice exhibit relative hyperinsulinaemia during fasting and postprandially [132]. However, exogenous PYY infusion had little effect on glucose-stimulated insulin in healthy humans [133].

4. Regional Differences in Nutrient Absorption and Gastrointestinal Hormone Secretion, and Associated Impact on Postprandial Glycemia and Appetite

4.1. Nutrient Absorption

The upper small intestine (duodenum and proximal jejunum) represents a major site of nutrient absorption. Given that the delivery of nutrients into the small intestine is controlled by gastric emptying, it is not surprising that the rate of nutrient absorption (such as glucose) is related directly to the rate of gastric emptying [134]. In the case of glucose, the maximum capacity of absorption of the upper small intestine approximates ~0.5 g/min per 30 cm [135]. Of note, glucose transporters (SGLT-1,

GLUT2 and GLUT5) are less abundant in the distal than proximal small intestine [9,136]. Accordingly, intra-ileal administration of glucose is associated with slower absorption than intraduodenal, in both healthy individuals and patients with T2DM [137]. Moreover, duodenal-jejunal bypass improves glucose tolerance, associated with a reduction in SGLT-1-mediated glucose absorption in both obese rats and T2DM patients [138–141]. Similarly, the expression of the majority of lipid transporters (e.g., FAT/CD36, FATP4 and NPC1L1) decreases from the duodenum and jejunum to the ileum in rodents [142–146], and fatty acid and cholesterol uptake is slower in the distal than proximal small intestine [146,147]. In mice, the ablation of FAT/CD36 and FATP4 is associated with impaired lipid absorption in the proximal [145,148], but not in the distal [145,149] small intestine. However, fatty acid transporters have been shown to be abundantly expressed in both proximal and distal small intestine in humans [150]. The expression of transporters of amino acids and peptides varies substantially along the gastrointestinal tract [16]. While the majority of digestive products of protein are absorbed in the proximal jejunum, a considerable proportion is also absorbed in other small intestinal segments [17]. Amino acid transporters are abundant in the distal jejunum and ileum [151], such that obese patients who have undergone Roux-en-Y gastric bypass (RYGB) exhibit accelerated uptake of amino acids [152]. The absorption of nutrients in the large intestine is minimal. Undigested nutrients are fermented by microbiota localised in the large intestine to produce SCFAs which can be absorbed passively across colonic mucosa.

4.2. Gastrointestinal Hormone Secretion

EECs secreting GIP, CCK, GLP-1 and PYY exhibit high regional specificity of distribution along the gastrointestinal tract. Their secretory profiles are, therefore, largely dependent on the region of the gut exposed to intraluminal stimuli. In response to meal ingestion, increments in plasma GIP and CCK usually occur earlier than those of GLP-1 and PYY [153], consistent with the proximal distribution of K- and I-cells, and distal predominance of L-cells. Studies employing intraduodenal infusion of nutrients at different rates that mimic the physiological range of gastric emptying have shown that the secretion of GIP and CCK increases in an approximately linear pattern with increasing rates of infusion in health, obesity and T2DM [154–161]. In obese and T2DM patients, both the GIP and CCK responses to oral meals are increased after Roux-en-Y gastric bypass [162,163], due probably to rapid gastric pouch emptying [164]. However, postprandial GIP secretion is decreased after biliopancreatic diversion, since this procedure bypasses the majority of K-cell rich regions of the small intestine [165,166]. By contrast, intraduodenal infusion of nutrients needs to exceed a threshold (e.g., ~2 kcal/min for glucose) for sufficient nutrient to escape proximal small intestinal absorption and stimulate more distal L-cells; accordingly, the GLP-1 response is minimal to intraduodenal glucose infusion at rates between 1–2 kcal/min but increases substantially in response to infusions of 3–4 kcal/min [155,158,159].

The extent to which nutrients are delivered to the more distal regions of the gut is dependent not only on their rate of entry to the small intestine but also on their digestion and absorption in the upper gut. For example, ablation or inhibition of SGLT-1 that reduces proximal intestinal glucose absorption augments the GLP-1 and PYY responses to oral glucose in rodents [167,168]. In humans, intestinal SGLT-1 inhibition (e.g., by GSK-1614235 [169] or licogliflozin [170]), while reducing GIP secretion, is associated with overall increased, albeit relatively delayed, responses of GLP-1 and PYY to carbohydrate meals. Similarly, malabsorption of carbohydrate induced by an α-glucosidase inhibitor (e.g., acarbose) was shown to increase GLP-1 and PYY secretion in both health and T2DM [171,172]. Alternatively, poorly absorbed carbohydrates, such as tagatose [27], xylose [173] and resistant starch [174], also can induce sustained secretion of GLP-1. Consistent with this principle, consumption of a small amount of tagatose or xylose as a "preload" has been shown to slow gastric emptying and improve the glycaemic response to the subsequent main meal by stimulating GLP-1 secretion in both health and T2DM [27,175]. Treatment with the lipase inhibitor, orlistat, however, has been reported to either increase [176] or decrease [177–179] postprandial GLP-1 secretion. These discrepancies may have reflected differences in the test meals (including the forms of dietary fat) and the associated impact of orlistat on their digestion between studies.

Compared with intraduodenal infusion, administration of nutrients directly into the jejunum or ileum is more effective at stimulating GLP-1 and PYY secretion [137,180–186]. Interestingly, intra-ileal infusion of glucose is also associated with a considerable, albeit relatively lower, GIP response than intraduodenal infusion in both healthy subjects and patients with T2DM [137,183], suggesting that a considerable number of EEC cells capable of secreting GIP are found even in the distal small intestine. The large intestine represents another major source of GLP-1 and PYY production. Microbial metabolites, including SCFAs and secondary bile acids, are known to stimulate GLP-1 and PYY secretion [47,187–193] and may also induce differentiation of stem cells towards L-cells [194]. Inhibition of ileal ASBT (by elobixibat), increasing the exposure of the large intestine to bile acids, is therefore associated with an increase in GLP-1 and PYY secretion in humans [195]. In both healthy individuals and patients with T2DM [196,197], rectal administration of primary bile acid, taurocholic acid (TCA), has also been shown to stimulate GLP-1 and PYY secretion in a dose-dependent manner, although the PYY response seems to be more robust than that of GLP-1.

4.3. Regulation of Postprandial Glycaemia and Appetite

As discussed, the upper gut coordinates the delivery of nutrients for intestinal digestion and absorption, and is primarily responsible for the release of GIP and CCK after meals, whereas the interaction of intraluminal nutrients and bioactive compounds with the distal gut gives rise to the secretion of both GLP-1 and PYY. These variations in nutrient absorption and gastrointestinal hormone secretion along the gastrointestinal tract are of major relevance to the regulation of postprandial glycaemia and appetite.

It is now widely recognised that the rate of gastric emptying represents a major determinant of the glycaemic profile in response to carbohydrates in both health and diabetes [198,199]. While obesity per se does not seem to have a major impact on gastric emptying [200], recent evidence suggests that gastric emptying in patients with "early-stage" uncomplicated type 1 and 2 diabetes is more rapid than in non-diabetic controls [199,201], which may predispose them to glucose intolerance. By contrast, in patients with longstanding diabetes who have poor glycaemic control and autonomic dysfunction, gastric emptying is often abnormally delayed [202]. Nevertheless, nutritional and/or pharmacological strategies that slow gastric emptying have been shown to attenuate postprandial glycaemic excursions in both type 1 and 2 diabetes [57,203–205]. However, it should be noted that the relationship between the rise in postprandial blood glucose and the gastric emptying rate is not necessarily linear. Intraduodenal glucose infusion at 2 kcal/min results in a much greater increase in blood glucose levels than 1 kcal/min in healthy humans, while minimal additional increase occurs in glycaemia at rates of 3 or 4 kcal/min [155,158,159], due probably to the increasing contribution of the distal gut to provide counter-regulation to glycaemic excursions.

In health, GIP contributes to approximately 50% of the incretin effect [206] and may serve to stabilise blood glucose by stimulating glucagon secretion during hypoglycaemia [87]. However, the loss of the insulinotropic effect of GIP in T2DM, and the potential for GIP to increase fat deposition, have rendered it an unappealing target for the management of T2DM. Recently, novel compounds with dual GIP and GLP-1 receptor agonism have been developed to treat T2DM, with promising glucose-lowering efficacy [96]. However, as mentioned earlier, the relative contribution of GIP receptor agonism to the overall metabolic benefits of these compounds remains unclear. The rapid release of CCK in response to meal ingestion is necessary for the digestion of complex macronutrients, particularly fat, so it represents a determinant of subsequent gastric emptying and appetite responses.

However, when nutrients are administered intraduodenally, a threshold of the caloric load is required to achieve suppression of appetite [207], indicative of a greater relevance of stimulating the distal gut to the control of appetite. Indeed, relative to the upper gut, the lower gut appears to be more effective at mediating postprandial glucose metabolism and suppressing appetite due to substantially augmented GLP-1 and PYY secretion. Recently, the comparative effects of the proximal and distal small intestine on postprandial glucose metabolism were evaluated using targeted intraluminal glucose infusion in both healthy individuals and patients with T2DM [137]. In both groups, intra-ileal administration of glucose (2 kcal/min over 60 min) was associated with substantially greater GLP-1 secretion, incretin effect and gastrointestinal-mediated glucose disposal (GIGD), when compared with intraduodenal infusion (Figure 3). That the absorption of glucose occurs at a lower rate in the ileum, probably because of fewer glucose transporters in the distal gut, may not only attenuate the glycaemic response to glucose infusion but also allow EECs to be stimulated over a longer duration than those in the proximal gut [137]. In a similar study setting, Poppitt and colleagues compared the effects of a small load of glucose (~0.65 kcal/min over 90 min), administered into either the ileum or the duodenum, on gastrointestinal hormone secretion, appetite and food intake in healthy subjects. In this study, ileal infusion of glucose-induced greater GLP-1 and PYY secretion and less food intake than did intraduodenal infusion [183]. Compared with oral ingestion or duodenal perfusion, delivering fat or protein into the ileum also induces a greater suppression of food intake in healthy humans [185,186,208]. Moreover, administration of a relatively small load of lauric acid (5 g; 20 kcal) in enterically coated pellets for release in the ileum and colon has been shown to stimulate sufficient GLP-1 secretion to improve the glycaemic response to a standardised breakfast and lunch in patients with T2DM [209]. Similarly, the ileocolonic delivery of mixed bile acids (1 g/day) increases GLP-1 secretion and reduces postprandial blood glucose levels in patients with obesity and T2DM during a 4-week treatment [210]. Alternatively, EEC stimuli can be delivered through rectal administration; rectal perfusion with TCA has been shown to stimulate GLP-1 and PYY secretion, and suppress appetite scores in health [196] and reduces energy intake and glycaemia in T2DM [197]. Accordingly, enhancing the exposure of the distal gut to nutrients, and associated bioactive compounds such as bile acids, either by pharmacological inhibition of nutrient digestion and absorption in the upper gut [171,172], surgical reconstruction of the gastrointestinal tract (such as Roux-en-Y gastric bypass) [211,212], or endoscopic implantation of a duodenal-jejunal bypass sleeve device [140,141], has been shown to improve blood glucose control in T2DM and reduce body weight in obesity. The causal links of these metabolic outcomes to GLP-1 and PYY signalling have been further validated in T2DM patients undergoing Roux-en-Y gastric bypass, in whom glucose tolerance is attenuated by the GLP-1 receptor antagonist exendin9-39) [213,214], while energy intake is increased with either GLP-1 receptor antagonism, or inhibition of PYY activation using a DPP-4 inhibitor [215].

In recognition that the gut microbiota are an essential regulator of the host energy metabolism [216], and that insulin resistance, obesity and T2DM are linked to dysbiosis [217], the role of the large intestinal bacteria in the regulation of glycaemia and food intake is now receiving increasing attention. While the mechanisms by which the gut microflora participate in the regulation of metabolic homeostasis remain incompletely understood, many of their metabolites are linked to gastrointestinal hormone secretion [218,219]. For example, SCFAs, including acetate, butyrate and propionate, have been shown to stimulate GLP-1 and PYY from colonic L-cells in a dose-dependent manner [187,188,192] and to enhance insulin secretion either directly or indirectly in both rodents and humans [187–192]. Oral supplementation with propionate and butyrate improves blood glucose control and promotes weight loss in rats [220]. In obese individuals, acute administration of inulin-propionate ester (10 g), designed to be released in the colon, was shown to increase postprandial GLP-1 and PYY concentrations and decrease energy intake, without affecting gastric emptying [191]. Moreover, the administration of inulin-propionate ester (10 g/day) over 24 weeks showed a tendency to reduce body weight in obese subjects [191]. However, this phenomenon is complicated by evidence of a central effect contributing to the suppression of energy intake after a single dose of colonic inulin-propionate ester, independent of changes in peripheral GLP-1 or PYY concentrations [221].

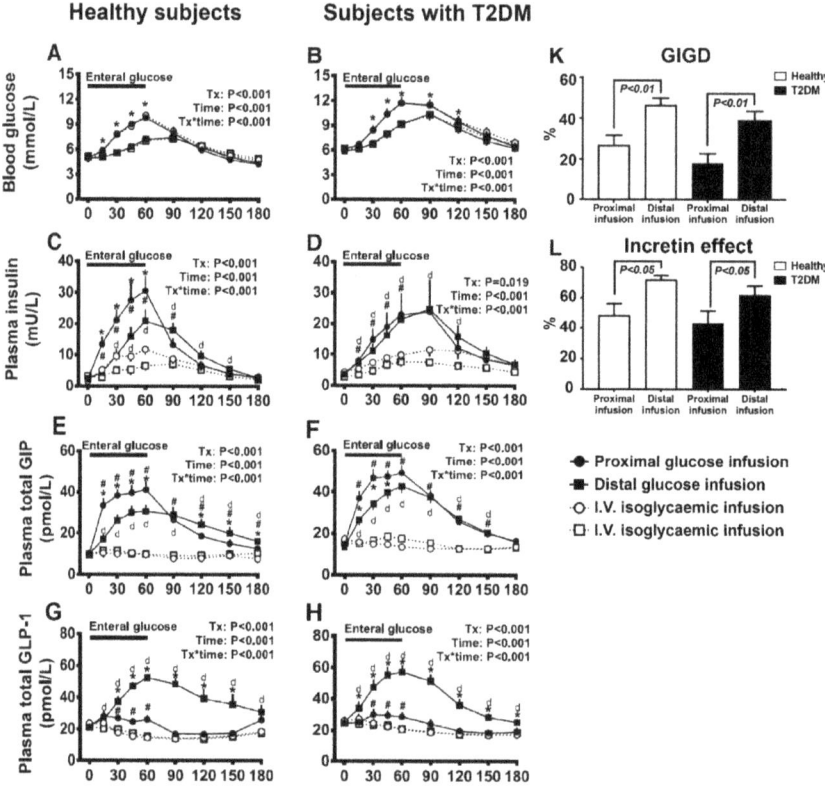

Figure 3. Comparative effects of proximal and distal small intestinal glucose exposure on glycaemia, incretin hormone secretion, and the incretin effect in both healthy individuals and patients with type 2 diabetes (T2DM) ($n = 10$ each). (**A,B**) Blood glucose levels, (**C,D**) plasma insulin, (**E,F**) plasma total glucose-dependent insulinotropic polypeptide (GIP), (**G,H**) plasma total glucagon-like peptide 1 (GLP-1), (**K**) Gastrointestinal-mediated glucose disposal (GIGD), and (**L**) Incretin effect. * $p < 0.05$ for proximal vs. distal enteral glucose infusion; # $p < 0.05$ for proximal enteral vs. corresponding i.v. glycaemic glucose infusion; d$p < 0.05$ for distal enteral vs. corresponding i.v. glycaemic glucose infusion. Data are mean ± SEM. (Figures are adapted from reference [137], with permission from Diabetes Care, 2019).

5. Summary

The gastrointestinal tract serves not only as the site of nutrient digestion and absorption but also as an endocrine organ secreting a variety of gastrointestinal hormones as a result of the complex interaction between ingested nutrients, bioactive compounds and EECs to regulate postprandial glucose metabolism and energy intake. Given the major difference in the distribution of EECs between the upper and lower gut, the load and delivery of nutrients, as well as the digestive processes in the gastrointestinal tract, have major implications on how these EECs are stimulated. Exposure of the upper gut to nutrients is associated with predominantly GIP and CCK release, whereas increasing the delivery of nutrients to the distal small intestine and colon is associated with augmented secretion of GLP-1 and PPY. These distal gut hormones appear more potent in mediating postprandial glucose metabolism and suppressing energy intake than those secreted from the proximal gut. Accordingly, the distal gut is becoming an appealing target for the management of T2DM and obesity, using nutritional, pharmacological or surgical approaches to increase its exposure to nutrients and other bioactive compounds. Future development in this area is likely to yield novel therapies for T2DM and obesity of high efficacy without the need for surgical procedures.

Author Contributions: C.X., K.L.J., C.K.R. and T.W. were all involved in the conception, design and writing of the manuscript. All authors have read and agreed to the published version of the manuscript.

Funding: The authors' work in this area is supported by the Australia National Health and Medical Research Council (NHMRC). C.X. is supported by a postgraduate scholarship from the China Scholarship Council. K.L.J. is supported by a University of Adelaide William T Southcott Research Fellowship. T.W. is supported by a Mid-Career Fellowship from The Hospital Research Foundation.

Acknowledgments: The Centre of Research Excellence (CRE) in Translating Nutritional Science to Good Health has been supported by The Hospital Research Foundation.

Conflicts of Interest: The authors declare no conflict of interest.

References

1. Steinert, R.E.; Feinle-Bisset, C.; Asarian, L.; Horowitz, M.; Beglinger, C.; Geary, N. Ghrelin, CCK, GLP-1, and PYY(3-36): Secretory controls and physiological roles in eating and glycemia in health, obesity, and after RYGB. *Physiol. Rev.* **2017**, *97*, 411–463. [CrossRef] [PubMed]
2. Gribble, F.M.; Reimann, F. Function and mechanisms of enteroendocrine cells and gut hormones in metabolism. *Nat. Rev. Endocrinol.* **2019**, *15*, 226–237. [CrossRef] [PubMed]
3. Phillips, L.K.; Deane, A.M.; Jones, K.L.; Rayner, C.K.; Horowitz, M. Gastric emptying and glycaemia in health and diabetes mellitus. *Nat. Rev. Endocrinol.* **2015**, *11*, 112–128. [CrossRef] [PubMed]
4. Iqbal, J.; Hussain, M.M. Intestinal lipid absorption. *Am. J. Physiol. Endocrinol. Metab.* **2009**, *296*, E1183–E1194. [CrossRef] [PubMed]
5. Erickson, R.H.; Kim, Y.S. Digestion and absorption of dietary protein. *Annu. Rev. Med.* **1990**, *41*, 133–139. [CrossRef]
6. Gray, G.M. Carbohydrate digestion and absorption. Role of the small intestine. *N. Engl. J. Med.* **1975**, *292*, 1225–1230. [CrossRef]
7. Song, P.; Onishi, A.; Koepsell, H.; Vallon, V. Sodium glucose cotransporter SGLT1 as a therapeutic target in diabetes mellitus. *Expert Opin. Ther. Targets* **2016**, *20*, 1109–1125. [CrossRef]
8. Wright, E.M.; Hirayama, B.A.; Loo, D.F. Active sugar transport in health and disease. *J. Intern. Med.* **2007**, *261*, 32–43. [CrossRef]
9. Balen, D.; Ljubojevic, M.; Breljak, D.; Brzica, H.; Zlender, V.; Koepsell, H.; Sabolic, I. Revised immunolocalization of the Na+-D-glucose cotransporter SGLT1 in rat organs with an improved antibody. *Am. J. Physiol. Cell Physiol.* **2008**, *295*, C475–C489. [CrossRef]
10. Thazhath, S.S.; Wu, T.; Young, R.L.; Horowitz, M.; Rayner, C.K. Glucose absorption in small intestinal diseases. *Expert Rev. Gastroenterol. Hepatol.* **2014**, *8*, 301–312. [CrossRef]
11. Gouyon, F.; Caillaud, L.; Carriere, V.; Klein, C.; Dalet, V.; Citadelle, D.; Kellett, G.L.; Thorens, B.; Leturque, A.; Brot-Laroche, E. Simple-sugar meals target GLUT2 at enterocyte apical membranes to improve sugar absorption: A study in GLUT2-null mice. *J. Physiol.* **2003**, *552*, 823–832. [CrossRef] [PubMed]
12. Davidson, N.O.; Hausman, A.M.; Ifkovits, C.A.; Buse, J.B.; Gould, G.W.; Burant, C.F.; Bell, G.I. Human intestinal glucose transporter expression and localization of GLUT5. *Am. J. Physiol.* **1992**, *262*, C795–C800. [CrossRef] [PubMed]
13. Abumrad, N.A.; Davidson, N.O. Role of the gut in lipid homeostasis. *Physiol. Rev.* **2012**, *92*, 1061–1085. [CrossRef] [PubMed]
14. Paalvast, Y.; de Boer, J.F.; Groen, A.K. Developments in intestinal cholesterol transport and triglyceride absorption. *Curr. Opin. Lipidol.* **2017**, *28*, 248–254. [CrossRef]
15. Carter, D.; Howlett, H.C.; Wiernsperger, N.F.; Bailey, C.J. Differential effects of metformin on bile salt absorption from the jejunum and ileum. *Diabetes Obes. Metab.* **2003**, *5*, 120–125. [CrossRef]
16. Broer, S. Amino acid transport across mammalian intestinal and renal epithelia. *Physiol. Rev.* **2008**, *88*, 249–286. [CrossRef]
17. Broer, S.; Fairweather, S.J. Amino acid transport across the mammalian intestine. *Compr. Physiol.* **2018**, *9*, 343–373. [CrossRef]

18. Daniel, H.; Zietek, T. Taste and move: Glucose and peptide transporters in the gastrointestinal tract. *Exp. Physiol.* **2015**, *100*, 1441–1450. [CrossRef]
19. Gill, S.; Chater, P.I.; Wilcox, M.D.; Pearson, J.P.; Brownlee, I.A. The impact of dietary fibres on the physiological processes of the large intestine. *Bioact. Carbohydr. Diet. Fibre* **2018**, *16*, 62–74. [CrossRef]
20. Scott, K.P.; Gratz, S.W.; Sheridan, P.O.; Flint, H.J.; Duncan, S.H. The influence of diet on the gut microbiota. *Pharm. Res.* **2013**, *69*, 52–60. [CrossRef]
21. Topping, D.L.; Clifton, P.M. Short-chain fatty acids and human colonic function: Roles of resistant starch and nonstarch polysaccharides. *Physiol. Rev.* **2001**, *81*, 1031–1064. [CrossRef] [PubMed]
22. Kreuch, D.; Keating, D.J.; Wu, T.; Horowitz, M.; Rayner, C.K.; Young, R.L. Gut mechanisms linking intestinal sweet sensing to glycemic control. *Front. Endocrinol. (Lausanne)* **2018**, *9*, 741. [CrossRef]
23. Wu, T.; Bound, M.J.; Standfield, S.D.; Bellon, M.; Young, R.L.; Jones, K.L.; Horowitz, M.; Rayner, C.K. Artificial sweeteners have no effect on gastric emptying, glucagon-like peptide-1, or glycemia after oral glucose in healthy humans. *Diabetes Care* **2013**, *36*, e202–e203. [CrossRef] [PubMed]
24. Jang, H.J.; Kokrashvili, Z.; Theodorakis, M.J.; Carlson, O.D.; Kim, B.J.; Zhou, J.; Kim, H.H.; Xu, X.; Chan, S.L.; Juhaszova, M.; et al. Gut-expressed gustducin and taste receptors regulate secretion of glucagon-like peptide-1. *Proc. Natl. Acad. Sci. USA* **2007**, *104*, 15069–15074. [CrossRef] [PubMed]
25. Mace, O.J.; Schindler, M.; Patel, S. The regulation of K- and L-cell activity by GLUT2 and the calcium-sensing receptor CasR in rat small intestine. *J. Physiol.* **2012**, *590*, 2917–2936. [CrossRef]
26. Gorboulev, V.; Schurmann, A.; Vallon, V.; Kipp, H.; Jaschke, A.; Klessen, D.; Friedrich, A.; Scherneck, S.; Rieg, T.; Cunard, R.; et al. Na(+)-D-glucose cotransporter SGLT1 is pivotal for intestinal glucose absorption and glucose-dependent incretin secretion. *Diabetes* **2012**, *61*, 187–196. [CrossRef]
27. Wu, T.; Zhao, B.R.; Bound, M.J.; Checklin, H.L.; Bellon, M.; Little, T.J.; Young, R.L.; Jones, K.L.; Horowitz, M.; Rayner, C.K. Effects of different sweet preloads on incretin hormone secretion, gastric emptying, and postprandial glycemia in healthy humans. *Am. J. Clin. Nutr.* **2012**, *95*, 78–83. [CrossRef]
28. Beglinger, S.; Drewe, J.; Schirra, J.; Goke, B.; D'Amato, M.; Beglinger, C. Role of fat hydrolysis in regulating glucagon-like Peptide-1 secretion. *J. Clin. Endocrinol. Metab.* **2010**, *95*, 879–886. [CrossRef]
29. Kuo, P.; Stevens, J.E.; Russo, A.; Maddox, A.; Wishart, J.M.; Jones, K.L.; Greville, H.; Hetzel, D.; Chapman, I.; Horowitz, M.; et al. Gastric emptying, incretin hormone secretion, and postprandial glycemia in cystic fibrosis–effects of pancreatic enzyme supplementation. *J. Clin. Endocrinol. Metab.* **2011**, *96*, E851–E855. [CrossRef]
30. Perano, S.J.; Couper, J.J.; Horowitz, M.; Martin, A.J.; Kritas, S.; Sullivan, T.; Rayner, C.K. Pancreatic enzyme supplementation improves the incretin hormone response and attenuates postprandial glycemia in adolescents with cystic fibrosis: A randomized crossover trial. *J. Clin. Endocrinol. Metab.* **2014**, *99*, 2486–2493. [CrossRef]
31. Edfalk, S.; Steneberg, P.; Edlund, H. Gpr40 is expressed in enteroendocrine cells and mediates free fatty acid stimulation of incretin secretion. *Diabetes* **2008**, *57*, 2280–2287. [CrossRef] [PubMed]
32. Lauffer, L.M.; Iakoubov, R.; Brubaker, P.L. GPR119 is essential for oleoylethanolamide-induced glucagon-like peptide-1 secretion from the intestinal enteroendocrine L-cell. *Diabetes* **2009**, *58*, 1058–1066. [CrossRef] [PubMed]
33. Sankoda, A.; Harada, N.; Iwasaki, K.; Yamane, S.; Murata, Y.; Shibue, K.; Thewjitcharoen, Y.; Suzuki, K.; Harada, T.; Kanemaru, Y.; et al. Long-chain free fatty acid receptor GPR120 mediates oil-induced GIP secretion through CCK in male mice. *Endocrinology* **2017**, *158*, 1172–1180. [CrossRef] [PubMed]
34. Poreba, M.A.; Dong, C.X.; Li, S.K.; Stahl, A.; Miner, J.H.; Brubaker, P.L. Role of fatty acid transport protein 4 in oleic acid-induced glucagon-like peptide-1 secretion from murine intestinal L cells. *Am. J. Physiol. Endocrinol. Metab.* **2012**, *303*, E899–E907. [CrossRef]
35. Sundaresan, S.; Shahid, R.; Riehl, T.E.; Chandra, R.; Nassir, F.; Stenson, W.F.; Liddle, R.A.; Abumrad, N.A. CD36-dependent signaling mediates fatty acid-induced gut release of secretin and cholecystokinin. *FASEB J.* **2013**, *27*, 1191–1202. [CrossRef]
36. Pais, R.; Gribble, F.M.; Reimann, F. Signalling pathways involved in the detection of peptones by murine small intestinal enteroendocrine L-cells. *Peptides* **2016**, *77*, 9–15. [CrossRef]
37. Jiang, Y.; Rose, A.J.; Sijmonsma, T.P.; Broer, A.; Pfenninger, A.; Herzig, S.; Schmoll, D.; Broer, S. Mice lacking neutral amino acid transporter B(0)AT1 (Slc6a19) have elevated levels of FGF21 and GLP-1 and improved glycaemic control. *Mol. Metab.* **2015**, *4*, 406–417. [CrossRef]

38. Clemmensen, C.; Jorgensen, C.V.; Smajilovic, S.; Brauner-Osborne, H. Robust GLP-1 secretion by basic L-amino acids does not require the GPRC6A receptor. *Diabetes Obes. Metab.* **2017**, *19*, 599–603. [CrossRef]
39. Trabelsi, M.S.; Daoudi, M.; Prawitt, J.; Ducastel, S.; Touche, V.; Sayin, S.I.; Perino, A.; Brighton, C.A.; Sebti, Y.; Kluza, J.; et al. Farnesoid X receptor inhibits glucagon-like peptide-1 production by enteroendocrine L cells. *Nat. Commun.* **2015**, *6*, 7629. [CrossRef]
40. Thomas, C.; Gioiello, A.; Noriega, L.; Strehle, A.; Oury, J.; Rizzo, G.; Macchiarulo, A.; Yamamoto, H.; Mataki, C.; Pruzanski, M.; et al. TGR5-mediated bile acid sensing controls glucose homeostasis. *Cell Metab.* **2009**, *10*, 167–177. [CrossRef]
41. Kuhre, R.E.; Wewer Albrechtsen, N.J.; Larsen, O.; Jepsen, S.L.; Balk-Moller, E.; Andersen, D.B.; Deacon, C.F.; Schoonjans, K.; Reimann, F.; Gribble, F.M.; et al. Bile acids are important direct and indirect regulators of the secretion of appetite- and metabolism-regulating hormones from the gut and pancreas. *Mol. Metab.* **2018**, *11*, 84–95. [CrossRef]
42. Tough, I.R.; Schwartz, T.W.; Cox, H.M. Synthetic G protein-coupled bile acid receptor agonists and bile acids act via basolateral receptors in ileal and colonic mucosa. *Neurogastroenterol. Motil.* **2020**, e13943. [CrossRef]
43. Xie, C.; Wang, X.; Young, R.L.; Horowitz, M.; Rayner, C.K.; Wu, T. Role of Intestinal Bitter Sensing in Enteroendocrine Hormone Secretion and Metabolic Control. *Front. Endocrinol. (Lausanne)* **2018**, *9*, 576. [CrossRef]
44. Wu, T.; Rayner, C.K.; Watson, L.E.; Jones, K.L.; Horowitz, M.; Little, T.J. Comparative effects of intraduodenal fat and glucose on the gut-incretin axis in healthy males. *Peptides* **2017**, *95*, 124–127. [CrossRef]
45. Ryan, A.T.; Luscombe-Marsh, N.D.; Saies, A.A.; Little, T.J.; Standfield, S.; Horowitz, M.; Feinle-Bisset, C. Effects of intraduodenal lipid and protein on gut motility and hormone release, glycemia, appetite, and energy intake in lean men. *Am. J. Clin. Nutr.* **2013**, *98*, 300–311. [CrossRef]
46. Jensen, C.Z.; Bojsen-Moller, K.N.; Svane, M.S.; Holst, L.M.; Hermansen, K.; Hartmann, B.; Wewer Albrechtsen, N.J.; Kuhre, R.E.; Kristiansen, V.B.; Rehfeld, J.F.; et al. Responses of gut and pancreatic hormones, bile acids, and fibroblast growth factor-21 differ to glucose, protein, and fat ingestion after gastric bypass surgery. *Am. J. Physiol. Gastrointest. Liver Physiol.* **2020**, *318*, G661–G672. [CrossRef]
47. Katsuma, S.; Hirasawa, A.; Tsujimoto, G. Bile acids promote glucagon-like peptide-1 secretion through TGR5 in a murine enteroendocrine cell line STC-1. *Biochem. Biophys. Res. Commun.* **2005**, *329*, 386–390. [CrossRef]
48. Andersen, A.; Lund, A.; Knop, F.K.; Vilsboll, T. Glucagon-like peptide 1 in health and disease. *Nat. Rev. Endocrinol.* **2018**, *14*, 390–403. [CrossRef]
49. Holst, J.J.; Albrechtsen, N.J.W.; Rosenkilde, M.M.; Deacon, C.F. Physiology of the incretin hormones, GIP and GLP-1-regulation of release and posttranslational modifications. *Compr. Physiol.* **2019**, *9*, 1339–1381. [CrossRef]
50. Wu, T.; Rayner, C.K.; Horowitz, M. Incretins. *Handb. Exp. Pharm.* **2016**, *233*, 137–171. [CrossRef]
51. Nauck, M.A.; Meier, J.J. Incretin hormones: Their role in health and disease. *Diabetes Obes. Metab.* **2018**, *20* (Suppl. 1), 5–21. [CrossRef]
52. Hare, K.J.; Vilsboll, T.; Asmar, M.; Deacon, C.F.; Knop, F.K.; Holst, J.J. The glucagonostatic and insulinotropic effects of glucagon-like peptide 1 contribute equally to its glucose-lowering action. *Diabetes* **2010**, *59*, 1765–1770. [CrossRef] [PubMed]
53. Maida, A.; Hansotia, T.; Longuet, C.; Seino, Y.; Drucker, D.J. Differential importance of glucose-dependent insulinotropic polypeptide vs glucagon-like peptide 1 receptor signaling for beta cell survival in mice. *Gastroenterology* **2009**, *137*, 2146–2157. [CrossRef]
54. Seghieri, M.; Rebelos, E.; Gastaldelli, A.; Astiarraga, B.D.; Casolaro, A.; Barsotti, E.; Pocai, A.; Nauck, M.; Muscelli, E.; Ferrannini, E. Direct effect of GLP-1 infusion on endogenous glucose production in humans. *Diabetologia* **2013**, *56*, 156–161. [CrossRef]
55. Nauck, M.A.; Niedereichholz, U.; Ettler, R.; Holst, J.J.; Orskov, C.; Ritzel, R.; Schmiegel, W.H. Glucagon-like peptide 1 inhibition of gastric emptying outweighs its insulinotropic effects in healthy humans. *Am. J. Physiol.* **1997**, *273*, E981–E988. [CrossRef]
56. Little, T.J.; Pilichiewicz, A.N.; Russo, A.; Phillips, L.; Jones, K.L.; Nauck, M.A.; Wishart, J.; Horowitz, M.; Feinle-Bisset, C. Effects of intravenous glucagon-like peptide-1 on gastric emptying and intragastric distribution in healthy subjects: Relationships with postprandial glycemic and insulinemic responses. *J. Clin. Endocrinol. Metab.* **2006**, *91*, 1916–1923. [CrossRef]

57. Jones, K.L.; Rigda, R.S.; Buttfield, M.D.M.; Hatzinikolas, S.; Pham, H.T.; Marathe, C.S.; Wu, T.; Lange, K.; Trahair, L.G.; Rayner, C.K.; et al. Effects of lixisenatide on postprandial blood pressure, gastric emptying and glycaemia in healthy people and people with type 2 diabetes. *Diabetes Obes. Metab.* **2019**, *21*, 1158–1167. [CrossRef]

58. Deane, A.M.; Nguyen, N.Q.; Stevens, J.E.; Fraser, R.J.; Holloway, R.H.; Besanko, L.K.; Burgstad, C.; Jones, K.L.; Chapman, M.J.; Rayner, C.K.; et al. Endogenous glucagon-like peptide-1 slows gastric emptying in healthy subjects, attenuating postprandial glycemia. *J. Clin. Endocrinol. Metab.* **2010**, *95*, 215–221. [CrossRef]

59. Lorenz, M.; Pfeiffer, C.; Steinstrasser, A.; Becker, R.H.; Rutten, H.; Ruus, P.; Horowitz, M. Effects of lixisenatide once daily on gastric emptying in type 2 diabetes–relationship to postprandial glycemia. *Regul. Pept.* **2013**, *185*, 1–8. [CrossRef]

60. Stevens, J.E.; Buttfield, M.; Wu, T.; Hatzinikolas, S.; Pham, H.; Lange, K.; Rayner, C.K.; Horowitz, M.; Jones, K.L. Effects of sitagliptin on gastric emptying of, and the glycaemic and blood pressure responses to, a carbohydrate meal in type 2 diabetes. *Diabetes Obes. Metab.* **2020**, *22*, 51–58. [CrossRef]

61. DeFronzo, R.A.; Okerson, T.; Viswanathan, P.; Guan, X.; Holcombe, J.H.; MacConell, L. Effects of exenatide versus sitagliptin on postprandial glucose, insulin and glucagon secretion, gastric emptying, and caloric intake: A randomized, cross-over study. *Curr. Med. Res. Opin.* **2008**, *24*, 2943–2952. [CrossRef] [PubMed]

62. Hsieh, J.; Longuet, C.; Baker, C.L.; Qin, B.; Federico, L.M.; Drucker, D.J.; Adeli, K. The glucagon-like peptide 1 receptor is essential for postprandial lipoprotein synthesis and secretion in hamsters and mice. *Diabetologia* **2010**, *53*, 552–561. [CrossRef] [PubMed]

63. Qin, X.; Shen, H.; Liu, M.; Yang, Q.; Zheng, S.; Sabo, M.; D'Alessio, D.A.; Tso, P. GLP-1 reduces intestinal lymph flow, triglyceride absorption, and apolipoprotein production in rats. *Am. J. Physiol. Gastrointest. Liver Physiol.* **2005**, *288*, G943–G949. [CrossRef]

64. Xiao, C.; Bandsma, R.H.; Dash, S.; Szeto, L.; Lewis, G.F. Exenatide, a glucagon-like peptide-1 receptor agonist, acutely inhibits intestinal lipoprotein production in healthy humans. *Arter. Thromb. Vasc. Biol.* **2012**, *32*, 1513–1519. [CrossRef]

65. Xiao, C.; Dash, S.; Morgantini, C.; Patterson, B.W.; Lewis, G.F. Sitagliptin, a DPP-4 inhibitor, acutely inhibits intestinal lipoprotein particle secretion in healthy humans. *Diabetes* **2014**, *63*, 2394–2401. [CrossRef] [PubMed]

66. Hjerpsted, J.B.; Flint, A.; Brooks, A.; Axelsen, M.B.; Kvist, T.; Blundell, J. Semaglutide improves postprandial glucose and lipid metabolism, and delays first-hour gastric emptying in subjects with obesity. *Diabetes Obes. Metab.* **2018**, *20*, 610–619. [CrossRef]

67. Holst, J.J. The physiology of glucagon-like peptide 1. *Physiol. Rev.* **2007**, *87*, 1409–1439. [CrossRef]

68. Plamboeck, A.; Veedfald, S.; Deacon, C.F.; Hartmann, B.; Wettergren, A.; Svendsen, L.B.; Meisner, S.; Hovendal, C.; Vilsboll, T.; Knop, F.K.; et al. The effect of exogenous GLP-1 on food intake is lost in male truncally vagotomized subjects with pyloroplasty. *Am. J. Physiol. Gastrointest. Liver Physiol.* **2013**, *304*, G1117–G1127. [CrossRef]

69. Krieger, J.P.; Arnold, M.; Pettersen, K.G.; Lossel, P.; Langhans, W.; Lee, S.J. Knockdown of GLP-1 receptors in vagal afferents affects normal food intake and glycemia. *Diabetes* **2016**, *65*, 34–43. [CrossRef]

70. Turton, M.D.; O'Shea, D.; Gunn, I.; Beak, S.A.; Edwards, C.M.; Meeran, K.; Choi, S.J.; Taylor, G.M.; Heath, M.M.; Lambert, P.D.; et al. A role for glucagon-like peptide-1 in the central regulation of feeding. *Nature* **1996**, *379*, 69–72. [CrossRef]

71. ten Kulve, J.S.; Veltman, D.J.; van Bloemendaal, L.; Barkhof, F.; Deacon, C.F.; Holst, J.J.; Konrad, R.J.; Sloan, J.H.; Drent, M.L.; Diamant, M.; et al. Endogenous GLP-1 mediates postprandial reductions in activation in central reward and satiety areas in patients with type 2 diabetes. *Diabetologia* **2015**, *58*, 2688–2698. [CrossRef] [PubMed]

72. Pratley, R.; Amod, A.; Hoff, S.T.; Kadowaki, T.; Lingvay, I.; Nauck, M.; Pedersen, K.B.; Saugstrup, T.; Meier, J.J. Oral semaglutide versus subcutaneous liraglutide and placebo in type 2 diabetes (PIONEER 4): A randomised, double-blind, phase 3a trial. *Lancet* **2019**, *394*, 39–50. [CrossRef]

73. Xu, F.; Lin, B.; Zheng, X.; Chen, Z.; Cao, H.; Xu, H.; Liang, H.; Weng, J. GLP-1 receptor agonist promotes brown remodelling in mouse white adipose tissue through SIRT1. *Diabetologia* **2016**, *59*, 1059–1069. [CrossRef] [PubMed]

74. Lynch, L.; Hogan, A.E.; Duquette, D.; Lester, C.; Banks, A.; LeClair, K.; Cohen, D.E.; Ghosh, A.; Lu, B.; Corrigan, M.; et al. iNKT cells induce FGF21 for thermogenesis and are required for maximal weight loss in GLP1 therapy. *Cell Metab.* **2016**, *24*, 510–519. [CrossRef]

75. Beiroa, D.; Imbernon, M.; Gallego, R.; Senra, A.; Herranz, D.; Villarroya, F.; Serrano, M.; Ferno, J.; Salvador, J.; Escalada, J.; et al. GLP-1 agonism stimulates brown adipose tissue thermogenesis and browning through hypothalamic AMPK. *Diabetes* **2014**, *63*, 3346–3358. [CrossRef]
76. Tomas, E.; Stanojevic, V.; McManus, K.; Khatri, A.; Everill, P.; Bachovchin, W.W.; Habener, J.F. GLP-1(32-36)amide pentapeptide increases basal energy expenditure and inhibits weight gain in obese mice. *Diabetes* **2015**, *64*, 2409–2419. [CrossRef]
77. Goldsmith, F.; Keenan, M.J.; Raggio, A.M.; Ye, X.; Hao, Z.; Durham, H.; Geaghan, J.; Jia, W.P.; Martin, R.J.; Ye, J.P. Induction of energy expenditure by sitagliptin is dependent on GLP-1 receptor. *PLoS ONE* **2015**, *10*, e0126177. [CrossRef]
78. Fukuda-Tsuru, S.; Kakimoto, T.; Utsumi, H.; Kiuchi, S.; Ishii, S. The novel dipeptidyl peptidase-4 inhibitor teneligliptin prevents high-fat diet-induced obesity accompanied with increased energy expenditure in mice. *Eur. J. Pharm.* **2014**, *723*, 207–215. [CrossRef]
79. Maciel, M.G.; Beserra, B.T.S.; Oliveira, F.C.B.; Ribeiro, C.M.; Coelho, M.S.; Neves, F.A.R.; Amato, A.A. The effect of glucagon-like peptide 1 and glucagon-like peptide 1 receptor agonists on energy expenditure: A systematic review and meta-analysis. *Diabetes Res. Clin. Pr.* **2018**, *142*, 222–235. [CrossRef]
80. Heruc, G.A.; Horowitz, M.; Deacon, C.F.; Feinle-Bisset, C.; Rayner, C.K.; Luscombe-Marsh, N.; Little, T.J. Effects of dipeptidyl peptidase IV inhibition on glycemic, gut hormone, triglyceride, energy expenditure, and energy intake responses to fat in healthy males. *Am. J. Physiol. Endocrinol. Metab.* **2014**, *307*, E830–E837. [CrossRef]
81. Xie, C.; Wang, X.; Jones, K.L.; Horowitz, M.; Sun, Z.; Little, T.J.; Rayner, C.K.; Wu, T. Role of endogenous glucagon-like peptide-1 enhanced by vildagliptin in the glycaemic and energy expenditure responses to intraduodenal fat infusion in type 2 diabetes. *Diabetes Obes. Metab.* **2020**, *22*, 383–392. [CrossRef] [PubMed]
82. Mortensen, K.; Christensen, L.L.; Holst, J.J.; Orskov, C. GLP-1 and GIP are colocalized in a subset of endocrine cells in the small intestine. *Regul. Pept.* **2003**, *114*, 189–196. [CrossRef]
83. Svendsen, B.; Pedersen, J.; Albrechtsen, N.J.; Hartmann, B.; Torang, S.; Rehfeld, J.F.; Poulsen, S.S.; Holst, J.J. An analysis of cosecretion and coexpression of gut hormones from male rat proximal and distal small intestine. *Endocrinology* **2015**, *156*, 847–857. [CrossRef] [PubMed]
84. Wu, T.; Rayner, C.K.; Jones, K.; Horowitz, M. Dietary effects on incretin hormone secretion. *Vitam Horm* **2010**, *84*, 81–110. [CrossRef] [PubMed]
85. Holst, J.J.; Gromada, J. Role of incretin hormones in the regulation of insulin secretion in diabetic and nondiabetic humans. *Am. J. Physiol. Endocrinol. Metab.* **2004**, *287*, E199–E206. [CrossRef] [PubMed]
86. Mentis, N.; Vardarli, I.; Köthe, L.D.; Holst, J.J.; Deacon, C.F.; Theodorakis, M.; Meier, J.J.; Nauck, M.A. GIP does not potentiate the antidiabetic effects of GLP-1 in hyperglycemic patients with type 2 diabetes. *Diabetes* **2011**, *60*, 1270–1276. [CrossRef] [PubMed]
87. Christensen, M.; Calanna, S.; Sparre-Ulrich, A.H.; Kristensen, P.L.; Rosenkilde, M.M.; Faber, J.; Purrello, F.; van Hall, G.; Holst, J.J.; Vilsboll, T.; et al. Glucose-dependent insulinotropic polypeptide augments glucagon responses to hypoglycemia in type 1 diabetes. *Diabetes* **2015**, *64*, 72–78. [CrossRef]
88. Bergmann, N.C.; Lund, A.; Gasbjerg, L.S.; Meessen, E.C.E.; Andersen, M.M.; Bergmann, S.; Hartmann, B.; Holst, J.J.; Jessen, L.; Christensen, M.B.; et al. Effects of combined GIP and GLP-1 infusion on energy intake, appetite and energy expenditure in overweight/obese individuals: A randomised, crossover study. *Diabetologia* **2019**, *62*, 665–675. [CrossRef]
89. Meier, J.J.; Goetze, O.; Anstipp, J.; Hagemann, D.; Holst, J.J.; Schmidt, W.E.; Gallwitz, B.; Nauck, M.A. Gastric inhibitory polypeptide does not inhibit gastric emptying in humans. *Am. J. Physiol. Endocrinol. Metab.* **2004**, *286*, E621–E625. [CrossRef]
90. Miyawaki, K.; Yamada, Y.; Ban, N.; Ihara, Y.; Tsukiyama, K.; Zhou, H.; Fujimoto, S.; Oku, A.; Tsuda, K.; Toyokuni, S.; et al. Inhibition of gastric inhibitory polypeptide signaling prevents obesity. *Nat. Med.* **2002**, *8*, 738–742. [CrossRef]
91. Naitoh, R.; Miyawaki, K.; Harada, N.; Mizunoya, W.; Toyoda, K.; Fushiki, T.; Yamada, Y.; Seino, Y.; Inagaki, N. Inhibition of GIP signaling modulates adiponectin levels under high-fat diet in mice. *Biochem. Biophys. Res. Commun.* **2008**, *376*, 21–25. [CrossRef] [PubMed]
92. Zhou, H.; Yamada, Y.; Tsukiyama, K.; Miyawaki, K.; Hosokawa, M.; Nagashima, K.; Toyoda, K.; Naitoh, R.; Mizunoya, W.; Fushiki, T.; et al. Gastric inhibitory polypeptide modulates adiposity and fat oxidation under diminished insulin action. *Biochem. Biophys. Res. Commun.* **2005**, *335*, 937–942. [CrossRef] [PubMed]

93. Hansotia, T.; Maida, A.; Flock, G.; Yamada, Y.; Tsukiyama, K.; Seino, Y.; Drucker, D.J. Extrapancreatic incretin receptors modulate glucose homeostasis, body weight, and energy expenditure. *J. Clin. Investig.* **2007**, *117*, 143–152. [CrossRef] [PubMed]
94. Boylan, M.O.; Glazebrook, P.A.; Tatalovic, M.; Wolfe, M.M. Gastric inhibitory polypeptide immunoneutralization attenuates development of obesity in mice. *Am. J. Physiol. Endocrinol. Metab.* **2015**, *309*, E1008–E1018. [CrossRef]
95. Asmar, M.; Asmar, A.; Simonsen, L.; Gasbjerg, L.S.; Sparre-Ulrich, A.H.; Rosenkilde, M.M.; Hartmann, B.; Dela, F.; Holst, J.J.; Bulow, J. The gluco- and liporegulatory and vasodilatory effects of glucose-dependent insulinotropic polypeptide (GIP) are abolished by an antagonist of the human GIP receptor. *Diabetes* **2017**, *66*, 2363–2371. [CrossRef]
96. Frias, J.P.; Nauck, M.A.; Van, J.; Kutner, M.E.; Cui, X.; Benson, C.; Urva, S.; Gimeno, R.E.; Milicevic, Z.; Robins, D.; et al. Efficacy and safety of LY3298176, a novel dual GIP and GLP-1 receptor agonist, in patients with type 2 diabetes: A randomised, placebo-controlled and active comparator-controlled phase 2 trial. *Lancet* **2018**, *392*, 2180–2193. [CrossRef]
97. Frias, J.P.; Bastyr, E.J., 3rd; Vignati, L.; Tschop, M.H.; Schmitt, C.; Owen, K.; Christensen, R.H.; DiMarchi, R.D. The sustained effects of a dual GIP/GLP-1 receptor agonist, NNC0090-2746, in patients with type 2 diabetes. *Cell Metab.* **2017**, *26*, 343–352. [CrossRef]
98. Bergmann, N.C.; Gasbjerg, L.S.; Heimburger, S.M.; Krogh, L.S.L.; Dela, F.; Hartmann, B.; Holst, J.J.; Jessen, L.; Christensen, M.B.; Vilsboll, T.; et al. No acute effects of exogenous glucose-dependent insulinotropic polypeptide on energy intake, appetite, or energy expenditure when added to treatment with a long-acting glucagon-like peptide 1 receptor agonist in men with type 2 diabetes. *Diabetes Care* **2020**, *43*, 588–596. [CrossRef]
99. Sykaras, A.G.; Demenis, C.; Cheng, L.; Pisitkun, T.; McLaughlin, J.T.; Fenton, R.A.; Smith, C.P. Duodenal CCK cells from male mice express multiple hormones including ghrelin. *Endocrinology* **2014**, *155*, 3339–3351. [CrossRef]
100. Little, T.J.; Doran, S.; Meyer, J.H.; Smout, A.J.; O'Donovan, D.G.; Wu, K.L.; Jones, K.L.; Wishart, J.; Rayner, C.K.; Horowitz, M.; et al. The release of GLP-1 and ghrelin, but not GIP and CCK, by glucose is dependent upon the length of small intestine exposed. *Am. J. Physiol. Endocrinol. Metab.* **2006**, *291*, E647–E655. [CrossRef]
101. Liddle, R.A.; Rushakoff, R.J.; Morita, E.T.; Beccaria, L.; Carter, J.D.; Goldfine, I.D. Physiological role for cholecystokinin in reducing postprandial hyperglycemia in humans. *J. Clin. Investig.* **1988**, *81*, 1675–1681. [CrossRef] [PubMed]
102. Ahren, B.; Holst, J.J.; Efendic, S. Antidiabetogenic action of cholecystokinin-8 in type 2 diabetes. *J. Clin. Endocrinol. Metab.* **2000**, *85*, 1043–1048. [CrossRef] [PubMed]
103. Horowitz, M.; Harding, P.E.; Maddox, A.F.; Wishart, J.M.; Akkermans, L.M.; Chatterton, B.E.; Shearman, D.J. Gastric and oesophageal emptying in patients with type 2 (non-insulin-dependent) diabetes mellitus. *Diabetologia* **1989**, *32*, 151–159. [CrossRef] [PubMed]
104. Reidelberger, R.D.; Hernandez, J.; Fritzsch, B.; Hulce, M. Abdominal vagal mediation of the satiety effects of CCK in rats. *Am. J. Physiol. Regul. Integr. Comp. Physiol.* **2004**, *286*, R1005–R1012. [CrossRef] [PubMed]
105. MacIntosh, C.G.; Morley, J.E.; Wishart, J.; Morris, H.; Jansen, J.B.; Horowitz, M.; Chapman, I.M. Effect of exogenous cholecystokinin (CCK)-8 on food intake and plasma CCK, leptin, and insulin concentrations in older and young adults: Evidence for increased CCK activity as a cause of the anorexia of aging. *J. Clin. Endocrinol. Metab.* **2001**, *86*, 5830–5837. [CrossRef] [PubMed]
106. Brennan, I.M.; Feltrin, K.L.; Horowitz, M.; Smout, A.J.; Meyer, J.H.; Wishart, J.; Feinle-Bisset, C. Evaluation of interactions between CCK and GLP-1 in their effects on appetite, energy intake, and antropyloroduodenal motility in healthy men. *Am. J. Physiol. Regul. Integr. Comp. Physiol.* **2005**, *288*, R1477–R1485. [CrossRef]
107. Brennan, I.M.; Little, T.J.; Feltrin, K.L.; Smout, A.J.; Wishart, J.M.; Horowitz, M.; Feinle-Bisset, C. Dose-dependent effects of cholecystokinin-8 on antropyloroduodenal motility, gastrointestinal hormones, appetite, and energy intake in healthy men. *Am. J. Physiol. Endocrinol. Metab.* **2008**, *295*, E1487–E1494. [CrossRef]
108. Beglinger, C.; Degen, L.; Matzinger, D.; D'Amato, M.; Drewe, J. Loxiglumide, a CCK-A receptor antagonist, stimulates calorie intake and hunger feelings in humans. *Am. J. Physiol. Regul. Integr. Comp. Physiol.* **2001**, *280*, R1149–R1154. [CrossRef]

109. de Krom, M.; van der Schouw, Y.T.; Hendriks, J.; Ophoff, R.A.; van Gils, C.H.; Stolk, R.P.; Grobbee, D.E.; Adan, R. Common genetic variations in CCK, leptin, and leptin receptor genes are associated with specific human eating patterns. *Diabetes* **2007**, *56*, 276–280. [CrossRef]
110. Lieverse, R.J.; Jansen, J.B.; Masclee, A.A.; Lamers, C.B. Satiety effects of a physiological dose of cholecystokinin in humans. *Gut* **1995**, *36*, 176–179. [CrossRef]
111. Habib, A.M.; Richards, P.; Rogers, G.J.; Reimann, F.; Gribble, F.M. Co-localisation and secretion of glucagon-like peptide 1 and peptide YY from primary cultured human L cells. *Diabetologia* **2013**, *56*, 1413–1416. [CrossRef] [PubMed]
112. Essah, P.A.; Levy, J.R.; Sistrun, S.N.; Kelly, S.M.; Nestler, J.E. Effect of macronutrient composition on postprandial peptide YY levels. *J. Clin. Endocrinol. Metab.* **2007**, *92*, 4052–4055. [CrossRef] [PubMed]
113. Brennan, I.M.; Luscombe-Marsh, N.D.; Seimon, R.V.; Otto, B.; Horowitz, M.; Wishart, J.M.; Feinle-Bisset, C. Effects of fat, protein, and carbohydrate and protein load on appetite, plasma cholecystokinin, peptide YY, and ghrelin, and energy intake in lean and obese men. *Am. J. Physiol. Gastrointest. Liver Physiol.* **2012**, *303*, G129–G140. [CrossRef] [PubMed]
114. Helou, N.; Obeid, O.; Azar, S.T.; Hwalla, N. Variation of postprandial PYY 3-36 response following ingestion of differing macronutrient meals in obese females. *Ann. Nutr. Metab.* **2008**, *52*, 188–195. [CrossRef] [PubMed]
115. Batterham, R.L.; Heffron, H.; Kapoor, S.; Chivers, J.E.; Chandarana, K.; Herzog, H.; Le Roux, C.W.; Thomas, E.L.; Bell, J.D.; Withers, D.J. Critical role for peptide YY in protein-mediated satiation and body-weight regulation. *Cell Metab.* **2006**, *4*, 223–233. [CrossRef]
116. Broberger, C.; Landry, M.; Wong, H.; Walsh, J.N.; Hokfelt, T. Subtypes Y1 and Y2 of the neuropeptide Y receptor are respectively expressed in pro-opiomelanocortin- and neuropeptide-Y-containing neurons of the rat hypothalamic arcuate nucleus. *Neuroendocrinology* **1997**, *66*, 393–408. [CrossRef]
117. Batterham, R.L.; Cowley, M.A.; Small, C.J.; Herzog, H.; Cohen, M.A.; Dakin, C.L.; Wren, A.M.; Brynes, A.E.; Low, M.J.; Ghatei, M.A.; et al. Gut hormone PYY3-36 physiologically inhibits food intake. *Nature* **2002**, *418*, 650–654. [CrossRef]
118. Abbott, C.R.; Small, C.J.; Kennedy, A.R.; Neary, N.M.; Sajedi, A.; Ghatei, M.A.; Bloom, S.R. Blockade of the neuropeptide Y Y2 receptor with the specific antagonist BIIE0246 attenuates the effect of endogenous and exogenous peptide YY(3-36) on food intake. *Brain Res.* **2005**, *1043*, 139–144. [CrossRef]
119. Guo, Y.; Ma, L.; Enriori, P.J.; Koska, J.; Franks, P.W.; Brookshire, T.; Cowley, M.A.; Salbe, A.D.; Delparigi, A.; Tataranni, P.A. Physiological evidence for the involvement of peptide YY in the regulation of energy homeostasis in humans. *Obesity (Silver Spring)* **2006**, *14*, 1562–1570. [CrossRef]
120. Stoeckel, L.E.; Weller, R.E.; Giddings, M.; Cox, J.E. Peptide YY levels are associated with appetite suppression in response to long-chain fatty acids. *Physiol. Behav.* **2008**, *93*, 289–295. [CrossRef]
121. Degen, L.; Oesch, S.; Casanova, M.; Graf, S.; Ketterer, S.; Drewe, J.; Beglinger, C. Effect of peptide YY3-36 on food intake in humans. *Gastroenterology* **2005**, *129*, 1430–1436. [CrossRef] [PubMed]
122. le Roux, C.W.; Borg, C.M.; Murphy, K.G.; Vincent, R.P.; Ghatei, M.A.; Bloom, S.R. Supraphysiological doses of intravenous PYY3-36 cause nausea, but no additional reduction in food intake. *Ann. Clin. Biochem.* **2008**, *45*, 93–95. [CrossRef] [PubMed]
123. Rangwala, S.M.; D'Aquino, K.; Zhang, Y.M.; Bader, L.; Edwards, W.; Zheng, S.; Eckardt, A.; Lacombe, A.; Pick, R.; Moreno, V.; et al. A long-acting PYY3-36 analog mediates robust anorectic efficacy with minimal emesis in nonhuman primates. *Cell Metab.* **2019**, *29*, 837–843. [CrossRef] [PubMed]
124. Savage, A.P.; Adrian, T.E.; Carolan, G.; Chatterjee, V.K.; Bloom, S.R. Effects of peptide YY (PYY) on mouth to caecum intestinal transit time and on the rate of gastric emptying in healthy volunteers. *Gut* **1987**, *28*, 166–170. [CrossRef]
125. Chelikani, P.K.; Haver, A.C.; Reidelberger, R.D. Comparison of the inhibitory effects of PYY(3-36) and PYY(1-36) on gastric emptying in rats. *Am. J. Physiol. Regul. Integr. Comp. Physiol.* **2004**, *287*, R1064–R1070. [CrossRef]
126. Moran, T.H.; Smedh, U.; Kinzig, K.P.; Scott, K.A.; Knipp, S.; Ladenheim, E.E. Peptide YY(3-36) inhibits gastric emptying and produces acute reductions in food intake in rhesus monkeys. *Am. J. Physiol. Regul. Integr. Comp. Physiol.* **2005**, *288*, R384–R388. [CrossRef]
127. Witte, A.B.; Gryback, P.; Holst, J.J.; Hilsted, L.; Hellstrom, P.M.; Jacobsson, H.; Schmidt, P.T. Differential effect of PYY1-36 and PYY3-36 on gastric emptying in man. *Regul. Pept.* **2009**, *158*, 57–62. [CrossRef]

128. Bottcher, G.; Ahren, B.; Lundquist, I.; Sundler, F. Peptide YY: Intrapancreatic localization and effects on insulin and glucagon secretion in the mouse. *Pancreas* **1989**, *4*, 282–288. [CrossRef]
129. Nieuwenhuizen, A.G.; Karlsson, S.; Fridolf, T.; Ahren, B. Mechanisms underlying the insulinostatic effect of peptide YY in mouse pancreatic islets. *Diabetologia* **1994**, *37*, 871–878. [CrossRef]
130. Lafferty, R.A.; Gault, V.A.; Flatt, P.R.; Irwin, N. Effects of 2 novel PYY(1-36) analogues, (P(3)L(31)P(34)) PYY(1-36) and PYY(1-36)(Lys(12)PAL), on pancreatic beta-cell function, growth, and survival. *Clin. Med. Insights Endocrinol. Diabetes* **2019**, *12*, 1179551419855626. [CrossRef]
131. Boey, D.; Heilbronn, L.; Sainsbury, A.; Laybutt, R.; Kriketos, A.; Herzog, H.; Campbell, L.V. Low serum PYY is linked to insulin resistance in first-degree relatives of subjects with type 2 diabetes. *Neuropeptides* **2006**, *40*, 317–324. [CrossRef] [PubMed]
132. Boey, D.; Lin, S.; Karl, T.; Baldock, P.; Lee, N.; Enriquez, R.; Couzens, M.; Slack, K.; Dallmann, R.; Sainsbury, A.; et al. Peptide YY ablation in mice leads to the development of hyperinsulinaemia and obesity. *Diabetologia* **2006**, *49*, 1360–1370. [CrossRef] [PubMed]
133. Ahrén, B.; Larsson, H. Peptide YY does not inhibit glucose-stimulated insulin secretion in humans. *Eur. J. Endocrinol.* **1996**, *134*, 362–365. [CrossRef] [PubMed]
134. Nguyen, N.Q.; Debreceni, T.L.; Burgess, J.E.; Bellon, M.; Wishart, J.; Standfield, S.; Malbert, C.H.; Horowitz, M. Impact of gastric emptying and small intestinal transit on blood glucose, intestinal hormones, glucose absorption in the morbidly obese. *Int. J. Obes. (Lond)* **2018**, *42*, 1556–1564. [CrossRef]
135. Duchman, S.M.; Ryan, A.J.; Schedl, H.P.; Summers, R.W.; Bleier, T.L.; Gisolfi, C.V. Upper limit for intestinal absorption of a dilute glucose solution in men at rest. *Med. Sci. Sports Exerc.* **1997**, *29*, 482–488. [CrossRef]
136. Yoshikawa, T.; Inoue, R.; Matsumoto, M.; Yajima, T.; Ushida, K.; Iwanaga, T. Comparative expression of hexose transporters (SGLT1, GLUT1, GLUT2 and GLUT5) throughout the mouse gastrointestinal tract. *Histochem. Cell Biol.* **2011**, *135*, 183–194. [CrossRef]
137. Zhang, X.; Young, R.L.; Bound, M.; Hu, S.; Jones, K.L.; Horowitz, M.; Rayner, C.K.; Wu, T. Comparative effects of proximal and distal small intestinal glucose exposure on glycemia, incretin hormone Ssecretion, and the incretin effect in health and type 2 diabetes. *Diabetes Care* **2019**, *42*, 520–528. [CrossRef]
138. Yan, S.; Sun, F.; Li, Z.; Xiang, J.; Ding, Y.; Lu, Z.; Tian, Y.; Chen, H.; Zhang, J.; Wang, Y.; et al. Reduction of intestinal electrogenic glucose absorption after duodenojejunal bypass in a mouse model. *Obes. Surg.* **2013**, *23*, 1361–1369. [CrossRef]
139. Jurowich, C.F.; Rikkala, P.R.; Thalheimer, A.; Wichelmann, C.; Seyfried, F.; Sander, V.; Kreissl, M.; Germer, C.T.; Koepsell, H.; Otto, C. Duodenal-jejunal bypass improves glycemia and decreases SGLT1-mediated glucose absorption in rats with streptozotocin-induced type 2 diabetes. *Ann. Surg.* **2013**, *258*, 89–97. [CrossRef]
140. de Jonge, C.; Rensen, S.S.; Verdam, F.J.; Vincent, R.P.; Bloom, S.R.; Buurman, W.A.; le Roux, C.W.; Schaper, N.C.; Bouvy, N.D.; Greve, J.W. Endoscopic duodenal-jejunal bypass liner rapidly improves type 2 diabetes. *Obes. Surg.* **2013**, *23*, 1354–1360. [CrossRef]
141. Koehestanie, P.; de Jonge, C.; Berends, F.J.; Janssen, I.M.; Bouvy, N.D.; Greve, J.W. The effect of the endoscopic duodenal-jejunal bypass liner on obesity and type 2 diabetes mellitus, a multicenter randomized controlled trial. *Ann. Surg.* **2014**, *260*, 984–992. [CrossRef] [PubMed]
142. Lobo, M.V.; Huerta, L.; Ruiz-Velasco, N.; Teixeiro, E.; de la Cueva, P.; Celdran, A.; Martin-Hidalgo, A.; Vega, M.A.; Bragado, R. Localization of the lipid receptors CD36 and CLA-1/SR-BI in the human gastrointestinal tract: Towards the identification of receptors mediating the intestinal absorption of dietary lipids. *J. Histochem. Cytochem.* **2001**, *49*, 1253–1260. [CrossRef]
143. Ockner, R.K.; Manning, J.A. Fatty acid-binding protein in small intestine. Identification, isolation, and evidence for its role in cellular fatty acid transport. *J. Clin. Investig.* **1974**, *54*, 326–338. [CrossRef]
144. Chen, M.; Yang, Y.; Braunstein, E.; Georgeson, K.E.; Harmon, C.M. Gut expression and regulation of FAT/CD36: Possible role in fatty acid transport in rat enterocytes. *Am. J. Physiol. Endocrinol. Metab.* **2001**, *281*, E916–E923. [CrossRef] [PubMed]
145. Nassir, F.; Wilson, B.; Han, X.; Gross, R.W.; Abumrad, N.A. CD36 is important for fatty acid and cholesterol uptake by the proximal but not distal intestine. *J. Biol. Chem.* **2007**, *282*, 19493–19501. [CrossRef] [PubMed]
146. Nguyen, D.V.; Drover, V.A.; Knopfel, M.; Dhanasekaran, P.; Hauser, H.; Phillips, M.C. Influence of class B scavenger receptors on cholesterol flux across the brush border membrane and intestinal absorption. *J. Lipid Res.* **2009**, *50*, 2235–2244. [CrossRef]

147. Wu, A.L.; Clark, S.B.; Holt, P.R. Transmucosal triglyceride transport rates in proximal and distal rat intestine in vivo. *J. Lipid Res.* **1975**, *16*, 251–257.
148. Nauli, A.M.; Nassir, F.; Zheng, S.; Yang, Q.; Lo, C.M.; Vonlehmden, S.B.; Lee, D.; Jandacek, R.J.; Abumrad, N.A.; Tso, P. CD36 is important for chylomicron formation and secretion and may mediate cholesterol uptake in the proximal intestine. *Gastroenterology* **2006**, *131*, 1197–1207. [CrossRef]
149. Shim, J.; Moulson, C.L.; Newberry, E.P.; Lin, M.H.; Xie, Y.; Kennedy, S.M.; Miner, J.H.; Davidson, N.O. Fatty acid transport protein 4 is dispensable for intestinal lipid absorption in mice. *J. Lipid Res.* **2009**, *50*, 491–500. [CrossRef]
150. Masson, C.J.; Plat, J.; Mensink, R.P.; Namiot, A.; Kisielewski, W.; Namiot, Z.; Fullekrug, J.; Ehehalt, R.; Glatz, J.F.; Pelsers, M.M. Fatty acid- and cholesterol transporter protein expression along the human intestinal tract. *PLoS ONE* **2010**, *5*, e10380. [CrossRef]
151. Mutch, D.M.; Anderle, P.; Fiaux, M.; Mansourian, R.; Vidal, K.; Wahli, W.; Williamson, G.; Roberts, M.A. Regional variations in ABC transporter expression along the mouse intestinal tract. *Physiol. Genom.* **2004**, *17*, 11–20. [CrossRef] [PubMed]
152. Bojsen-Moller, K.N.; Jacobsen, S.H.; Dirksen, C.; Jorgensen, N.B.; Reitelseder, S.; Jensen, J.E.; Kristiansen, V.B.; Holst, J.J.; van Hall, G.; Madsbad, S. Accelerated protein digestion and amino acid absorption after Roux-en-Y gastric bypass. *Am. J. Clin. Nutr.* **2015**, *102*, 600–607. [CrossRef] [PubMed]
153. Dirksen, C.; Graff, J.; Fuglsang, S.; Rehfeld, J.F.; Holst, J.J.; Madsen, J.L. Energy intake, gastrointestinal transit, and gut hormone release in response to oral triglycerides and fatty acids in men with and without severe obesity. *Am. J. Physiol. Gastrointest. Liver Physiol.* **2019**, *316*, G332–G337. [CrossRef] [PubMed]
154. Little, T.J.; Feltrin, K.L.; Horowitz, M.; Smout, A.J.; Rades, T.; Meyer, J.H.; Pilichiewicz, A.N.; Wishart, J.; Feinle-Bisset, C. Dose-related effects of lauric acid on antropyloroduodenal motility, gastrointestinal hormone release, appetite, and energy intake in healthy men. *Am. J. Physiol. Regul. Integr. Comp. Physiol.* **2005**, *289*, R1090–R1098. [CrossRef]
155. Pilichiewicz, A.N.; Chaikomin, R.; Brennan, I.M.; Wishart, J.M.; Rayner, C.K.; Jones, K.L.; Smout, A.J.; Horowitz, M.; Feinle-Bisset, C. Load-dependent effects of duodenal glucose on glycemia, gastrointestinal hormones, antropyloroduodenal motility, and energy intake in healthy men. *Am. J. Physiol. Endocrinol. Metab.* **2007**, *293*, E743–E753. [CrossRef]
156. Hutchison, A.T.; Feinle-Bisset, C.; Fitzgerald, P.C.; Standfield, S.; Horowitz, M.; Clifton, P.M.; Luscombe-Marsh, N.D. Comparative effects of intraduodenal whey protein hydrolysate on antropyloroduodenal motility, gut hormones, glycemia, appetite, and energy intake in lean and obese men. *Am. J. Clin. Nutr.* **2015**, *102*, 1323–1331. [CrossRef]
157. Wu, T.; Zhang, X.; Trahair, L.G.; Bound, M.J.; Little, T.J.; Deacon, C.F.; Horowitz, M.; Jones, K.L.; Rayner, C.K. Small intestinal glucose delivery affects the lowering of blood glucose by acute vildagliptin in type 2 diabetes. *J. Clin. Endocrinol. Metab.* **2016**, *101*, 4769–4778. [CrossRef]
158. Ma, J.; Pilichiewicz, A.N.; Feinle-Bisset, C.; Wishart, J.M.; Jones, K.L.; Horowitz, M.; Rayner, C.K. Effects of variations in duodenal glucose load on glycaemic, insulin, and incretin responses in type 2 diabetes. *Diabet Med.* **2012**, *29*, 604–608. [CrossRef]
159. Trahair, L.G.; Horowitz, M.; Rayner, C.K.; Gentilcore, D.; Lange, K.; Wishart, J.M.; Jones, K.L. Comparative effects of variations in duodenal glucose load on glycemic, insulinemic, and incretin responses in healthy young and older subjects. *J. Clin. Endocrinol. Metab.* **2012**, *97*, 844–851. [CrossRef]
160. Pilichiewicz, A.N.; Papadopoulos, P.; Brennan, I.M.; Little, T.J.; Meyer, J.H.; Wishart, J.M.; Horowitz, M.; Feinle-Bisset, C. Load-dependent effects of duodenal lipid on antropyloroduodenal motility, plasma CCK and PYY, and energy intake in healthy men. *Am. J. Physiol. Regul. Integr. Comp. Physiol.* **2007**, *293*, R2170–R2178. [CrossRef]
161. Wu, T.; Rayner, C.K.; Horowitz, M. Inter-regulation of gastric emptying and incretin hormone secretion: Implications for postprandial glycemic control. *Biomark. Med.* **2016**, *10*, 1167–1179. [CrossRef] [PubMed]
162. Laferrere, B.; Heshka, S.; Wang, K.; Khan, Y.; McGinty, J.; Teixeira, J.; Hart, A.B.; Olivan, B. Incretin levels and effect are markedly enhanced 1 month after Roux-en-Y gastric bypass surgery in obese patients with type 2 diabetes. *Diabetes Care* **2007**, *30*, 1709–1716. [CrossRef] [PubMed]

163. Dirksen, C.; Jorgensen, N.B.; Bojsen-Moller, K.N.; Kielgast, U.; Jacobsen, S.H.; Clausen, T.R.; Worm, D.; Hartmann, B.; Rehfeld, J.F.; Damgaard, M.; et al. Gut hormones, early dumping and resting energy expenditure in patients with good and poor weight loss response after Roux-en-Y gastric bypass. *Int. J. Obes.* **2013**, *37*, 1452–1459. [CrossRef] [PubMed]

164. Nguyen, N.Q.; Debreceni, T.L.; Bambrick, J.E.; Bellon, M.; Wishart, J.; Standfield, S.; Rayner, C.K.; Horowitz, M. Rapid gastric and intestinal transit is a major determinant of changes in blood glucose, intestinal hormones, glucose absorption and postprandial symptoms after gastric bypass. *Obesity* **2014**, *22*, 2003–2009. [CrossRef]

165. Mingrone, G.; Nolfe, G.; Gissey, G.C.; Iaconelli, A.; Leccesi, L.; Guidone, C.; Nanni, G.; Holst, J.J. Circadian rhythms of GIP and GLP1 in glucose-tolerant and in type 2 diabetic patients after biliopancreatic diversion. *Diabetologia* **2009**, *52*, 873–881. [CrossRef]

166. Salinari, S.; Bertuzzi, A.; Asnaghi, S.; Guidone, C.; Manco, M.; Mingrone, G. First-phase insulin secretion restoration and differential response to glucose load depending on the route of administration in type 2 diabetic subjects after bariatric surgery. *Diabetes Care* **2009**, *32*, 375–380. [CrossRef]

167. Powell, D.R.; Smith, M.; Greer, J.; Harris, A.; Zhao, S.; DaCosta, C.; Mseeh, F.; Shadoan, M.K.; Sands, A.; Zambrowicz, B.; et al. LX4211 increases serum glucagon-like peptide 1 and peptide YY levels by reducing sodium/glucose cotransporter 1 (SGLT1)-mediated absorption of intestinal glucose. *J. Pharm. Exp. Ther.* **2013**, *345*, 250–259. [CrossRef]

168. Oguma, T.; Nakayama, K.; Kuriyama, C.; Matsushita, Y.; Yoshida, K.; Hikida, K.; Obokata, N.; Tsuda-Tsukimoto, M.; Saito, A.; Arakawa, K.; et al. Intestinal sodium glucose cotransporter 1 inhibition enhances glucagon-like peptide-1 secretion in normal and diabetic rodents. *J. Pharm. Exp. Ther.* **2015**, *354*, 279–289. [CrossRef]

169. Dobbins, R.L.; Greenway, F.L.; Chen, L.; Liu, Y.; Breed, S.L.; Andrews, S.M.; Wald, J.A.; Walker, A.; Smith, C.D. Selective sodium-dependent glucose transporter 1 inhibitors block glucose absorption and impair glucose-dependent insulinotropic peptide release. *Am. J. Physiol. Gastrointest. Liver Physiol.* **2015**, *308*, G946–G954. [CrossRef]

170. He, Y.L.; Haynes, W.; Meyers, C.D.; Amer, A.; Zhang, Y.; Mahling, P.; Mendonza, A.E.; Ma, S.; Chutkow, W.; Bachman, E. The effects of licogliflozin, a dual SGLT1/2 inhibitor, on body weight in obese patients with or without diabetes. *Diabetes Obes. Metab.* **2019**, *21*, 1311–1321. [CrossRef]

171. Qualmann, C.; Nauck, M.A.; Holst, J.J.; Orskov, C.; Creutzfeldt, W. Glucagon-like peptide 1 (7-36 amide) secretion in response to luminal sucrose from the upper and lower gut. A study using alpha-glucosidase inhibition (acarbose). *Scand. J. Gastroenterol.* **1995**, *30*, 892–896. [CrossRef] [PubMed]

172. Zheng, M.Y.; Yang, J.H.; Shan, C.Y.; Zhou, H.T.; Xu, Y.G.; Wang, Y.; Ren, H.Z.; Chang, B.C.; Chen, L.M. Effects of 24-week treatment with acarbose on glucagon-like peptide 1 in newly diagnosed type 2 diabetic patients: A preliminary report. *Cardiovasc. Diabetol.* **2013**, *12*, 73. [CrossRef] [PubMed]

173. Vanis, L.; Hausken, T.; Gentilcore, D.; Rigda, R.S.; Rayner, C.K.; Feinle-Bisset, C.; Horowitz, M.; Jones, K.L. Comparative effects of glucose and xylose on blood pressure, gastric emptying and incretin hormones in healthy older subjects. *Br. J. Nutr.* **2011**, *105*, 1644–1651. [CrossRef] [PubMed]

174. Crapo, P.A.; Reaven, G.; Olefsky, J. Plasma glucose and insulin responses to orally administered simple and complex carbohydrates. *Diabetes* **1976**, *25*, 741–747. [CrossRef]

175. Wu, T.; Bound, M.J.; Zhao, B.Y.R.; Standfield, S.D.; Bellon, M.; Jones, K.L.; Horowitz, M.; Rayner, C.K. Effects of a D-xylose preload with or without sitagliptin on gastric emptying, glucagon-like peptide-1, and postprandial glycemia in type 2 diabetes. *Diabetes Care* **2013**, *36*, 1913–1918. [CrossRef]

176. Damci, T.; Yalin, S.; Balci, H.; Osar, Z.; Korugan, U.; Ozyazar, M.; Ilkova, H. Orlistat augments postprandial increases in glucagon-like peptide 1 in obese type 2 diabetic patients. *Diabetes Care* **2004**, *27*, 1077–1080. [CrossRef]

177. Ellrichmann, M.; Kapelle, M.; Ritter, P.R.; Holst, J.J.; Herzig, K.H.; Schmidt, W.E.; Schmitz, F.; Meier, J.J. Orlistat inhibition of intestinal lipase acutely increases appetite and attenuates postprandial glucagon-like peptide-1-(7-36)-amide-1, cholecystokinin, and peptide YY concentrations. *J. Clin. Endocrinol. Metab.* **2008**, *93*, 3995–3998. [CrossRef]

178. Enc, F.Y.; Ones, T.; Akin, H.L.; Dede, F.; Turoglu, H.T.; Ulfer, G.; Bekiroglu, N.; Haklar, G.; Rehfeld, J.F.; Holst, J.J.; et al. Orlistat accelerates gastric emptying and attenuates GIP release in healthy subjects. *Am. J. Physiol. Gastrointest. Liver Physiol.* **2009**, *296*, G482–G489. [CrossRef]

179. O'Donovan, D.; Horowitz, M.; Russo, A.; Feinle-Bisset, C.; Murolo, N.; Gentilcore, D.; Wishart, J.M.; Morris, H.A.; Jones, K.L. Effects of lipase inhibition on gastric emptying of, and on the glycaemic, insulin and cardiovascular responses to, a high-fat/carbohydrate meal in type 2 diabetes. *Diabetologia* **2004**, *47*, 2208–2214. [CrossRef]
180. Chaikomin, R.; Wu, K.L.; Doran, S.; Meyer, J.H.; Jones, K.L.; Feinle-Bisset, C.; Horowitz, M.; Rayner, C.K. Effects of mid-jejunal compared to duodenal glucose infusion on peptide hormone release and appetite in healthy men. *Regul. Pept.* **2008**, *150*, 38–42. [CrossRef]
181. Wu, T.; Thazhath, S.S.; Marathe, C.S.; Bound, M.J.; Jones, K.L.; Horowitz, M.; Rayner, C.K. Comparative effect of intraduodenal and intrajejunal glucose infusion on the gut-incretin axis response in healthy males. *Nutr. Diabetes* **2015**, *5*, e156. [CrossRef] [PubMed]
182. Rigda, R.S.; Trahair, L.G.; Little, T.J.; Wu, T.; Standfield, S.; Feinle-Bisset, C.; Rayner, C.K.; Horowitz, M.; Jones, K.L. Regional specificity of the gut-incretin response to small intestinal glucose infusion in healthy older subjects. *Peptides* **2016**, *86*, 126–132. [CrossRef] [PubMed]
183. Poppitt, S.D.; Shin, H.S.; McGill, A.T.; Budgett, S.C.; Lo, K.; Pahl, M.; Duxfield, J.; Lane, M.; Ingram, J.R. Duodenal and ileal glucose infusions differentially alter gastrointestinal peptides, appetite response, and food intake: A tube feeding study. *Am. J. Clin. Nutr* **2017**, *106*, 725–735. [CrossRef] [PubMed]
184. Mangan, A.M.; Al Najim, W.; McNamara, N.; Martin, W.P.; Antanaitis, A.; Bleil, S.B.; Kent, R.M.; le Roux, C.W.; Docherty, N.G. Effect of macronutrient type and gastrointestinal release site on PYY response in normal healthy subjects. *J. Clin. Endocrinol. Metab.* **2019**, *104*, 3661–3669. [CrossRef]
185. Maljaars, P.W.; Symersky, T.; Kee, B.C.; Haddeman, E.; Peters, H.P.; Masclee, A.A. Effect of ileal fat perfusion on satiety and hormone release in healthy volunteers. *Int. J. Obes.* **2008**, *32*, 1633–1639. [CrossRef]
186. van Avesaat, M.; Troost, F.J.; Ripken, D.; Hendriks, H.F.; Masclee, A.A. Ileal brake activation: Macronutrient-specific effects on eating behavior? *Int. J. Obes.* **2015**, *39*, 235–243. [CrossRef]
187. Christiansen, C.B.; Gabe, M.B.N.; Svendsen, B.; Dragsted, L.O.; Rosenkilde, M.M.; Holst, J.J. The impact of short-chain fatty acids on GLP-1 and PYY secretion from the isolated perfused rat colon. *Am. J. Physiol. Gastrointest. Liver Physiol.* **2018**, *315*, G53–G65. [CrossRef]
188. Tolhurst, G.; Heffron, H.; Lam, Y.S.; Parker, H.E.; Habib, A.M.; Diakogiannaki, E.; Cameron, J.; Grosse, J.; Reimann, F.; Gribble, F.M. Short-chain fatty acids stimulate glucagon-like peptide-1 secretion via the G-protein-coupled receptor FFAR2. *Diabetes* **2012**, *61*, 364–371. [CrossRef]
189. Psichas, A.; Sleeth, M.L.; Murphy, K.G.; Brooks, L.; Bewick, G.A.; Hanyaloglu, A.C.; Ghatei, M.A.; Bloom, S.R.; Frost, G. The short chain fatty acid propionate stimulates GLP-1 and PYY secretion via free fatty acid receptor 2 in rodents. *Int. J. Obes.* **2015**, *39*, 424–429. [CrossRef]
190. Freeland, K.R.; Wolever, T.M. Acute effects of intravenous and rectal acetate on glucagon-like peptide-1, peptide YY, ghrelin, adiponectin and tumour necrosis factor-alpha. *Br. J. Nutr.* **2010**, *103*, 460–466. [CrossRef]
191. Chambers, E.S.; Viardot, A.; Psichas, A.; Morrison, D.J.; Murphy, K.G.; Zac-Varghese, S.E.; MacDougall, K.; Preston, T.; Tedford, C.; Finlayson, G.S.; et al. Effects of targeted delivery of propionate to the human colon on appetite regulation, body weight maintenance and adiposity in overweight adults. *Gut* **2015**, *64*, 1744–1754. [CrossRef] [PubMed]
192. Canfora, E.E.; van der Beek, C.M.; Jocken, J.W.E.; Goossens, G.H.; Holst, J.J.; Olde Damink, S.W.M.; Lenaerts, K.; Dejong, C.H.C.; Blaak, E.E. Colonic infusions of short-chain fatty acid mixtures promote energy metabolism in overweight/obese men: A randomized crossover trial. *Sci. Rep.* **2017**, *7*, 2360. [CrossRef] [PubMed]
193. Christiansen, C.B.; Trammell, S.A.J.; Wewer Albrechtsen, N.J.; Schoonjans, K.; Albrechtsen, R.; Gillum, M.P.; Kuhre, R.E.; Holst, J.J. Bile acids drive colonic secretion of glucagon-like-peptide 1 and peptide-YY in rodents. *Am. J. Physiol. Gastrointest. Liver Physiol.* **2019**, *316*, G574–G584. [CrossRef]
194. Petersen, N.; Reimann, F.; Bartfeld, S.; Farin, H.F.; Ringnalda, F.C.; Vries, R.G.; van den Brink, S.; Clevers, H.; Gribble, F.M.; de Koning, E.J. Generation of L cells in mouse and human small intestine organoids. *Diabetes* **2014**, *63*, 410–420. [CrossRef] [PubMed]
195. Rudling, M.; Camilleri, M.; Graffner, H.; Holst, J.J.; Rikner, L. Specific inhibition of bile acid transport alters plasma lipids and GLP-1. *BMC Cardiovasc Disord.* **2015**, *15*, 75. [CrossRef] [PubMed]
196. Wu, T.; Bound, M.J.; Standfield, S.D.; Gedulin, B.; Jones, K.L.; Horowitz, M.; Rayner, C.K. Effects of rectal administration of taurocholic acid on glucagon-like peptide-1 and peptide YY secretion in healthy humans. *Diabetes Obes. Metab.* **2013**, *15*, 474–477. [CrossRef] [PubMed]

197. Adrian, T.E.; Gariballa, S.; Parekh, K.A.; Thomas, S.A.; Saadi, H.; Al Kaabi, J.; Nagelkerke, N.; Gedulin, B.; Young, A.A. Rectal taurocholate increases L cell and insulin secretion, and decreases blood glucose and food intake in obese type 2 diabetic volunteers. *Diabetologia* **2012**, *55*, 2343–2347. [CrossRef]
198. Marathe, C.S.; Rayner, C.K.; Jones, K.L.; Horowitz, M. Relationships between gastric emptying, postprandial glycemia, and incretin hormones. *Diabetes Care* **2013**, *36*, 1396–1405. [CrossRef]
199. Watson, L.E.; Xie, C.; Wang, X.; Li, Z.; Phillips, L.K.; Sun, Z.; Jones, K.L.; Horowitz, M.; Rayner, C.K.; Wu, T. Gastric emptying in patients with well-controlled type 2 diabetes compared with young and older control subjects without diabetes. *J. Clin. Endocrinol. Metab.* **2019**, *104*, 3311–3319. [CrossRef]
200. Seimon, R.V.; Brennan, I.M.; Russo, A.; Little, T.J.; Jones, K.L.; Standfield, S.; Wishart, J.M.; Horowitz, M.; Feinle-Bisset, C. Gastric emptying, mouth-to-cecum transit, and glycemic, insulin, incretin, and energy intake responses to a mixed-nutrient liquid in lean, overweight, and obese males. *Am. J. Physiol. Endocrinol. Metab.* **2013**, *304*, E294–E300. [CrossRef]
201. Perano, S.J.; Rayner, C.K.; Kritas, S.; Horowitz, M.; Donaghue, K.; Mpundu-Kaambwa, C.; Giles, L.; Couper, J.J. Gastric Emptying Is More Rapid in Adolescents With Type 1 Diabetes and Impacts on Postprandial Glycemia. *J. Clin. Endocrinol. Metab.* **2015**, *100*, 2248–2253. [CrossRef] [PubMed]
202. Jones, K.L.; Horowitz, M.; Wishart, J.M.; Maddox, A.F.; Harding, P.E.; Chatterton, B.E. Relationships between gastric-emptying, intragastric meal distribution and blood-glucose concentrations in diabetes-mellitus. *J. Nucl. Med.* **1995**, *36*, 2220–2228. [PubMed]
203. Watson, L.E.; Phillips, L.K.; Wu, T.; Bound, M.J.; Checklin, H.L.; Grivell, J.; Jones, K.L.; Clifton, P.M.; Horowitz, M.; Rayner, C.K. A whey/guar "preload" improves postprandial glycaemia and glycated haemoglobin levels in type 2 diabetes: A 12-week, single-blind, randomized, placebo-controlled trial. *Diabetes Obes. Metab.* **2019**, *21*, 930–938. [CrossRef] [PubMed]
204. Ghazi, T.; Rink, L.; Sherr, J.L.; Herold, K.C. Acute metabolic effects of exenatide in patients with type 1 diabetes with and without residual insulin to oral and intravenous glucose challenges. *Diabetes Care* **2014**, *37*, 210–216. [CrossRef] [PubMed]
205. Wu, T.; Little, T.J.; Bound, M.J.; Borg, M.; Zhang, X.; Deacon, C.F.; Horowitz, M.; Jones, K.L.; Rayner, C.K. A protein preload enhances the glucose-lowering efficacy of vildagliptin in type 2 diabetes. *Diabetes Care* **2016**, *39*, 511–517. [CrossRef]
206. Vilsbøll, T.; Krarup, T.; Madsbad, S.; Holst, J.J. Both GLP-1 and GIP are insulinotropic at basal and postprandial glucose levels and contribute nearly equally to the incretin effect of a meal in healthy subjects. *Regul. Pept.* **2003**, *114*, 115–121. [CrossRef]
207. Alleleyn, A.M.; van Avesaat, M.; Troost, F.J.; Masclee, A.A. Gastrointestinal nutrient infusion site and eating behavior: Evidence for a proximal to distal gradient within the small intestine? *Nutrients* **2016**, *8*, 117. [CrossRef]
208. Maljaars, P.W.; Peters, H.P.; Kodde, A.; Geraedts, M.; Troost, F.J.; Haddeman, E.; Masclee, A.A. Length and site of the small intestine exposed to fat influences hunger and food intake. *Br. J. Nutr.* **2011**, *106*, 1609–1615. [CrossRef]
209. Ma, J.; Checklin, H.L.; Wishart, J.M.; Stevens, J.E.; Jones, K.L.; Horowitz, M.; Meyer, J.H.; Rayner, C.K. A randomised trial of enteric-coated nutrient pellets to stimulate gastrointestinal peptide release and lower glycaemia in type 2 diabetes. *Diabetologia* **2013**, *56*, 1236–1242. [CrossRef]
210. Calderon, G.; McRae, A.; Rievaj, J.; Davis, J.; Zandvakili, I.; Linker-Nord, S.; Burton, D.; Roberts, G.; Reimann, F.; Gedulin, B.; et al. Ileo-colonic delivery of conjugated bile acids improves glucose homeostasis via colonic GLP-1-producing enteroendocrine cells in human obesity and diabetes. *EBioMedicine* **2020**, *55*, 102759. [CrossRef]
211. Fruhbeck, G. Bariatric and metabolic surgery: A shift in eligibility and success criteria. *Nat. Rev. Endocrinol.* **2015**, *11*, 465–477. [CrossRef] [PubMed]
212. Rubino, F.; Schauer, P.R.; Kaplan, L.M.; Cummings, D.E. Metabolic surgery to treat type 2 diabetes: Clinical outcomes and mechanisms of action. *Annu. Rev. Med.* **2010**, *61*, 393–411. [CrossRef] [PubMed]
213. Jørgensen, N.B.; Dirksen, C.; Bojsen-Møller, K.N.; Jacobsen, S.H.; Worm, D.; Hansen, D.L.; Kristiansen, V.B.; Naver, L.; Madsbad, S.; Holst, J.J. The exaggerated glucagon-like peptide-1 response is important for the improved β-cell function and glucose tolerance after Roux-en-Y gastric bypass in patients with type 2 diabetes. *Diabetes* **2013**, *62*, 3044–3052. [CrossRef] [PubMed]

214. Svane, M.S.; Bojsen-Moller, K.N.; Nielsen, S.; Jorgensen, N.B.; Dirksen, C.; Bendtsen, F.; Kristiansen, V.B.; Hartmann, B.; Holst, J.J.; Madsbad, S. Effects of endogenous GLP-1 and GIP on glucose tolerance after Roux-en-Y gastric bypass surgery. *Am. J. Physiol. Endocrinol. Metab.* **2016**, *310*, E505–E514. [CrossRef]
215. Svane, M.S.; Jorgensen, N.B.; Bojsen-Moller, K.N.; Dirksen, C.; Nielsen, S.; Kristiansen, V.B.; Torang, S.; Wewer Albrechtsen, N.J.; Rehfeld, J.F.; Hartmann, B.; et al. Peptide YY and glucagon-like peptide-1 contribute to decreased food intake after Roux-en-Y gastric bypass surgery. *Int. J. Obes.* **2016**, *40*, 1699–1706. [CrossRef]
216. Nicholson, J.K.; Holmes, E.; Kinross, J.; Burcelin, R.; Gibson, G.; Jia, W.; Pettersson, S. Host-gut microbiota metabolic interactions. *Science* **2012**, *336*, 1262–1267. [CrossRef]
217. Seck, E.H.; Senghor, B.; Merhej, V.; Bachar, D.; Cadoret, F.; Robert, C.; Azhar, E.I.; Yasir, M.; Bibi, F.; Jiman-Fatani, A.A.; et al. Salt in stools is associated with obesity, gut halophilic microbiota and Akkermansia muciniphila depletion in humans. *Int. J. Obes.* **2019**, *43*, 862–871. [CrossRef]
218. Canfora, E.E.; Meex, R.C.R.; Venema, K.; Blaak, E.E. Gut microbial metabolites in obesity, NAFLD and T2DM. *Nat. Rev. Endocrinol.* **2019**, *15*, 261–273. [CrossRef]
219. Wahlstrom, A.; Sayin, S.I.; Marschall, H.U.; Backhed, F. Intestinal crosstalk between bile acids and microbiota and its impact on host metabolism. *Cell Metab.* **2016**, *24*, 41–50. [CrossRef]
220. De Vadder, F.; Kovatcheva-Datchary, P.; Goncalves, D.; Vinera, J.; Zitoun, C.; Duchampt, A.; Backhed, F.; Mithieux, G. Microbiota-generated metabolites promote metabolic benefits via gut-brain neural circuits. *Cell* **2014**, *156*, 84–96. [CrossRef]
221. Byrne, C.S.; Chambers, E.S.; Alhabeeb, H.; Chhina, N.; Morrison, D.J.; Preston, T.; Tedford, C.; Fitzpatrick, J.; Irani, C.; Busza, A.; et al. Increased colonic propionate reduces anticipatory reward responses in the human striatum to high-energy foods. *Am. J. Clin. Nutr.* **2016**, *104*, 5–14. [CrossRef] [PubMed]

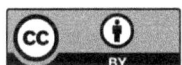

© 2020 by the authors. Licensee MDPI, Basel, Switzerland. This article is an open access article distributed under the terms and conditions of the Creative Commons Attribution (CC BY) license (http://creativecommons.org/licenses/by/4.0/).

MDPI
St. Alban-Anlage 66
4052 Basel
Switzerland
Tel. +41 61 683 77 34
Fax +41 61 302 89 18
www.mdpi.com

Pharmaceutics Editorial Office
E-mail: pharmaceutics@mdpi.com
www.mdpi.com/journal/pharmaceutics

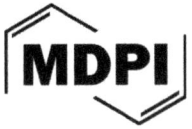

www.ingramcontent.com/pod-product-compliance
Lightning Source LLC
LaVergne TN
LVHW070428100526
838202LV00014B/1550